Flexible Sigmoidoscopy
Techniques and Utilization

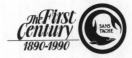

Flexible Sigmoidoscopy

Techniques and Utilization

Edited by

Melvin Schapiro, M.D. ———————————

Associate Clinical Professor of Medicine
University of California Center for the Health Sciences
University of California at Los Angeles
Los Angeles, California
Director of Gastrointestinal Diagnostic Unit
Valley Presbyterian Hospital
Van Nuys, California

Glen A. Lehman, M.D. ———————————

Professor of Medicine
Division of Gastroenterology/Hepatology
Indiana University School of Medicine
Indianapolis, Indiana

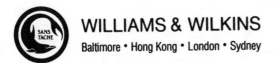

WILLIAMS & WILKINS

Baltimore • Hong Kong • London • Sydney

Editor: Michael G. Fisher
Associate Editor: Carol Eckhart
Copy Editor: Melisse Andrews
Designer: Saturn Graphics
Illustration Planner: Ray Lowman
Production Coordinator: Charles E. Zeller

Copyright © 1990
Williams & Wilkins
428 East Preston Street
Baltimore, Maryland 21202, USA

Acknowledgments

The authors gratefully acknowledge the support of the Olympus Corporation, Medical Instrument Division, Lake Success, New York and Boehringer Ingelheim Pharmaceuticals, Inc., Ridgefield, Connecticut in preparing the color atlas section of this book.

Accurate indications, adverse reactions, and dosage schedules for drugs are provided in this book, but it is possible that they may change. The reader is urged to review the package information data of the manufacturers of the medications mentioned.

Printed in the United States of America

Library of Congress Cataloging-in-Publication Data
Flexible sigmoidoscopy—Techniques and Utilization
  Includes index.
  1. Sigmoidoscopy. I. Schapiro, Melvin. II. Lehman, Glen A.
RC804.S47F57 1989   617'.5547   88-33813
ISBN 0-683-04909-7

90 91 92 93
1 2 3 4 5 6 7 8 9 10

Foreword

It is now well recognized that the widespread use of flexible sigmoidoscopy has largely superceded the use of rigid instruments. However, there have been no comprehensive publications dealing exclusively with flexible sigmoidoscopy. This book edited by Schapiro and Lehman addresses this need in fine fashion. The editors have assembled an impressive list of contributors who have authored 17 chapters covering 220 pages. Some key topics covered include: anatomy and physiology of the anus, rectum, and left colon; indications and contraindications of flexible sigmoidoscopy and comparison with rigid sigmoidoscopy, colonoscopy, and barium enema; instruments and associated equipment with special attention to length of the various instruments; patient preparation; techniques; recognition of diseases of the anus, rectum, and sigmoid colon as identified by the proctologic examination; infectious diseases as identified at flexible sigmoidoscopy; colorectal biopsy; complications of flexible sigmoidoscopy; screening for colorectal cancer in average and high risk patients; cost considerations in the use of flexible sigmoidoscopy; and training in flexible sigmoidoscopy and quality assurance.

Thus, the book provides a truly comprehensive treatise on flexible sigmoidoscopy and a uniform and appropriate emphasis on practical considerations. The book will be most useful to primary care physicians such as general internists and family physicians and to resident physicians. The book also could be useful reading for medical students. It seems clear that this book will be of service to the medical profession, to students, and its patients.

Norton J. Greenberger, M.D.

Contributors

Philip A. Christiansen, M.D.
Professor of Medicine
Division of Gastroenterology/Hepatology
Indiana University Medical Center
Indianapolis, Indiana

Thomas L. Gross, M.D.
Staff Physician
Methodist Hospital
Indianapolis, Indiana

Robert H. Hawes, M.D.
Assistant Professor of Medicine
Division of Gastroenterology/Hepatology
Indiana University Medical Center
Indianapolis, Indiana

Glen A. Lehman, M.D.
Professor of Medicine
Division of Gastroenterology/Hepatology
Indiana University Medical Center
Indianapolis, Indiana

Sidney Niemark, M.D.
Chief of Gastrointestinal Endoscopy
St. Mary's Hospital
West Palm Beach, Florida

K. W. O'Connor, M.D.
Clinical Associate Professor of Medicine
Indiana University Medical Center
Staff Physician
St. Vincent Hospital
Indianapolis, Indiana

David C. Pound, M.D.
Assistant Professor of Medicine
Division of Gastroenterology/Hepatology
Indiana University Medical Center
Indianapolis, Indiana

Douglas K. Rex, M.D.
Assistant Professor of Medicine
Division of Gastroenterology/Hepatology
Indiana University Medical Center
Indianapolis, Indiana

Melvin Schapiro, M.D.
Associate Clinical Professor of Medicine
University of California Center for the Health Sciences
University of California at Los Angeles
Los Angeles, California
Director of Gastrointestinal Diagnostic Unit
Valley Presbyterian Hospital
Van Nuys, California

Theodore R. Schrock, M.D.
Professor of Surgery
Department of Surgery
University of California Medical Center
San Francisco, California

Norman Sohn, M.D., F.A.C.S.
Associate Surgeon
Lenox Hill Hospital
New York City, New York
Clinical Assistant Professor of Surgery
New York Medical College
Valhalla, New York

Christina M. Surawicz, M.D.
Associate Professor of Medicine
Harborview Medical Center
University of Washington
Seattle, Washington

Francis J. Tedesco, M.D.
Professor of Medicine
Medical College of Georgia
Augusta, Georgia

John Trocino, R.N., G.I.A.
Chief Technologist
Endoscopic Laser Unit
Medical Center of Tarzana
Tarzana, California

Jerome D. Waye, M.D.
Clinical Professor of Medicine
Columbia University
New York, New York

Sidney J. Winawer, M.D.
Clinical Professor of Medicine
Cornell University
Chief Gastroenterology Service
Memorial Sloan Kettering Cancer Center
New York, New York

Contents

Overview of Colorectal Cancer
Sidney J. Winawer, M.D.

INTRODUCTION

Colorectal cancer, with the exception of skin cancer, is one of the three most frequently found lethal cancers in the United States. The incidence of more than 160,000 new cases, along with the high 5-year mortality rate of over 50%, has stimulated interest in approaches using new concepts and new technology (1). It has become apparent that in addition to the average-risk patients (women and men age 40 or older) there are subgroups in the population at increased risk for this cancer. These include patients who have had a prior colon cancer and patients with adenomas, ulcerative colitis, female genital cancer, a family history of familial polyposis, Gardner's syndrome, or the nonpolyposis inherited colon cancer family syndromes. Although considerable work remains in the identification of these high-risk groups, a clearer picture exists today of the spectrum of risk for colorectal cancer. The past decade has also witnessed major technical advances, including new fecal occult blood tests and the evolution of flexible endoscopes. The application of contrast radiologic techniques is better understood (2,3).

EPIDEMIOLOGY AND ETIOLOGY

Adenocarcinoma of the colon is more prevalent in developed countries. The incidence of this carcinoma is high in North America and Europe and low in South America, Africa, and Asia. The United States has one of the highest rates for colorectal cancer in the world. Migrants to a particular geographic area assume the colorectal cancer risk for that area. This is illustrated by the observation of a higher incidence among blacks who have migrated to the United States as compared to those who have remained in Africa. Puerto Ricans who have migrated to the mainland have the risk of those on the mainland. First- and second-generation Japanese migrating to Hawaii and the mainland of the United States assume the risk of their new country. In the United States, the incidence of colorectal cancer is higher in the North than in the South, in urban areas as compared to rural areas, and in whites as compared to blacks. There is a slightly higher risk among certain occupations, such as automobile factory workers and woodworkers (4).

Although the geographic distribution of rectal cancer is fairly similar to that of colon cancer, rectal cancer and colon cancer may not be the same epidemiologically and etiologically. There is male predominance in rectal cancer, whereas the male-female ratio is approximately equal in colon cancer. In addition, there are some variations in the ratio of incidence rates of rectal to colon cancer from country to country.

The distinction between rectal cancer and colon cancer is complicated because of a change in the anatomic distribution, with a more proximal migration of colorectal cancer. Approximately 55% of colon cancers are in the distal 25 cm of bowel today, whereas 30 years ago it was approximately 75%. The incidence for colorectal cancer has been fairly stable in some countries, such as England and Wales, but has been increasing slowly in other countries, such as the United States and Denmark. The increase in incidence in the

Table 1.1.
Anatomic Distribution of Colorectal Cancers
Modified from the Third National Cancer Survey
(26,598 Patients)

Site	Percentage of Cancers
Rectum	22%
Sigmoid	32%
Descending colon	6%
Transverse colon	11%
Ascending colon	9%
Cecum	12.5%
Unspecified & appendix	7.5%

United States may reflect increases in subgroups of the population, such as those in the South, blacks, and those living in rural areas. In other countries, such as Japan, increases have been occurring substantially in the past decade, perhaps reflecting a westernization of the diet (Table 1.1) (2).

There are variations in incidence rates for colorectal cancer within populations. In addition to the above-mentioned variations based on race and residence, there are also variations related to religious persuasion. There is, for example, increased risk among Jews but a decreased risk among Seventh Day Adventists.

Migrant studies strongly suggest that environmental factors, especially diet, are important in the etiology of colon cancer. In populations where colorectal cancer is low in incidence, there is also a low incidence of other colonic diseases, including appendicitis, adenomas, diverticulosis, and ulcerative colitis. This has been noticed in the South African Bantu and other African populations whose diets contain more fiber and less refined carbohydrate. One suggested mechanism of high-fiber diets is the rapid intestinal transit time produced by fiber such that any potential carcinogen remains in contact with the mucosa for a shorter period of time. It has also been suggested that fiber increases intraluminal bulk and thereby dilutes carcinogens that are normally ingested. A direct association between increased fat and animal protein intake, particularly present in the Western diet, and the rising incidence of colon cancer has also been suggested. In Japan, for example, the intake of fat, mostly unsaturated, provides 10% of the caloric intake, whereas in the United States fat intake represents about 40% of the total caloric intake. It has been suggested that the Western diet with its high fat and beef content favors the establishment of bacterial flora with enzymes such as β-glucuronidase and azoreductase. This causes increased metabolism of neutral and acid sterols to carcinogenic and co-carcinogenic metabolites. Studies have also shown that mutagens present in feces, including nitrosamide, are increased in individuals on high-beef diets. A reduction in mutagenicity and in levels of nitrosamide in the stool has been noted in patients on ascorbic acid and α-tocopherol. More recent evidence also strongly suggests that fatty acids and bile acids have an irritative effect on the colonic mucosa, resulting in high cellular proliferation and high risk for polyps and cancer. This is seen in groups eating the usual high-fat Western diet and is not seen in vegetarians. Supplemental oral calcium may lower this risk. The relationship of diet to colorectal cancer, regarding the association between diet and neoplastic transformation, requires further study (5,6).

Other factors have been examined regarding the etiology of colorectal cancer. The role of alcohol, mainly beer, in the etiology of large bowel cancer has been an interesting issue. Studies have suggested a correlation of beer drinking with colon and rectal cancer in several countries. The mechanism for carcinogenic action of beer has been speculative. It has been suggested that beer may interact with the diet to influence either the fecal flora or the fecal sterol concentration. Some evidence has been suggested that events of reproductive life have an influence on a woman's subsequent risk of developing colon cancer. It has been suggested that the events accompanying pregnancy may protect against the development of colon cancer through a decrease of bile acid secretion. Data from several studies suggest that very low serum cholesterol, although associated with very low mortality from coronary heart disease, may be associated with some increase in subsequent risk and mortality from various types of cancer, including colorectal cancer. This may be related to the promotion effect of bile acids on colon carcinogens. At present, the data are insufficient to make any definite conclusions regarding the causal relationship between low cholesterol and cancer. Cholecystectomy has also been implicated in large bowel cancer, particularly of the ascending colon, probably by allowing increased bile acid promotion of carcinogens. The relationship is not proven, and the increased risk is small if present (4–6).

A high intake of cruciferous vegetables has been suggested to be protective against large bowel cancer, the protective effect being attributed to certain indoles in the vegetables and also to their high-fiber content. Case control studies have also shown a negative association between the frequency of the use of vegetables and colorectal cancer, especially those vegetables with low concentrations of vitamin A. There is some suggestive evidence of the possible protective effect of retinol and carotene against cancer, including colorectal cancer. Several antioxidants, including ascorbic acid and selenium, are also said to have a protective effect against cancer, especially colorectal cancer (4–6).

TRENDS IN ANATOMIC LOCATION

Countries subject to a high incidence of colon cancer demonstrate a relatively higher frequency of sigmoid cancers, whereas in lower risk countries cancers of the cecum and ascending colon predominate. A recent analysis of colorectal carcinoma reported by the Connecticut Tumor Registry from 1940 through 1973 demonstrated that the proportion of right colon lesions increased gradually from 13 to 22%. During the 30-year period of the survey, age-adjusted cancer incidence increased 2.4 times in the ascending colon and 1.7 times in the sigmoid colon. The most significant increases above the rectosigmoid occurred in the men and women who were older than 65 years at the time of diagnosis. During the calendar period 1970 to 1973, the incidence per 100,000 of carcinoma of the ascending colon and cecum in men over 65 years of (93.4) exceeded that reported in women (85.3) (2).

The cancer incidence data from the Surveillance, Epidemiology and End Results (SEER) program in the United States for the period 1973 to 1976 indicated that the distribution by subsites within the large intestine was rectum (22%), rectosigmoid (10%), sigmoid colon (25%), descending colon (6%), transverse colon including flexures (13%), ascending colon (8%), cecum (15%), and appendix (1%). These data would suggest that routine digital and flexible sigmoidoscopy in general practice would detect 50 to 60% of all new cases of colorectal cancer (Table 1.1) (2).

PERSONAL RISK FACTORS

Age

The age-specific incidence rates of both colon and rectal cancer rise steadily from about age 10 to 84. There is a decline in rates in the 85+ group, probably representing incomplete ascertainment. The rate of increase in incidence

Table 1.2.
Colorectal Cancer Risk Factors

Risk Status	Factor
Standard risk	Age over 40 (both men and women)
High risk	Inflammatory bowel disease
	History of female genital or breast cancer
	History of colon cancer or adenoma
	Peutz-Jeghers' syndrome
	Familial polyposis syndromes
	Family cancer syndromes
	Hereditary site-specific colon cancer
	History of juvenile polyps
	Immunodeficiency disease

is rather steady until age 70 to 75. In data from the Third National Cancer Survey, age-specific incidence rates for males and females of both black and white populations were similar for colon cancer, particularly from ages 30 to 65, reflecting converging trends in colon cancer among blacks and whites in the United States. Rectal cancer incidence rates increase slowly after age 70 and decline after age 85. Average age-specific mortality rates in the United States from 1950 to 1969 appear to reach a plateau for blacks of both sexes, beginning at age 65, but this may largely represent reporting and classification errors (Table 1.2) (2).

During the 3 years of the Third National Cancer Survey, in which a population of 21,003,451 was surveyed, there were nine cases of cancer of the colon and one of cancer of the rectum in children under 15 years of age. Twenty cases of cancer of the colon, one of cancer of the rectum, and one of cancer of the rectosigmoid occurred in the 15- to 19-year-old age group. The corresponding average annual age-specific incidence rates for large intestinal cancer are 0.6 per million under age 15 and 4.5 per million for ages 15 through 19. These figures are higher than estimates based on mortality rates from large bowel cancer in persons under age 20 derived from national death certificate data. The average annual mortality rate for colorectal cancer under age 15 was 0.2 per million (50 deaths during the period from 1960 to 1968) and 2.3 per million for ages 15 to 19 (76 deaths between 1965 and 1968). The incidence of colorectal tumors among blacks under age 20 is 1.6 times that of whites of the same age group. Mortality rates have been three to four times as high among blacks under age 20 as among white children in the same age group.

Colorectal neoplasms in children differ from those in adults in several ways. They may be more often located in the colon; a higher percentage are associated with identifiable predisposing factors; and the histologic pattern differs from that in adults. Among 76 children with colorectal cancer, who were identified by hospital survey, familial polyposis occurred in 5.3%, ulcerative colitis in 3.9%, and granulomatous colitis in 1.3%. Thus, 10.5% of pediatric patients with colorectal cancer had known of predisposing diseases, and other children came from families that may represent so-called "cancer families."

Between one-third and one-half of children with colorectal cancer have mucinous adenocarcinomas compared with adults, in whom this histologic type occurs in only about 5 to 8%. The aggressive character of colloid or mucinous tumors contributes to the overall poor survival of young patients with cancer of the large intestine. Only 11% of patients under age 30 with colloid carcinoma of the large intestine survived 5 years, whereas in the older age groups with colloid cancers the 5-year survival rate was 37%.

Sex

The rank order of large bowel cancer incidence and mortality in men as compared with women is closely correlated in most countries. This is true for colon cancer and rectal cancer when considered separately. Correlations between selected environmental variables and colon cancer mortality rates are similar for males and females, though less so for rectal cancer. The sex ratios of colon cancer and rectal cancer differ, with rectal cancer being distinctly more common among males in most countries, whereas colonic cancer affects both sexes at rather similar rates. In the United States, colon cancer rates are slightly higher for white males, whereas the rates are nearly equal for black males and black females. Among young patients with colon and rectal cancer, males predominate (4).

Prior Colorectal Cancers

Patients who have had colorectal cancer are at increased risk for subsequent colorectal cancer if they have been cured of the first cancer. This has been defined as a metachronous lesion, or one that occurs at a time later than the original lesion. This concept is different from recurrent carcinoma, which occurs in patients who have not been cured of their original lesion and return with evidence of spread of their cancer to adjacent or distant sites. Patients with an index colorectal cancer are also at risk for an additional colorectal cancer at the time of their index lesion. This is defined as the synchronous lesion, occurring at the same time as the index cancer. It is therefore important in approaching patients with colorectal cancer to be cognizant of these additional risk factors, not only for a subsequent time frame but also for the immediate time frame when the diagnosis is made and the treatment plan is established. These concepts will have important bearing on the use of currently available diagnostic techniques to evaluate the entire colon at the time of initial diagnosis. The frequency of metachronous cancers is between 5 and 10% in patients who have had an index colorectal cancer. The frequency of synchronous cancers ranges from 1.5 to 5% in patients with an index colorectal cancer (7–9).

Prior Colorectal Cancers

Associated benign and malignant neoplasms in individuals with colorectal cancer include breast (21%); gynecologic (16%); genitourinary (11%); and other regions of the gastrointestinal tract (9%). These patients experience an early age of onset of colorectal cancer.

Single and Multiple Sporadic Colorectal Adenomas

The presence of one or more adenomas occurs in the majority of all individuals in the general population by age 60. Kindreds have been reported that show an association of single and multiple adenomas with adenocarcinomas, thus suggesting a genetic susceptibility. There is overwhelming evidence that most, if not all, adenocarcinomas of the colon arise from preexisting adenomas. Male-female distribution of adenocarcinomas and the frequency distribution related to age of adenomas correlates well with that of adenocarcinomas. The anatomic distribution of adenomas parallels that of adenocarcinomas, and the geographic distribution of adenomas is similar to that of adenocarcinomas. Countries at high risk for adenocarcinomas of the colon are also at high risk for adenomas of the colon. In addition, there is increasing evidence that as adenomas of the colon grow in size, the likelihood of premalignant dysplasia and the likelihood of carcinoma being found in the adenoma increases. The likelihood of carcinoma in adenoma is related to pathology, but the histology is related to size. Whereas most adenomas under 1 cm in size are tubular, most adenomas (75%) of 2 cm in size or over feature a villous component. The villous component is considered to be the histologic feature most related to malignancy within the adenoma (8–12).

The likelihood of carcinoma being found in an adenoma is 1% for adenomas of 1 cm or less, approximately 10% for adenomas between 1 and 2 cm, and over 25% in adenomas over 2 cm in size. For adenomas greater than 3 to 5 cm in size, a frequency of 55% carcinoma in the polyp has been reported. Anatomic distribution of the adenomas relates also to potential for malignancy, the adenomas in the distal descending colon and sigmoid having a greater frequency of dysplasia and malignancy than those elsewhere in the colon. This correlates well with the greatest distribution of colorectal cancer in the descending colon and the rectosigmoid area. As one would expect, the risk of carcinoma is greater in those patients with multiple adenomas of the colon. In one study, the risk of invasive carcinoma overall was 8% when one adenoma was present; 10% when two adenomas were present; and 14% when three or more were present. Until very recently, diminutive polyps (0.5 cm in size or less) had been considered to be hyperplastic. However, in recent years colonoscopic polypectomy data indicated that a substantial proportion of these polyps are true adenomas. The diminutive adenomas can be dysplastic, have villous features, have carcinoma in situ, and rarely contain invasive cancer (8–13).

Adenomas also occur with increased frequency in patients with an index invasive cancer. In some studies, the frequency is as high as 50%. This observation is quite important because these synchronous adenomas may harbor malignancy at that time or may evolve into additional adenocarcinomas years after a curative resection has been performed.

There is considerable evidence that strongly relates the adenoma to the carcinoma. Residual adenomatous tissue has been found in a significant percentage (20%) of adenocarcinomas of the colon that have been removed. Presumably, the growth of the adenocarcinoma has destroyed residual preexisting adenoma. If adenocarcinoma arose de novo without preexisting adenomas, they should be detectable at this early small stage as pure adenocarcinomas of a very small size (under 1 cm and possibly under 0.5 cm). However, with use of screening techniques and colonoscopy, the very small carcinomas of 0.5 to 1 cm are still not found except within preexisting adenomas. There are animal observations that form the basis for the theory of de novo carcinomas. Clinically, there have been occasional cases of convincing de novo cancer without a documented prior adenoma. However, these are rare exceptions rather than the rule. Other evidence of the relationship of adenomas to adenocarcinomas includes (a) the reduction in risk in patients in whom search and removal of adenomas has been performed on a regular basis and (b) the increased risk for adenocarcinoma in those patients in whom adenomas are present but not removed (8,12).

Inflammatory Bowel Disease

Ulcerative colitis of long standing is a risk factor for colorectal cancer. The number of colorectal cancers in the United States associated with ulcerative colitis is approximately 1000 per year. Approximately one-third of deaths related to chronic ulcerative colitis are due to colorectal cancer, which occurs at an overall incidence of 7 to 11 times greater in patients with chronic ulcerative colitis than in the general population. The magnitude of the cancer risk in ulcerative colitis reported from large research centers has been challenged by recent reports from community hospitals. The risk of cancer in ulcerative colitis can be related to two recognized variables: the duration of active colitis and the anatomic extent of colonic involvement by the pathologic process. In adults the risk begins to rise after 7 years, and 20% of the patients with cancer and chronic ulcerative colitis develop their malignancies between 7 and 10 years from onset of the colitis. Pancolitis carries a greater risk than colitis confined to the left side of the colon where risk appears later—approximately 15 years after onset. Colitis limited to the rectosigmoid has only minimal risk, and ulcerative proctitis appears to have no increased risk for cancer at all. In recent years a small subgroup of about 10 to 15% of patients with long-standing chronic ulcerative colitis has been identified by biopsy as having dysplasia in their colonic mucosa. When severe dysplasia is found, approximately one-half of patients will be found to have cancer at that time; with moderate dysplasia, approximately one-third of the patients will have cancer. The type of dysplasia that is most related to carcinoma is severe dysplasia of the nodular or villous type. About 80% of patients with chronic ulcerative colitis and colorectal cancer have dysplasia on biopsy. There are many difficulties in histologic interpretation and dysplastic changes may be patchy. The demonstration of dysplasia has potential value in identifying these patients with ulcerative colitis who are at greater risk for colorectal cancer, although recently this biologic indicator has been increasingly challenged in terms of its sensitivity and specificity.

Thus, there is considerable controversy regarding the concept and terminology in dysplasia. Some pathologists are beginning to use the terms low-grade and high-grade dysplasia instead of moderate and severe. The category of mild dysplasia is being omitted. Patients with granulomatous colitis are also at higher risk for colorectal cancer than the general population, but the risk is considerably less than with chronic ulcerative colitis. In these patients the risk is also related to the duration of the disease (14–17).

Familial Polyposis

Familial polyposis is characterized by the development of large numbers of adenomatous polyps throughout the entire colon and rectum. Carcinomas eventually develop in all affected individuals. The cancers occur with highest frequency in the distal colon, a distribution that is similar to that of colorectal cancer in the general population. The disease is an autosomal dominant genetic defect, affecting each generation, and is expressed phenotypically about 80% of the time. The disease has occurred among Caucasians, Orientals, Arabs, West Indians, American and African blacks, and Native Americans. Analysis of age at onset of disease is an important determinant in the identification of familial predisposition (18).

Gardner's Syndrome

Gardner's syndrome, a variant of familial polyposis, is an autosomal dominant disorder showing a high degree of penetrance. Adenomatous polyps of the colon (and occasionally of the small intestine and stomach) are formed. There is a propensity for development of adenocarcinoma in these adenomas. It is a clinical diagnosis. The incidence of the syndrome is lower than familial polyposis and is estimated at one in 14,000 births. Adenomatosis of the large intestine, multiple osteomata of the skull and mandible, multiple epidermoid cysts, and soft tissue tumors of the skin were reported by Gardner in 1951. New observations have shown impacted teeth, early dental caries, abnormal bones (mandible and tibia), and desmoid tumors (abdominal wall and small intestinal mesentery). It should be noted that an epidermoid cyst, uncommon before the age of puberty, may indicate polyposis.

Other possibly associated lesions include carcinomas of the thyroid; carcinoma of the ampulla of Vater, duodenum, and adrenal glands; adenomas of the small intestine; carcinoma in situ of the gallbladder; carcinoid tumors of the small intestine; tumors of the brain and central nervous system; and lymphoid polyps of the ileum. Gene expression is variable, with some persons having the various manifestations of the major triad of Gardner's syndrome and others with hereditary polyposis having only intestinal neoplasms. The incidence of Gardner's syndrome among families in which more than one member has polyposis has been estimated at 14 to 18%. Only one or several family members may have obvious clinical manifestations of the disease. Abnormalities of epidermal cells and fibroblasts can be observed in family members lacking clinical manifestations of disease. It is not yet clear whether features of the syndrome result from one dominant gene or from two or more genes. There are questions also about the number, nature, and location of polyps in polyposis patients showing manifestations of Gardner's syndrome as compared with those with the typical non-Gardner familial polyposis. In terms of pathogenesis, the syndrome described by Gardner could represent the full manifestation of a spectrum of pathologic changes affecting all patients with multiple polyposis. It is possible that a single mutation may be responsible for most of the various associated syndromes. On that basis, Gardner's syndrome would include all adenomatous polyposis, with subsidiary lesions expressed in different degrees (18).

Turcot's Syndrome

This syndrome has been described by Turcot as polyposis coli associated with malignant tumors of the central nervous system. In this study, two family members, a boy and a girl with polyposis, died from medulloblastoma of the spinal cord and a cerebral tumor, respectively. Several other similar instances have been reported and may be examples of the tumor association found in Gardner's syndrome.

Peutz-Jeghers' Syndrome

Peutz-Jeghers' syndrome, an additional autosomal dominant inherited disease with variable expression, was first described by Peutz in 1921 and later elaborated on by Jeghers and colleagues. In this disease, pigmented spots often appear on the lips and buccal mucosa and also on the dorsal aspect of the hands and feet. Dozens of intestinal tumors are found throughout the gastrointestinal tract and can intussuscept and obstruct the small intestine. These are usually not as numerous as those seen in familial polyposis. Because of their composition (normal intestinal epithelium and abnormal amounts and arrangements of smooth muscle), they are considered hamartomas. Juvenile polyps are similar, except for the smooth muscle arrangement. The tumors originally were considered benign, without high potential for malignancy. However, more than 15 cases of cancer (stomach, duodenum, and colon) have been reported, and adenomas have been found to coexist with the hamartomatous lesions. Most patients have been under the age of 40. In this disease, when carcinoma of the colon develops, it is believed to arise from the adenomas.

Juvenile Polyps

Although juvenile polyps occur indiscriminately throughout the gastrointestinal tract, they are seen more often in the large intestine. They are not precancerous, and surgery is not necessarily required. Average onset of the disease is at 6 years of age. It has been diagnosed earlier, often in infants. The main symptom is bleeding, which can be accompanied by severe anemia, hypoproteinemia, malnutrition, and retarded development. Found singly or in small numbers, the polyps consist of normal mucosal epithelium in irregular glandular patterns, surrounded by an increased amount of lamina propria. The mucous glands may be cystic and distended. Hemorrhage and secondary inflammation are additional symptoms. Some tumors have exhibited the combined characteristics of juvenile polyps and adenomas. Adenomatous tumors have been discovered in rare patients with multiple juvenile polyps (juvenile polyposis), and a higher incidence of colon carcinomas may occur in family members. Thirty-seven cases of juvenile polyposis were recorded in 28 families. In six of these, more than one member was affected, and in one case, the disease spanned three generations. Most cases have been solitary rather than familial.

Familial Colon Cancer without Polyposis

Findings in recent years indicate that familial associations in colon cancer are higher than in control groups, suggesting that inherited factors may play a role in the genesis of colorectal cancer. Criteria for a familial syndrome associated with cancer of the large intestine include (a) increased numbers of all types of adenocarcinomas in affected patients, especially colonic and endometrial carcinomas; (b) early age of cancer development as compared with that noted from the same organ sites in the general population; (c) a tendency to multiple primary malignant neoplasms in affected persons; and (d) segregation ratios consistent with an autosomal mode of inheritance (Fig. 1.1) (19).

Many other kindreds with site-specific colon lesions also have been reported. In this type of familial cancer only colorectal cancer is present. Lynch's reports on family "R" (19) seemed consistent with findings on this disease observed in Europe and the United States over the past 20 years. Colon cancer risk in the "R" family segregated with ratios consistent with that of a single autosomal dominant gene with complete penetrance. All but one of 33 family members with cancer of the gastrointestinal tract had a parent with the same disease. The family as a whole showed a high risk (50%) for devel-

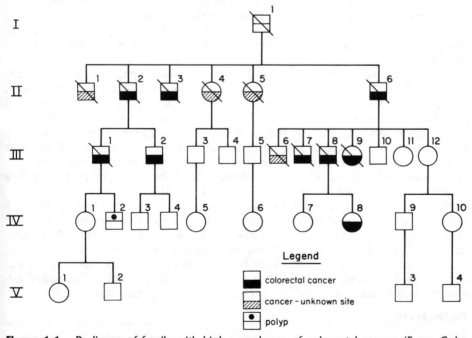

Figure 1.1. Pedigree of family with high prevalence of colorectal cancer. (From: Colorectal Cancer: Essentials for Primary Care Physicians. Winawer S, Editor. Produced by Health Learning Systems. Bloomfield, NJ)

opment of primary malignant neoplasms of the colon. Along with many cancer family parents, Lynch's "R" family revealed a strong tendency toward developing cancer of the proximal colon; the mean frequency is higher in this group than in either patients with familial polyposis or the general population. The figure for proximal colon cancer is three to four times that for site distribution of colon cancer among familial polyposis coli patients.

Most cases of colorectal cancer are "sporadic." They fit into no defined or suggested genetic syndrome. Defining any risk of colon cancer based on family history is a difficult task. Because cancer develops during the lifetime of one in four persons in the United States, a history of cancer in close relatives is not unusual. Thirty percent of patients in the general population will have one first-degree relative with cancer; 20% will have two or more first-degree relatives with cancer. In addition, because both adenomas and carcinomas of the colon and rectum appear in the later decades of life, demonstration of a genetic factor in sporadic cancer poses a difficult problem, made even more complex by the influence of environmental factors.

Despite these obstacles it is becoming clear that common cancers of human beings have familial tendencies. These tendencies, though not compelling, are suggestive enough to place some populations in "high-risk" categories with regard to screening. In general, the risk of the same neoplasm developing in a close relative of a cancer patient is about three times greater than would be expected in the general population. For colon, breast, and some childhood tumors there is an even greater risk. In families in which tumors develop at a younger than usual age or at multiple sites, the risk in first-degree relatives may be 20 to 30 times greater than in the general population (18,19).

In a cancer detection program at the M.D. Anderson Hospital, the criteria for entry was the presence of colon cancer in two relatives. Sigmoidoscopy and air-contrast barium enemas were performed. Cancer of the colon was detected in 2.7% in all ages studied and in 3.7% in cases over 35 years of age. This exceeds the detection rate of cancer in the general population, where the rate of detection is one in 1000. This demonstrates that a relevant family history may guide risk estimation and screening procedures for colorectal cancer.

In another investigation, the family histories of all patients with colon cancer were studied. In 218 male first-degree relatives of 123 index cases of colon cancer, 25 had colon cancer. The expected number was 4.5. In women, 212 first-degree relatives of index cases had 22 recorded cancers of the colon, with 6.3 expected. Among 352 first-degree relatives of 29 index cases, the observed incidence of carcinoma of the large bowel was 42; expected incidence was 11.65. The difference between the observed incidence and the expected incidence was probably caused by an increased incidence of polyps in families where a history of polyps or cancer had been noted.

Macklin studied 145 patients with colon cancer. In the 1369 first-degree relatives, 78 colon cancers were seen, whereas 27.2 were expected. The difference is highly significant. Woolf studied 763 first-degree relatives of 242 probands with colonic carcinoma. Twenty-six carcinomas were seen. In the control group, eight were noted. This too is a significant difference. A recent study from Utah demonstrated that a significant proportion of "sporadic" adenomas and hence "sporadic" cancers are genetically determined (18).

PATHOLOGY

Size

The size of the primary tumor appears to have little relationship to prognosis. In fact, the opposite has been observed, in that large size may be associated with a good prognosis. Several authors have pointed to the unique feature in colon cancer of some very large bulky tumors that have few, if any, lymph node metastases and that carry a correspondingly better 5-year outlook.

Location

Carcinomas of the abdominal colon generally have a reasonably good prognosis. Cancers of the rectum have a significantly poorer prognosis in virtually every major surgical series. This poor outlook is almost entirely associated with cancers of the low or distal rectum (0 to 5 cm from the anal verge), as cancers of the mid- or upper rectum seem to have a similar prognosis, if not identical outlook, as do rectosigmoid or sigmoid lesions. The reasons for this difference in survival are multiple. From the standpoint of natural history, cancers of the lower rectum naturally spread both to hypogastric lymph nodes along the pelvic side walls and to mesorectal lymph nodes along the superior hemorrhoidal artery. From the standpoint of therapy, the vascular pelvic dissection that is required to extirpate all lymph nodes associated with the potential spread of rectal cancer is a challenging operation that rarely is accomplished. As a result of both the natural course of the disease and the operative limitations of pelvic dissections, treatment failures and recurrent pelvic disease frequently complicate the subsequent course of rectal cancer after resection. The combined end result is a significantly poorer outlook for rectal cancers. Some series have demonstrated an advantage for right-sided lesions. Other series have, in fact, experienced a poorer outlook for right-sided lesions (and ascending colon cancers in particular), leaving this issue unresolved.

Gross Configuration

Carcinomas of the large bowel generally assume one of four shapes: exophytic, ulcerative, infiltrative, or annular. To the extent that there are variations, almost all primary lesions assume one of these configurations. It is unclear whether these are all independent shapes or whether some represent later stages of evolution, that is, ulcerative, as in the case of polypoid, or annular, as in the case of infiltrative. Rarely does site influence configuration. Exceptions include the cecum, where large polypoid carcinomas are common and may become large enough to obstruct the small bowel by size alone. Exophytic or polypoid lesions project into the lumen. Whereas ulceration may be present, this is by no means uniformly seen. On the other hand, focal ulceration may be the gross indication of malignancy in an otherwise benign-appearing adenoma. The exophytic carcinoma frequently will have arisen in an adenoma, and a significant portion of the mass may still be nonmalignant polyp.

The shape of the cancer, whether polypoid on a stalk or sessile, has been related to prognosis. Sessile or infiltrative lesions carry a worse prognosis than do the stalked variety. On cut sections the tumor usually invades all layers of the bowel wall, exaggerating the gross features of each individual layer, whether due to infiltration or to secondary edema. The extent of circumferential involvement becomes important, in relation to both symptoms and prognosis. Infiltrating or annular carcinomas cause obstructive symptoms, changes in bowel habits, and bleeding. Annular carcinomas are probably the end product of the infiltrating type of cancer. These tumors are responsible for clinical colonic obstruction. Such tumors are associated with a poorer prognosis, with an overall 5-year survival of less than 30%. Ulcerating carcinomas may originate as polypoid tumors, but with continued infection and necrosis the luminal component is gradually eroded. The malignant ulcer may have a clean grayish-pink nodular base that is easily biopsied for a histologic diagnosis, or it may have a necrotic lining with or without a significant pericolic inflammation. Such cancers will occasionally perforate. Free perforation with peritonitis generally carries an ominous prognosis that is at least as bad as obstruction.

Histology

The histologic features that are related to prognosis include degree of differentiation (histologic or cytologic grade); degree of mural penetration; presence or absence of lymph node involvement; character of leading tumor margin; lymphatic, venous, or perineural infiltration; presence of an associated inflammatory response; extranodal mesenteric implants; extramesenteric nodal involvement; presence or absence of involved surgical margins; and adjacent organ involvement.

Histologic grading as a tool for assessing tumor differentiation is a useful prognostic indicator. Most pathologists use either a numbering system (1 to 3 or 4) or a series of descriptive terms, such as *well, moderately well, poorly differentiated, undifferentiated,* or *anaplastic.* These systems are generally interchangeable. The poorly differentiated category may include a few cases showing minimal ability to form glandular structures, which would be included in the grade 4 category. These differences rest in part on whether the grading system is more cytologically oriented or oriented toward a description of gland-forming structures, the latter being simpler to use. Well-differentiated tumors consist of those tumors that are nearly to fully composed of gland-forming structures, with nuclei showing polarity and basal orientation. Moderately differentiated tumors are predominantly glandular but may demonstrate some loss of polarity and nuclear orientation. There may be some tendency for tumor cells to form solid nuclear orientation or solid nests. Poorly differentiated tumors are those in which the tendency to form sheets and nests outweighs the glandular elements. When the glandular structures disappear, the tumor is considered undifferentiated. The majority of colorectal tumors fit into such a grading scheme. Nevertheless, sampling errors result, and grading must reflect an examination of the entire resected tumor. Grading cannot be based on biopsies alone. There may be nearly a 50% rate of error in ascribing the label of poor differentiation to rectal tumor by assessment of the preoperative biopsy alone, since biopsies are not representative of the entire cancer. Variants of undifferentiated carcinoma such as signet-ring cell carcinoma or mucinous carcinoma carry a particularly poor prognosis. There is an unusually high incidence of mucinous adenocarcinomas in young patients, especially adolescents. The role of mucin in the particularly poor prognosis in rectal lesions is unknown. Separation of tissue planes, disruption of vascular integrity, tumor glycocalix abetting the process of metastasis, as well as immunologic protection, have all been suggested. The mucin produced by tumors is histochemically different from the mucin of normal benign colonic epithelium. Reports continue to characterize the changes in mucin production associated with colonic malignancy. As yet, these changes elude practical value as markers with specific prognostic information. Recent studies have demonstrated that tumor cell deoxyribonucleic acid (DNA) content may be a better reflection of tumor grade, which is more accurately associated with prognosis. Chromatin content of an aneuploid or heteroploid nature was associated with poor prognosis independent of stage. These findings have now been extended to observations of nuclear ribonucleic acid (RNA) content as well.

Carcinomas, which are epithelial in origin, spread directly into and through the bowel wall. The degrees of transmural spread are recorded as one of the

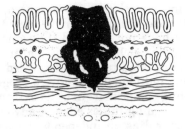

Stage A:
Invasion of the muscle only.

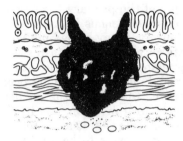

Stage B:
Invasion to the serosa.

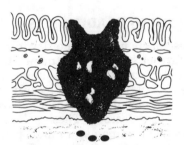

Stage C:
Invasion through the serosa
and involvement of regional
lymph nodes.

Figure 1.2. Stages of colorectal cancer (Dukes' staging).

two prime features of all large bowel cancer staging methods. (See Fig. 1.2.)
Severe epithelial dysplasia, carcinoma in situ, intramucosal carcinoma, and
severe atypia are all terms indicating restriction of the cancer to the epithelial
layer of origin. The lack of systemic or nodal spread from carcinoma in situ
is attributable to the lack of lymphatic vessels in the epithelial stroma. Invasive carcinoma (requiring therapeutic resection for potential spread of disease) is defined as cancer that has penetrated or invaded the muscularis mucosa. Invasion of the submucosa, muscularis propria, serosa, or perirectal fat
constitutes varying degrees of penetration that are recognized in the classic
staging methods. Further degrees of direct extension include adherence, invasion, and/or fistula formation to or involving an adjacent organ. Every abdominal or retroperitoneal organ is vulnerable to direct involvement.

The presence or absence of lymph node involvement is the second prime
feature of all staging methods. The prognostic significance of nodal metastases is critical. In general, the survival rate of patients with nodal metastases is half that of patients without nodal disease. Correlations regarding
survival have been made with level of nodal involvement as well as with the
number of involved lymph nodes. The quality of mesenteric lymph node examination varies from institution to institution and from specimen to speci-

men. Whereas routine serial sectioning is probably unwarranted, the value of serial sections of the entire lymph node has been demonstrated. Whereas extracapsular lymph node metastases have not received the same attention in large bowel cancer as in breast cancer, such pathologic features are generally in association with poorly differentiated tumors of guarded prognosis. This feature probably carries the same individual or additive prognostic significance either as an aggressive leading tumor margin or as extranodal mesenteric implants. The character of the leading tumor edge or advancing margin has also been correlated with survival as an independent variable. The significance of venous invasion is another factor of clear-cut importance that has been demonstrated repeatedly in the literature. The frequency of vein invasion rises with depth of penetration of the primary tumor and the presence of lymph node metastases. The effect of venous invasion on survival is significant. In its absence, the 5-year survival may be as high as 73% and in its presence, 41%. However, in patients without node metastases, intramural venous invasion is not a significant prognostic factor. Lymphatic invasion in invasive carcinoma in the absence of nodal metastases has not been of proven prognostic significance and has been noted to relate to the incidence of local tumor recurrence. The frequency of perineural invasion may be a function of tumor grade. Survival is influenced to the same degree as in venous invasion, and perineural venous lymphatic invaison seems to be additive prognostic factors.

CHARACTERISTICS OF CANCERS ARISING IN ADENOMAS

Carcinoma must penetrate the muscularis mucosa in order to metastasize. In-situ cancer therefore requires no further surgical treatment. Any invasive carcinoma in a sessile adenoma should be treated by resection. Controversy exists, however, over the management of carcinoma arising in pedunculated adenomas. Pedunculated adenomas are removable by cautery snare, whether by rigid protocosigmoidoscopy or flexible endoscopy. These polyps may demonstrate carcinoma in situ, microinvasive carcinoma (a minor penetration of the muscularis mucosa), stromal invasion (above the level of normal colonic mucosa), or invasion of the stalk. The cautery line may be involved by cancer or be free. Lymphatic invasion may be present in stromal or stalk invasion. Recent papers strongly suggest that with the exception of carcinomas deeply involving the stalk or those with an involved or unclear cautery line, further resection of the colon usually is not necessary, unless the cancer is poorly differentiated or shows lymphatic or vascular space involvement. The usual risk of lymph node metastases from a lesion that has not yet penetrated the bowel wall is less than 1%, rising to 5% with bowel wall invasion (20).

CLINICAL FEATURES

Cancers of the rectum and colon grow and obstruct, ulcerate and bleed, invade and cause pain, and, less commonly, perforate into an adjacent organ or the peritoneal space. The clinical features present in an individual patient are determined by the biologic growth characteristics of the cancer and by its location in the colon. Rectal bleeding is a symptom most often associated with cancers in the left side of the colon and cancers in the rectum. The passage of red blood sometimes mixed with darker blood clots is a common development, but the bleeding is usually not massive. With cancers in the right side of the colon, however, bleeding may be slow, and the blood mixed with bowel contents may be occult. However, patients gradually become iron deficient and anemic because of blood loss. They may present with symptoms such as weakness, dizziness, congestive heart failure, angina, or claudication. If right-sided colon cancers bleed more rapidly, they may be a source of melena. A severe hemorrhage may produce a reddish, maroon stool. Bleeding from colon cancer tends to be intermittent, with symptom-free intervals when no blood may be detected. Anorexia and weight loss are common in advanced colon cancer. The anorexia is intensified by partially obstructing lesions that may cause cramping abdominal pain associated with meals. Weakness and malaise may be related to anemia but are often an indication of advanced and metastatic disease. Metastases from colon cancer will produce symptoms, depending on the areas affected. Local invasion of the peritoneum or retroperitoneum may produce localized abdominal or back pain. Neurologic signs and pelvic and sciatic pain may result from invasion of the lumbosacral plexus, spine, and pelvis. Ascites, bowel obstruction, and ileus may develop from intra-abdominal tumor spread. Right upper quadrant mass, pain, and jaundice will result from liver metastases. Pulmonary metastases may be a cause of cough and dyspnea.

DIAGNOSIS

The early symptoms of colorectal cancer may be intermittent and subtle. Initial mild symptoms tend to be overlooked or regarded as unimportant by patient and physician alike. Nonneoplastic conditions may produce similar clinical pictures, but in high-risk patients or average-risk patients over 40 years of age, these symptoms should be approached with the possibility of colon cancer in mind. Other common causes for bright-red rectal bleeding include hemorrhoids, diverticulosis, angiodysplasia, colitis, and adenomatous polyps. The character and severity of rectal bleeding does not help distinguish benign from malignant disease. Hemorrhoids or fissures in-ano frequently produce a small amount of blood noted on the toilet tissue, but rectal cancer may cause the same symptom. Profuse bleeding is more likely due to angiodysplasia, diverticulosis, or inflammatory bowel disease but may also emanate from an ulcerated carcinoma. A single episode of such bleeding may occur as the only symptom of the cancer. Changes in bowel habits, with constipation, crampy pain, and narrowed stool caliber, may result from diverticulosis as well as cancer involving the left colon. It is often difficult to determine if a localized peritoneal abscess is due to a perforated diverticulum or to a cancer. Inflammatory bowel disease or infectious colitis may cause bleeding, tenesmus, urgency, and diarrhea, but colorectal cancer must be a consideration. In most patients with irritable bowel syndrome, a careful history will document long-standing symptoms. However, although patients with irritable bowel syndrome do not seem to have a higher incidence of colon cancer, they certainly still may develop this malignancy. In patients with known irritable bowel, a sudden worsening or change in the nature of their symptoms suggests the possibility of colon cancer. Digital examination of the rectum may detect an unsuspected mass lesion. Thus, the digital rectal examination becomes a crucial part of the physical examination and should not be omitted without reason. Colon cancers that become large and bulky, usually right-sided in location, may produce a palpable abdominal mass. Metastatic spread to the liver may cause hepatomegaly, and the liver may feel hard and nodular and be slightly tender. Peritoneal metastases may cause ascites, and peripheral lymphadenopathy may represent metastatic spread. Weight loss, cachexia, pallor, and jaundice suggest advanced disease.

LABORATORY

Laboratory tests are of limited help in diagnosing and evaluating patients with colon cancer. Tests that document iron deficiency anemia and occult blood in the stool suggest the diagnosis of colon cancer. A complete blood count typically would show low hemoglobin and hematocrit and low mean corpuscular hemoglobin concentration. Blood smears would be hypochromic and microcytic in appearance. Serum iron would be low and iron-binding capacity high. A bone marrow would show absent iron stores. Occult blood in the stool may be tested at the time of rectal examination using a guaiac-impregnated slide. A positive test suggests the diagnosis of cancer, but bleeding from cancer may be intermittent, and a single negative test does not rule out the disease. Hypoalbuminemia suggests malnutrition and advanced disease. Abnormal levels of liver enzymes may represent hepatic metastases, and elevated blood urea nitrogen (BUN) and creatinine may be due to blockage of the ureters by retroperitoneal or pelvic diseases. Carcinoembryonic antigen (CEA) is a glycoprotein with a molecular weight of approximately 200,000. It was first described by Gold and Freedman in 1965, followed by the development of a radioimmunoassay in 1969 that could detect serum level in nanogram amounts. Further experiments have shown CEA to be a complex and heterogeneous material that exists on peripheral cell membranes, from which it is shed into surrounding body fluids. It is catabolized in the circulation and in the liver and partially excreted into the bile. Commercially available radioimmunoassays have a sensitivity of 0.5 mg per ml and are sensitive and reproducible tests, with some interlaboratory variations (2,7). When first described it appeared that CEA would be a tumor-specific test for colon cancer that would enable early diagnosis in asymptomatic patients. This has proved not to be the case. CEA has been found to be elevated in the blood in patients with a variety of malignancies, including gastric, pancreatic, lung, breast, and bladder cancers. In addition, CEA was identified in the tissues of many normal organs, and benign conditions of these organs can produce serum elevations. CEA elevations are common in smokers, in active cirrhosis, in pancreatitis, and in inflammatory bowel disease. In screening large populations for colon cancer, CEA was found to have a false-positive rate of 15% and false-negative rate of 40 to 60% in nonmetastatic disease. Thus, the test lacks both the specificity and the sensitivity to allow for screening. Moreover, patients with elevated CEA tended to be those with more advanced cancer. A majority of asymptomatic patients with early stages of disease have normal CEA values in their blood. The CEA test may have some value in estimating prognosis, in judging progression, and in indicating recurrence after surgery.

PREVENTION

General Principles and Definitions

For improved survival, a desirable goal is earlier diagnosis. This concept fits into the current emphasis on preventive measures for cancer in general and for colorectal cancer specifically. Prevention can be defined as primary or secondary. Primary prevention is the identification of factors, either genetic or environmental, responsible for colorectal cancer and its eradication. Secondary prevention may be defined as early detection of colorectal cancer prior to its more advanced, devastating, and fatal consequences, as well as detection and eradication of premalignant disease before its transformation into cancer. The goal in secondary prevention is to reduce the mortality from colorectal cancer in the entire group targeted for this approach. This is an important concept and must be distinguished from survival of those patients identified as having a premalignant or malignant lesion. It is obviously important to identify such individuals, and our goal is, of course, for these individuals to have a long survival free of disease. However, if our approach fails to identify a significantly large number of people in this group, and they go on to develop their disease in the usual manner with the usual mortality, then the approach is a failure. Effective mortality reduction for colorectal cancer or the population targeted by a secondary prevention approach requires methods that are successful in identifying the majority of patients developing the disease at an early stage. It is also important to keep this in mind in evaluating results of programs. Reports of improved survival in detected cases represent only one part of the overall picture (3). A secondary approach to the prevention of colorectal cancer encompasses several concepts. The first concept is the prompt recognition of symptoms suggesting colorectal cancer and application of an aggressive approach using all presently available diagnostic techniques to uncover the neoplastic problem. It is preferable to make a diagnosis in the presymptomatic stage, but we must also take a new look at our approach to symptomatic patients. There are many delays in the health care system in arriving at diagnosis in patients with symptoms of colorectal cancer. Prompt use of endoscopy and adequate barium enemas could probably reduce the diagnostic delay in many patients. In many instances, aggressive search of the colon in patients with symptoms of colorectal neoplasia would uncover premalignant adenomas. Their removal could provide protection for the evolution of colorectal cancer. It has been reported from some centers that radical cancer surgery in patients presenting at a symptomatic stage could result in better survival than following lesser operations for cancer. Asymptomatic patients can be approached with screening or case-finding techniques. *Screening* is defined as an approach to a large population, and *case finding* is defined as an approach to individual patients and small groups within the framework of the health care system. These screening or case-finding approaches should be varied depending on whether the patients are at average risk or in one of the high-risk groups.

Fecal Occult Blood Testing

The testing of stools for the presence of occult blood as an early indicator of gastrointestinal malignancy is an old concept. In past years patients were asked to bring one or more stool samples in without any dietary restriction for testing with guaiac solution. There was no quality control of the stability of the reagents used. This approach was soon discarded because of the high percentage of false positives and false negatives. Benzidine was used in a similar manner but discarded because of extremely high sensitivity, which resulted in a high percentages of false positives with unnecessary diagnostic workups of patients. Hematest® (Orthotoluidine) was shown not to be reproducible for clinical screening. The guaiac test for occult blood in the stool was reintroduced by Greegor in the late 1960s. In this approach the patient smeared two samples of stool per day for a total of six smears over 3 days onto a smear slide. Using this approach, Greegor reported detection of colorectal cancers in several patients at an early pathologic stage. The nature of the reaction of the guaiac test is not well understood. The current guaiac paper slide test consists of filter paper impregnated with guaiac, which undergoes phenolic oxidation in the presence of hemoglobin in the stool, and hydrogen peroxide in the test reagent. The guaiac consists of a group of heterogeneous compounds present in varying proportions and with different stages of purity, depending on the processing of the guaiac before impregnation of the paper. The positive reaction produced by hemoglobin is a result of its pseudoperoxidase activity, which interacts with the hydrogen peroxide, resulting in the phenolic oxidation of the guaiac, changing it to blue. Anything having peroxidase activity, such as fresh fruit and uncooked vegetables, can produce a positive reaction. Agents that interfere with the oxidation reaction, such as ascorbic acid, may produce a false-negative reaction in the presence of hemo-

Table 1.3.
Application of Fecal Occult Blood Test

Not applicable	Patients with symptoms suggesting colorectal neoplasia
	Patients with familial polyposis or Gardner's syndrome
	Patients with ulcerative colitis
As primary screen or case finding	Asymptomatic average-risk men and women over age 50; suggestive family history over age 40
As adjunctive interval test	Patients with past history of adenoma
	Patients with past history of colorectal cancer
	Strong history of family cancer syndrome

globin. A positive test, therefore, can be positive from nonhuman hemoglobin present in foods such as meat, from human hemoglobin lost as physiologic blood loss of no consequence, or from lesions such as adenomas and cancers. Sufficient quantities of blood lost anywhere in the GI tract can lead to a positive test (Table 1.3) (21–29).

There are five controlled trials studying the possible usefulness of the stool blood test in screening for colorectal cancer. A trial was started in 1975 by Memorial Sloan-Kettering Cancer Center (MSKCC) and Strang Clinic to evaluate the stool occult blood test for detection of colorectal cancer in conjunction with proctosigmoidoscopic examination in the setting of comprehensive preventive medical examinations. At the Preventive Medicine Institute-Strang Clinic, health-conscious people received self-paid comprehensive medical examinations, with emphasis on cancer detection. Patients over age 40 who came to the clinic were enrolled and allocated to the study and control groups based on date of enrollment. All 21,756 participants underwent a comprehensive examination that included a general physical examination, a health history questionnaire, and 25 cm proctosigmoidoscopy. Patients assigned to the study group were also offered stool blood testing; control patients were not. It was found that the incorporation of the stool blood test in the Strang Clinic routine was feasible and that approximately 75% of patients were willing to prepare their slides at the time of their enrollment in the program. Participation in the following years dropped sharply, primarily because most patients failed to return to Strang Clinic for rescreening. When offered the opportunity to mail in their test slides, with no charge for the service, only a small fraction complied. The overall rate of positive tests was 1.7% with non-hydrated slides and was strongly age dependent. The rate of positivity was higher for patients who had not had periodic sigmoidoscopic examination in previous years. The predictive value of the test for adenomas or cancer combined was 30% and was also strongly age dependent, greatest on first screen and poor under age 50. Thus, it was clear that the greatest yield of neoplasms from the stool blood test will result from screening people over age 50 who have not been examined for several years. More than 75% of the patients with a positive stool blood test underwent diagnostic procedures within a year after their tests. The barium enema missed 25% of the lesions found through colonoscopy. The sensitivity for the stool blood test for cancer was estimated at 70% and specificity at 98%. A distinct stage difference was observed with respect to those cancers found on the first screen, and the prevalence cases in those patients not having prior screens at the clinic. The screened group had 65% of Dukes' A or B cancers compared to 33% in the control group (Table 1.4) (22).

Table 1.4.
Early Results of Controlled Trials of Colorectal Cancer Screening Using Stool Blood Tests[a]

	Cohort Size	Positivity Rate (%)	Predictive Value (%) (Adenomas & Cancer)	Dukes' A & B Cancers (%)	
				Screened Group	Control Group
Göteborg, Sweden	27,000	1.9	22	65	33
Nottingham, England	150,000	2.1	53	90	40
New York, USA	22,000	1.7	30	65	33
Minnesota, USA	48,000	2.4	31	78	35
Odense, Denmark	62,000	1.0	58	81	55

[a]This table is derived from multiple sources and summarizes mainly nonhydrated slide data, although hydrated slides also have been used in a phase of some programs. The staging is from initial screening. See text and references for details.

A second controlled trial evaluating stool occult blood testing was initiated at the University of Minnesota. In this study, 48,000 participants age 50 and older were randomly allocated into one of three study groups: those who were offered stool blood testing each year, those who were offered slides every other year, and a control group. Compliance with slide preparation was 75%, and the overall rate of slide positivity was 2.4%. Of patients with positive tests who underwent diagnostic evaluation, 31% had either adenomas or cancer of the colon or rectum, 78% of which were Dukes' A or B. This study is now in a rescreening and follow-up stage. The single-column barium enema had a poor sensitivity and was discontinued, and colonoscopy was considered extremely important (23). A controlled trial was started more recently in England with asymptomatic individuals identified from family doctor registries and allocated randomly to test and control groups. The first test group (10,253) had a 39% compliance with stool blood tests, resulting in 2.1% positive tests for nonhydrated slides, with a predictive value for adenomas and cancer of 40%, and a Dukes' A and B staging of cancers. Sensitivity was estimated at 80% and specificity at 98% for the 2-year period. The group is now undergoing follow-up and further screening. A fourth controlled trial of screening is in progress in Sweden and involves 27,700 inhabitants of Göteborg, ages 60 to 64. The rate of positivity in the screened group was 1.9%, using nonhydrated slides. In the initial screen, 65% of the cancers were Dukes' A or B compared to 33% in the control group. The estimated sensitivity for cancer was 52%, which may reflect the method for interpretation of the slide test since the positive rate of 1.9% is extremely low for a first screen of an older age group. Additional trials have been planned or just recently initiated, and additional data will be forthcoming. The trials thus far appear to have similar rates of positive slide tests for nonhydrated slides (1.7 to 4.0%), similar predictive values for adenoma and cancer (22 to 40%), and a shift to earlier Dukes' staging (65 to 90% Dukes' A and B). However, the compliance has ranged from a low of 39 to 80% for the first screen, with variable acceptance of subsequent screening. All data indicate an improved clinical sensitivity for cancers but loss of specificity when slides were hydrated. The sensitivity of the nonhydrated slide has been estimated to be 70 to 80%, with one study reporting 52% sensitivity associated with a low rate of positive slide tests. Complete evaluation of the colon is clearly necessary, and colonoscopy is favored as part of the diagnostic workup, but not uniformly as the initial step. As yet survival data are not available but can be expected to be favorable given the stage improvement. Mortality data will be forthcoming within the next few years from those programs having complete follow-up and mortality review. It will be important to see whether identification of colonic adenomas and their removal will be associated with a reduced incidence of colon cancer in these patients. The percentage of patients with colon adenomas detected by a single screen with stool blood testing is small. Identification and removal of a significant proportion of larger prevalent adenomas probably will require several screens and use of colonoscopy as the diagnostic tool. Furthermore, the impact of this on colorectal cancer incidence and mortality would require a fairly long period of time to determine given the natural history of colorectal cancer and its evolution from adenomas (26).

Sigmoidoscopy

The effectiveness of sigmoidoscopy as a screening test has not been well studied, but some valuable data are available that suggest effectiveness. In a Memorial Sloan-Kettering Cancer Center/Strang Clinic program more than 26,000 mostly asymptomatic patients underwent a total of 47,091 rigid examinations, with 58 cancers detected (9). Of these 58 cancers, 81% were Dukes' A and B, and the 15-year survival was 90%. This was an uncontrolled study with follow-up data only on the cancer cases. Studies evaluating the efficacy of periodic Multiphasic Health Checkup in the Northern California Kaiser-Permanente program indicated a reduced mortality from colorectal cancer in a group having rigid sigmoidoscopy as part of their checkup. This mortality reduction was reconfirmed in a 16-year follow-up. Adenomas are detected by sigmoidoscopy at a higher frequency than carcinomas. The frequency of polyps detected by sigmoidoscopy has varied from 2 to 30%, and approximately half are true adenomas. The first encounter has a higher yield than the subsequent encounter, since it uncovers prevalent rather than incident disease. The yield increases with age and in the presence of high-risk factors, especially a family history of colorectal cancer or adenomas. One study has addressed the value of sigmoidoscopy in the control of rectosigmoid cancer by identification and removal of polyps (10). Periodic rigid sigmoidoscopy was performed in 18,000 patients over a 25-year period, and all polyps were removed. Only 14 rectal cancers were detected during this period, which was 15% of that expected in the state of Minnesota during this period of time. The study was uncontrolled, and the pathology of the removed polyps and the completeness of follow-up were not reported. These studies have used rigid sigmoidoscopy. There are no controlled trials in progress evaluating long-term benefit of newer flexible endoscopes (29).

General Guidelines

An important issue is what our current professional posture should be toward colorectal cancer screening (see Chapter 15). This issue should be viewed within the context of the larger issue of how to improve survival of patients with or at risk for colorectal cancer. We have seen exciting conceptual and technologic developments in a relatively short period of time that have enhanced our ability to control this disease. There is a clearer understanding of the importance of identifying and removing premalignant adenomas; the nature of synchronous and metachronous lesions; risk factors, especially familial; and the value of anatomic surgical resection. There are now available accurate diagnostic tests and the ability to remove most adenomas without the need for major surgery. Appropriate application of these concepts and techniques to symptomatic patients and those with increased risk can have a significant impact. Should screening be added to these developments to provide additional benefit? Certain mathematical projections based on available data, especially from controlled trials, can be provided for physicians who have elected to screen asymptomatic people in their practice. Approximately 2% of patients will have a positive test, and one out of three of these people will have an adenoma or cancer on further workup. This yield is comparable to that found in high risk groups. Unfortunately, approximately 30% of the cancers will be missed by one screening. Within this framework, proctosigmoidoscopy once every three to five years and stool blood testing annually beginning at age 50 may be the most reasonable approach to detect early colorectal cancer and adenomas. Rigid sigmoidoscopy should be used if this is the only available expertise, but flexible sigmoidoscopy would be better accepted by the patient and have a higher yield of neoplastic lesions. Diagnostic workup of patients with a positive screening test should include evaluation of the entire colon by either colonoscopy, double contrast barium enema with flexible sigmoidoscopy, or both. Colonoscopy provides the opportunity for polypectomy in addition to its diagnostic capability. Appropriate study of the upper gastrointestinal (UGI) tract should be at the discretion of the physician in each patient. The American Cancer Society (ACS) and the International Workgroup on Colorectal Cancer (now the World Health Organization [WHO] Collaborating Center for the Prevention of Colorectal Cancer) have supported guidelines such as the above; other groups such as the Canadian Cancer Society and the International Union Against Cancer (UICC) have not (30,31).

The National Cancer Institute (NCI) has recently developed and reported working guidelines for the early detection of cancers at multiple sites, including the colon. Their guidelines agree with those of the ACS and the WHO Collaborating Center. In developing these guidelines, the NCI noted the decreasing mortality rate in spite of the rising incidence of colorectal cancer and attributed this to early detection and improved treatment (32). All organizations recommending early detection strategies include both sigmoidoscopy, preferably flexible, and stool blood testing. In addition, the recommendation is for case finding by physicians of individuals seeking health checkups. There is insufficient evidence, nor is it desirable, to encourage mass population screening.

High-risk patients require an individualized approach. Those with a family history of familial polyposis or Gardner's syndrome need to have an annual sigmoidoscopy beginning in their teens to determine if they are affected. Adenomas in the affected family member will appear in the rectosigmoid as well as in the remainder of the colon. On the other hand, members of families with the family cancer syndrome tend to have a more proximal distribution of the adenomas and cancer and thus need to have an entire colon examination periodically. Colonoscopy is the preferred examination, since adenomas will be the most frequent finding and can be removed at the same time. Individuals with a lesser family history of colorectal cancer, such as those with a single affected first-degree relative, can be reasonably screened with the same approach as for average-risk patients, but it is felt that the screening should begin at an earlier age, perhaps age 40. Colonoscopy and double contrast barium enema have also been suggested as a result of a recent report using a mathematical model (33). The more aggressive approach would have to be individualized considering the large number of people at increased risk because of a single first-degree relative with colorectal cancer. Recent evidence strongly suggests that "sporadic" colon cancer probably is inherited to a large extent but presently is unidentifiable because of low expression and lack of sensitive biomarkers (34–36). The decision whether to employ the more aggressive approach in people with a family history short of the family cancer syndrome would also rest on the number of family members affected as well as their age of diagnosis. Patients with ulcerative colitis involving the entire colon of more than 7 years' duration, or with left-sided colitis of 15 years duration, should have periodic colonoscopy with search for cancers and biopsies for dysplasia either every year or every 2 years. The interval has not been well established. Patients having an adenoma removed need to have their colons examined for synchronous adenomas and need to be in a long-term surveillance program to search periodically for metachronous adenomas. Colonoscopy every 3 years after initial clearing colonoscopies is adequate for the majority of such patients, but there are individual considerations such as multiple polyps, large sessile polyps and malignant polyps, which would alter the approach (37).

Considerably more data are needed regarding risk factors, screening tests, patient acceptance, and physician attitudes. Concepts of risk are evolving rapidly, especially in regard to those at risk because of genetic transmission of the disease. It is possible that a much greater proportion of colorectal cancers and adenomas have a genetic basis. Studies are underway to test the hypothesis that a significant proportion of colorectal cancer is caused by a dominant gene with low penetrance (21). Classification of the genetic basis of colorectal cancer and a better understanding of who the high-risk patients are would allow for more effective application of screening and would help resolve the major problems of patient acceptance of these preventive approaches. Improved identification of high-risk patients could also result from the studies examining the phenotypic expression of neoplastic predisposition, as observed in abnormalities of cell proliferation, maturation, and repair.

The introduction of screening requires an understanding of natural history; the availability of facilities for diagnosis and optimal treatment; a defined policy about the indications for treatment; and the application of a screening test that is acceptable, effective, and efficient. Interest in colorectal cancer screening research over the past 10 years has stimulated interest in colorectal cancer in general. Whenever screening is introduced into a community, a major educational benefit results. It stimulates discussions and reduces denial about lifestyle and diet, elucidates the public health importance of colorectal cancer, and increases awareness of the nature of significant warning signs that should compel medical attention. It begins to erode the fear of disabling colostomy, reduces anxiety, enables more reassuring discussions of treatment options, and emphasizes principles of optimal surgical management. It focuses attention on risk factors such as polyps and family history and the need for lifetime, periodic follow-up of high-risk patients.

We now have a new understanding of the risks and natural history of colorectal cancer. We have techniques for earlier detection, improved diagnosis and treatment, and guidelines for appropriate follow-up. It is clear that we need and await more data and better tools. New developments in technology over the past 10 years will influence performance of screening tests and may dictate changes in approach. Current examples of this are the flexible sigmoidoscopy and the HemoQuant test, and further developments in biochemical and immunologic assays could radically alter available opportunities. It is also clear that preventive approaches must in the future include primary intervention. However, we, as physicians, have a responsibility to communicate advancing frontiers of knowledge to our colleagues, and collectively we should communicate to the public a positive message regarding the progress that has been made in the prevention and control of colorectal cancer (38,39).

References

1. American Cancer Society, Inc. Cancer facts and figures. New York: American Cancer Society, 1982.

2. Schottenfeld D, Winawer SJ. Large intestine. In: Schottenfeld D, Fraumeni J Jr., eds. Cancer, epidemiology and prevention. Philadelphia: W.B. Saunders, 1982:703–727.
3. Winawer SJ, Sherlock P, Schottenfeld D, et al. Screening for colon cancer. Gastroenterology 1976;70:783–789.
4. Doll R. General epidemiologic considerations in etiology of colorectal cancer. In: Winawer SJ, Schottenfeld D, Sherlock P, eds. Progress in cancer research and therapy. Vol. 13. Colorectal cancer: Prevention, epidemiology and screening. New York: Raven Press, 1980:3–12.
5. Burkitt DP. Fiber in the etiology of colorectal cancer. In: Winawer SJ, Schottenfeld D, Sherlock P, eds. Progress in cancer research and therapy. Vol. 13. Colorectal cancer: Prevention, epidemiology and screening. New York: Raven Press, 1980:13–18.
6. Weisburger JH, Reddy BS, Spingarn NE, et al. Current views on the mechanisms involved in the etiology of colorectal cancer. In: Winawer SJ, Schottenfeld D, Sherlock P, eds. Progress in cancer research and therapy. Vol. 13. Colorectal cancer: Prevention, epidemiology and screening. New York: Raven Press, 1980:19–41.
7. Sherlock P, Lipkin M, Winawer SJ. The prevention of colon cancer: A combined clinic and basic science seminar. Am J Med 1980;68:917–931.
8. Morson BC. Genesis of colorectal cancer. Clin Gastroenterol 1976;5:505–525.
9. Heald RJ, Bussey HJR. Clinical experience at St. Mark's Hospital with multiple synchronous cancers of the colon and rectum. Dis Colon Rectum 1975;18:6.
10. Schottenfeld D, Berg JW, Vitsky B. Incidence of multiple primary cancers: II. Index cancers arising in the stomach and lower digestive system. JNCI 1969;42:77.
11. Ekelund GR. Cancer risk with single and multiple adenomas: Synchronous and metachronous tumors. In: Winawer SJ, Schottenfeld D, Sherlock P, eds. Progress in cancer research and therapy. Vol. 13. Colorectal cancer: Prevention, epidemiology and screening. New York: Raven Press, 1980:151–155.
12. Sherlock P, Lipkin M, Winawer SJ. Predisposing factors in colon carcinoma. Adv Intern Med 1975;20:121–150.
13. Shinya H. Colonoscopy: Diagnosis and treatment of colonic diseases. New York: Igaku-Shoin, 1982.
14. Devroede G. Risk of cancer in inflammatory bowel disease. In: Winawer SJ, Schottenfeld D, Sherlock P, eds. Progress in cancer research and therapy. Vol. 13. Colorectal cancer: Prevention, epidemiology and screening. New York: Raven Press, 1980:325–334.
15. Lennard-Jones JW, Morson BC, Ritchie JK, et al. Cancer in colitis: Assessment of the individual risk by clinical and histological criteria. Gastroenterology 1977;73:1280.
16. Levin B, Riddell RH, Frank P, et al. Evaluation of cancer risk in chronic ulcerative colitis: University of Chicago experience. In: Winawer SJ, Schottenfeld D, Sherlock P, eds. Progress in cancer research and therapy. Vol. 13. Colorectal cancer: Prevention, epidemiology and screening. New York: Raven Press, 1980:381–385.
17. Waye JD. The role of colonoscopy in surveillance for patients with ulcerative colitis. In: Winawer SJ, Schottenfeld D, Sherlock P, eds. Progress in cancer research and therapy. Vol. 13. Colorectal cancer: Prevention, epidemiology and screening. New York: Raven Press, 1980.
18. Kussin SZ, Lipkin M, Winawer SJ. Inherited colon cancer: Clinical implications. Am J Gastroenterol 1979;72:448–457.
19. Lynch HT, Lynch PM, Lynch JF. Analysis of genetics of inherited colon cancer. In: Winawer SJ, Schottenfeld D, Sherlock P, eds. Progress in cancer research and therapy. Vol. 13. Colorectal cancer: Prevention, epidemiology and screening. New York: Raven Press, 1980:117–131.
20. Haggitt RC, Glotzbach RE, Soffer EE, et al. Prognostic factors in colorectal carcinomas arising in adenomas. Gastroenterology 1985;89(2):328–336.
21. Winawer SJ, Fleisher M, Baldwin M, et al. Current status of fecal occult blood testing in screening for colorectal cancer. New York: American Cancer Society, Inc., 1982.
22. Winawer SJ, Andrews M, Flehinger B, et al. Progress report on controlled trial of fecal occult blood testing for the detection of colorectal neoplasia. Cancer 1980;45:2959–2964.
23. Gilbertsen VA, McHugh R, Schuman L, et al. The earlier detection of colorectal cancers: A preliminary report on the results of the occult blood study. Cancer 1980;45:2899–2901.
24. MacRae FA, James D, St. John B. Relationship between patterns of bleeding and hemoccult sensitivity in patients with colorectal cancers of adenoma. Gastroenterology 1982;82(5):891–898.
25. MacRae FA, James D, St. John B, et al. Optimal dietary conditions for hemoccult testing. Gastroenterology 1982;82(5):899–903.

26. Simon J. Occult blood screening for colorectal carcinoma: A critical review. Gastroenterology 1985;88:820–837.
27. Ahlquist DA, McGill DB, Schwartz S, et al. HemoQuant, a new quantitative assay for fecal hemoglobin. Ann Intern Med 1984;101:297–302.
28. Winchester DP, Sylvester J, Maher ML. Risks and benefits of mass screening for colorectal neoplasia with the stool guaiac test. Ca-A Cancer Journal for Clinicians 1983;33:333–343.
29. Third International Symposium on Colorectal Cancer. Ca-A Cancer Journal for Clinicians 1984;34:130–176.
30. American Cancer Society. Guidelines for the cancer-related checkup: Recommendations and rationale. Ca-A Cancer Journal for Clinicians 1980;30(4):208–223.
31. Winawer SJ (chairman). Report of the international workgroup on colorectal cancer. Geneva, January 1980.
32. National Cancer Institute, Early Detection Branch, Division of Cancer Prevention and Control. Working guidelines for early cancer detection, 1987.
33. Eddy DM, Nugent FW, Eddy JF, et al. Screening for colorectal cancer in a high-risk population: Results of a mathematical model. Gastroenterology 1987;92:682–692.
34. Burt RW, Bishop DT, Cannon LA, Dowdle MA, Lee RG, Skolnick MH. Dominant inheritance of adenomatous colonic polyps and colorectal cancer. NEJM 1985;312:1540–1544.
35. Bodmer WF, Bailey CJ, Bodmer J, et al. Localization of the gene for familial adenomatous polyposis on chromosome 5. Nature 1987;328:614–616.
36. Solomon E, Voss R, Hall V, et al. Chromosome 5 allele loss in human colorectal carcinomas. Nature 1987;328:616–619.
37. Winawer SJ, Ritchie MT, Diaz BJ, et al. The National Polyp Study: Aims and organization. In: Rozen P, Winawer SJ, eds. Secondary prevention of colorectal cancer. Basel: Karger, 1986:216–225.
38. Winawer SJ. Screening for colorectal cancer. In: DeVita VT, Hellman S, Rosenberg SA, eds. Cancer: Principles and practice of oncology. 2nd ed. Updates 1987; 1(6).
39. Winawer SJ, Kerner, JF. Sigmoidoscopy: Case finding vs. screening. Gastroenterology 1988;95:527–529.

2

Anatomy and Physiology of the Anus, Rectum, and Left Colon

Theodore R. Schrock, M.D.

ANATOMY

Divisions

The large intestine extends continuously from the ileocecal valve to the anal verge (Fig. 2.1). Anatomic divisions are based on embryologic origin and position within the abdomen (1,2). The *right colon,* derived from the midgut, consists of the cecum, ascending colon, hepatic flexure, and proximal transverse colon. Its blood supply comes from the superior mesenteric artery by way of ileocolic and middle colic branches. The *left colon* develops from the hindgut. It includes the distal transverse colon, splenic flexure, descending colon, and sigmoid colon. Arterial blood flows directly from the aorta through the inferior mesenteric artery.

The rectum also derives from the hindgut (Fig. 2.2). It joins the anal canal, which develops from the proctodeum. The rectum receives arterial blood from the inferior mesenteric artery and from branches of the internal iliac arteries entering bilaterally. The anal canal also receives blood from terminal branches of the internal iliac arteries.

Anatomic divisions of the large intestine are not sharply defined, and one portion connects with another over a distance of several centimeters. Nevertheless, during flexible sigmoidoscopy it is important to visualize the location of the instrument tip with respect to anatomic divisions, relationships of each portion of bowel with other structures, and risks of injury that result from these relationships (3).

These anatomic divisions will be discussed further in the sequence with which they are encountered during flexible sigmoidoscopy, that is from distal to proximal.

Anal Canal

The perineal skin is typical hair-bearing skin with sebaceous, sweat, and apocrine glands. At the anal verge (anal orifice), marked by corrugated skin, the anal canal actually begins (4). The anal canal is 4 cm long, points toward the umbilicus, and is collapsed into a slit in the resting state (Fig. 2.3). Because the anal canal is collapsed, it cannot be fully viewed from above, for example through a retroflexed flexible sigmoidoscope.

The lower two centimeters of the anal canal are lined by thin, pale, stratified squamous epithelium (anoderm). This modified skin contains no hair follicles, sebaceous glands, or sweat glands. About two centimeters above the anal verge is an important landmark called the dentate (pectinate) line. Tiny tooth-like projections of tissue (anal papillae) appear like a serrated fringe. Transverse flaps of skin (anal valves) overlie pits termed anal crypts. An anal gland extends deeply from each crypt into the underlying tissue and is the origin of most anorectal abscesses and fistulas. The columns of Morgagni are longitudinal gatherings of mucosa at the top of the dentate line.

The epithelium from the dentate line upward is cuboidal or transitional for

25

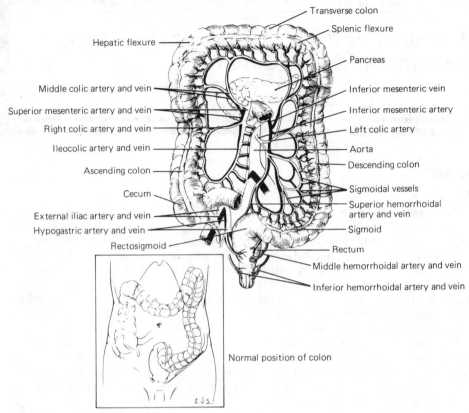

Figure 2.1. Anatomic divisions and blood supply of the large intestine. The veins are shown in black. The usual configuration of the colon is shown in the insert. Reproduced, with permission, from Way LW: *Current Surgical Diagnosis and Treatment,* 8th edition, copyright Appleton & Lange, 1988.

about 1 cm, and above that point typical columnar epithelium of the rectum is encountered.

The anal canal fuses with the rectum over a distance of several centimeters, but usually a landmark termed the anorectal ring marks the upper border of the anal canal about 4 cm from the anal verge. The anorectal ring is the fusion of puborectalis and external sphincter muscles (1). It is easily palpable: It is the point at which the rectal lumen curves posteriorly, and the examining finger hooks over the puborectalis sling that pulls the anorectal junction anteriorly. The direction of insertion of an instrument, initially toward the umbilicus, must be changed at the anorectal ring so the tip will head posteriorly.

The internal anal sphincter is the rounded, thickened lower terminus of the circular muscle layer of the gut (5). It is autonomically innervated. A pronounced sulcus (intersphincteric groove) is often visible and invariably palpable just at or inside the anal verge (Fig. 2.2). This groove separates the internal from the external sphincter, a continuous sheet of striated skeletal muscle surrounding the anal canal (1,5). The internal sphincter is involuntary, but the external sphincter is contracted voluntarily. Although the external sphincter is sometimes divided into various portions, these distinctions are not important clinically. The external sphincter fuses superiorly with the

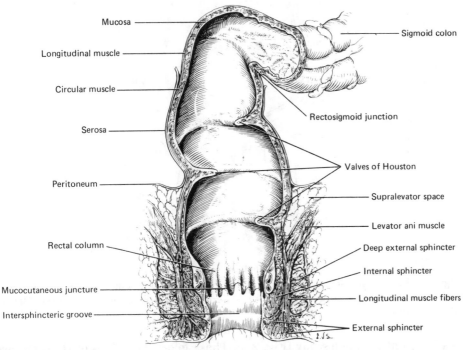

Mucosa

Longitudinal muscle

Circular muscle

Serosa

Peritoneum

Rectal column

Mucocutaneous juncture

Intersphincteric groove

Sigmoid colon

Rectosigmoid junction

Valves of Houston

Supralevator space

Levator ani muscle

Deep external sphincter

Internal sphincter

Longitudinal muscle fibers

External sphincter

Figure 2.2. Anatomy of the rectum and anus. Reproduced, with permission, from Way LW: Current Surgical Diagnosis and Treatment, 8th edition, copyright Appleton & Lange, 1988.

puborectalis portion of the levator ani muscle group. This fusion creates the anorectal ring described above. The external sphincter is deficient anteriorly but is very strong laterally and posteriorly.

The levator ani muscles can be divided into four parts (5). The puborectalis sling is the most medial of these muscles. It arises from the pubis, encircles the rectum, and pulls the anorectal junction forward. Just laterally is the pubococcygeus, which runs from the pubis to the coccyx. Further laterally is the iliococcygeus, and most lateral is the ischiococcygeus. Together the levators ani form a continuous sheet of striated muscle comprising a sort of diaphragm that is of great importance in supporting pelvic viscera. The levators have central defects for the rectum and urogenital structures. Recently a number of anatomic and physiologic abnormalities have been grouped under the heading of "disorders of the pelvic floor" to emphasize the importance of normal structure and function of this area.

Rectum

The rectum begins about 4 cm above the anal verge and extends to the rectosigmoid junction, approximately 16 cm above the anal verge. The rectum therefore is approximately 12 cm long, and it can be divided into distal, middle, and proximal portions. The anterior pelvis peritoneal reflection (pouch of Douglas) is about 7 cm above the anal verge; the rectum below that point is extraperitoneal (Fig. 2.4). Above the peritoneal reflection, the anterior and lateral portions of the rectum are intraperitoneal, and the posterior aspect is extraperitoneal. These points are important to remember in assessing the risks of biopsy or polypectomy in the rectum.

The rectum has three lateral curves that correspond with folds of the rectal

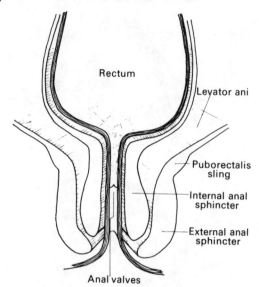

Figure 2.3. Transverse section showing the slit-like configuration of the anal canal at rest. From Goligher J. Surgery of the Anus, Rectum and Colon, 5th ed. London: Baillière Tindall, 1984.

wall seen at sigmoidoscopy (Fig. 2.5). These folds, the valves of Houston, are important landmarks in the lumen. About one-half of people have the so-called normal configuration of two valves on the left and one on the right. The middle (right) rectal valve corresponds closely with the anterior pelvic peritoneal reflection, a critical landmark during rectal procedures. A biopsy of the anterior or lateral wall above the middle valve of Houston has a risk

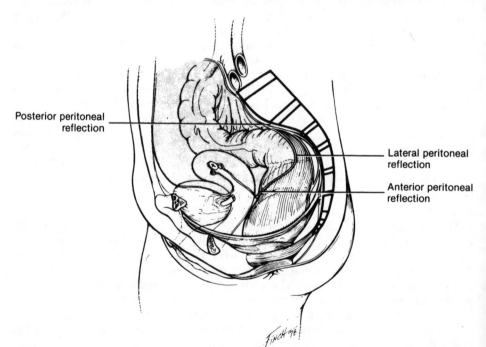

Figure 2.4. Relationship of the rectum to the peritoneum.

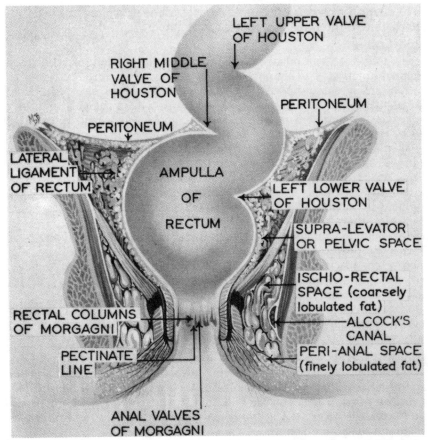

LEFT UPPER VALVE
OF HOUSTON

RIGHT MIDDLE
VALVE OF
HOUSTON

PERITONEUM

PERITONEUM

LATERAL
LIGAMENT
OF RECTUM

AMPULLA

OF

RECTUM

LEFT LOWER VALVE
OF HOUSTON

SUPRA-LEVATOR
OR PELVIC SPACE

ISCHIO-RECTAL
SPACE (coarsely
lobulated fat)

ALCOCK'S
CANAL

RECTAL COLUMNS
OF MORGAGNI

PECTINATE
LINE

PERI-ANAL SPACE
(finely lobulated fat)

ANAL VALVES
OF MORGAGNI

Figure 2.5. Coronal section showing the lateral curves of the rectum and the valves of Houston. From Goligher J. Surgery of the Anus, Rectum and Colon, 5th edition. London: Baillière Tindall, 1984.

of perforation into the peritoneal cavity, and below that point perforation results in extraperitoneal contamination by rectal contents, a serious but less catastrophic complication. Valves of Houston normally are thin and sharp, but they become thickened and blunted by inflammation. Valves may hide a small lesion from endoscopic view, and the superior surfaces of these folds must be examined.

In addition to these lateral curves, the rectum is curved posteriorly to lie in close proximity to the sacrum (Fig. 2.4). The anorectal angle produced by the anorectal ring is thought to be of some importance for continence (6).

The rectum is supported by the lateral ligaments, broad bands of connective tissue containing fat. Vessels, nerves, and lymph nodes extend from the rectal wall to the pelvis on both sides. The endopelvic fascia of Waldeyer supports the rectum posteriorly (1). Anteriorly the rectum is attached to the urogenital viscera, and of course the pelvic muscular floor is an important supporting structure. The rectum and the anal canal are surrounded by potential spaces in which infections can arise (Fig. 2.5).

At its upper end the rectum merges with the sigmoid colon at an ill-defined zone called the rectosigmoid junction. Here the longitudinal muscle changes from a continuous coat to a gathering into three discrete bundles (taeniae coli). The sigmoid mesocolon appears and appendices epiploicae are seen. Above the rectosigmoid, the intestinal wall is sacculated.

Sigmoid Colon

The sigmoid colon extends from the rectosigmoid junction into the descending-sigmoid junction. The sigmoid is a loop of variable length, extremely long and redundant in some individuals, short and contracted in others. The sigmoid is about 40 cm in length on average. It lies within the pelvis, mostly on the left side. The sigmoid is free to move in most people within constraints caused by tethering at both ends, but disease or operative scarring may fix it firmly in place in the pelvis. Diverticular disease and gynecologic surgical procedures commonly result in immobility of the sigmoid; the fixation may be so marked that progress of a flexible sigmoidoscope is impaired.

Peritoneum surrounds the sigmoid colon except in the mesocolic side, so the sigmoid is suspended in the peritoneal cavity. Most perforations of the sigmoid colon therefore are intraperitoneal.

The rectosigmoid junction is angulated in most patients, and the sigmoid drops into the pelvis. This angulation must be negotiated by examining instruments. The presence of a rectosigmoid sphincter was postulated long ago, and recently physiologic studies have given some support to this concept (2). Certainly the sigmoid has a smaller lumen than the rectum.

The sigmoid colon has prominent haustra. In the presence of diverticular disease, haustra may be exaggerated so that examination is difficult. Diverticula themselves are seen readily during flexible sigmoidoscopy.

Descending Colon, Splenic Flexure, and Transverse Colon

The descending colon runs proximally for about 30 cm from the descending-sigmoid junction to the splenic flexure. Some anatomists refer to the "iliac" colon as the portion between the iliac crest and the sigmoid colon; in the United States the term *descending colon* generally applies to all of the colon from sigmoid to splenic flexure.

The descending colon is retroperitoneal. Perforation directly anteriorly may penetrate through the posterior parietal peritoneum into the peritoneal cavity, but most perforations are confined to the retroperitoneal space.

The splenic flexure is an angulation of varying acuteness where the descending colon becomes the distal transverse colon. There are attachments between the splenic flexure and the spleen and between the splenic flexure and the diaphragm. Directly posteriorly Gerota's fascia separates the mesocolon from the kidney. The splenic flexure can be very high and sharp, or it may be much blunter. Chronic inflammatory bowel disease typically contracts the colon and straightens this flexure.

The distal transverse colon lies very close to the greater curvature of the stomach. The greater omentum drapes over the surface of the transverse colon; flimsy avascular attachments between omentum and colon are divided easily during colectomy. The transverse colon is suspended in the peritoneal cavity on its mesocolon. Below the transverse colon and mesocolon is the small intestine. Above it lies the lesser sac.

Blood Supply

The inferior mesenteric artery arises from the abdominal aorta and supplies the left colon and upper rectum (1,2). The left colic branch from the inferior mesenteric supplies the splenic flexure area, the transverse colon, and the proximal descending colon (Fig. 2.1). Sigmoidal branches from the inferior mesenteric artery supply the descending colon and sigmoid. The inferior mesenteric continues caudad as the superior hemorrhoidal artery, passing across the sacral promontory to enter the mesorectum posterior to the rectum. Collaterals are formed with the superior mesenteric artery in the splenic flexure area, and collateral also develops from the internal iliac (hypogastric) arteries. The middle hemorrhoidal arteries arise bilaterally from anterior divisions of the internal iliac and run medially in the lateral ligaments of the rectum. The inferior hemorrhoidal arteries derive from the internal pudendals and pass through Alcock's canal. These vessels anastomose with the branches from above.

Veins accompany the corresponding arteries. They drain into the liver through the portal vein or into the systemic circulation by way of the hypogastric veins. Lymphatic drainage from the submucous and subserous layers of the bowel wall passes into collecting channels and through lymph nodes that accompany the blood vessels.

Innervation

The left colon is supplied by sympathetic fibers arising in L1-3. These nerves synapse in paravertebral ganglia and travel with the inferior mesenteric arterials to the colon and rectum. Parasympathetic nerves to the left colon derive from S2-4. These fibers emerge from the spinal cord as the nervi erigentes, which form the pelvic plexus, and branches are sent to the transverse, descending, sigmoid, and upper rectum.

Somatic innervation of the anoderm and perianal skin accounts for the extreme sensitivity of this area to painful stimuli. Motor nerves to the internal sphincter are autonomic, but the voluntarily contracting external sphincter and levators ani are somatically innervated by branches from the inferior hemorrhoidal and fourth sacral nerves.

Nerve supply to erectile tissue of the penis derives from nerves that also travel to the anorectum. Injuries to these neural structures during operations to excise the rectum may cause sexual or bladder dysfunction.

PHYSIOLOGY

The small intestine digests food and absorbs nutrients. The residue entering the colon consists mainly of undigested plant cell walls (fiber). In the colon electrolytes and water are extracted, and the liquid feces are solidified. The left colon stores the waste until defecation is convenient.

The primary functions of the colon are absorption, secretion, motility, and intraluminal digestion (7). These interrelated functions are discussed separately.

Absorption

From 1 to 2 liters of water enter the colon each day as ileal effluent. This material is dessicated during colonic transit, and only 100 to 200 ml of water is excreted in stool (Table 2.1). The maximal absorptive capacity of the large intestine is 5 to 6 liters per day. Maximal capacity depends on the rate at which fluid enters the cecum, and in steady state infusion experiments the values are even higher. This reserve absorptive capacity prevents incapacitating diarrhea in healthy people. Formed feces contain about 30% solids and 70% water. Bacteria make up almost 50% of the solid wastes, and the remainder is food residue and desquamated epithelium (2).

Sodium absorption is an active process against a concentration gradient and against an electrical gradient (7). Mineralocorticoids and glucocorticoids enhance absorption of sodium and water, and antidiuretic hormone diminishes absorption of these substances in the colon. Normally sodium absorption is so efficient that as little as 5 mEq daily in the diet is sufficient. Colectomy increases minimum requirements to 80 to 100 mEq daily. There are segmental differences in the mode of absorption, and capacity to absorb di-

Table 2.1.

Mean Values for Electrolyte and Water Balance in the Normal Colon. A plus (+) Sign Indicates Absorption from the Colonic Lumen; a Minus (−) Sign Indicates Secretion into the Lumen.

	Ileal Effluent		Fecal Fluid		Colonic Absorption (per 24 h)	
	Concentration (mEq/L)	Quantity (per 24 h)	Concentration (mEq/L)	Quantity (per 24 h)	Normal	Maximal Capacity
Na$^+$	120	180 mEq	30	2 mEq	+178 mEq	+400 mEq
K$^+$	6	10 mEq	67	5 mEq	+5 mEq	−45 mEq
Cl$^-$	67	100 mEq	20	1.5 mEq	+98 mEq	+500 mEq
HCO$_3^-$	40	60 mEq	50	4 mEq	+56 mEq	
H$_2$O		1500 mL		100 mL	+1400 mL	+5000 mL

Reproduced, with permission, from Way LW: *Current Surgical Diagnosis and Treatment*, 8th edition, copyright Appleton & Lange, 1988.

minishes as waste moves distally. The cecum and right colon absorb sodium and water more rapidly than does the distal large intestine, and the rectal mucosa absorbs poorly.

Potassium enters feces by passive diffusion and by secretion in mucus. Colonic mucus contains 45 mEq of potassium; lesions that secrete excessive mucous may lead to hypokalemia (7).

Chloride is absorbed actively in exchange for bicarbonate. Volatile fatty acids are generated by bacterial enzymatic action on polysaccharides that reach the colon undigested. This fermentation process is physiologically important. There is some evidence that volatile fatty acids are required for normal absorption of sodium and water, and they may help regulate other metabolic functions of the large intestine by acting as mucosal nutrients (7). Not all volatile fatty acids are absorbed from the colon, and the remaining ones are the major osmotic force in fecal water in healthy individuals. Water enters the lumen through the mucosa to dilute the high osmolality created by fatty acids.

The nonrenal fraction of urea generated in humans each day is probably degraded to ammonia by the action of urease in colonic mucosa. The colon is able to absorb some vitamins, amino acids, and bile acids. Normally only a small amount of nutrients reaches the colon, however.

Secretion

The colon can secrete fluid as well as absorb it. Absorption and secretion are opposite poles of the transport process. Because the healthy colon absorbs more than 90% of the water entering the cecum, diarrhea can result from even small defects in colonic absorption. This is probably the mechanism of diarrhea in ulcerative colitis. Secretion of sufficient degree to produce diarrhea can result from the effects of malabsorbed bile acids on colonic mucosa. The mechanism is similar to that evoked by ricinoleic acid, the active ingredient in castor oil.

Intraluminal Digestion

Perhaps 10 to 20% of ingested starch passes unabsorbed into the colon, where bacterial fermentation converts it to short-chain volatile fatty acids as described above. This mechanism provides calories at least to the mucosa and perhaps to the entire body. Sugars also are metabolized in the colon in patients who malabsorb carbohydrate, but this mechanism probably has little significance in healthy people.

Motility

Complex mechanisms govern movement of ileal effluent through the colon (7–10). Propulsion through the colon is normally slow, allowing prolonged time for chyme to remain in contact with mucosa and thus facilitate absorption. Although most portions of the large intestine are capable of both storage and propulsion of contents, most of the absorption occurs in the right colon and in a healthy individual, and storage is a principal function of the transverse colon. Contents arriving at the rectum are stored only briefly before defecation occurs.

Myoelectrical Activity

Although the small intestine participates in regular cycles of interdigestive migrating electrical complexes in the fasting state, these electrical impulses apparently do not propagate into the colon. Myoelectrical recordings at very slow frequencies have been described in the distal colon and rectum, but recent data challenges the validity of these earlier reports, and much remains to be learned about myoelectrical activity in this portion of the bowel.

Eating produces a group of alterations in colonic myoelectrical activity collectively termed the gastrocolic response. There is a motor response as well as an electrical one; motor activity is most convincingly demonstrated in the distal colon where mass movements are increased and the urge to defecate may be perceived.

The mid-transverse colon is the site of a proposed pacemaker (7). Propagation in the orad direction retards transit and improves absorption. Distal propagation from the pacemaker facilitates propulsion of luminal contents toward the rectum.

Colonic Pressure

The proposed mid-colonic pacemaker generates muscular contractions that raise pressures to accompany propagating electrical waves. Very high pressures can be generated in the sigmoid colon. In the rectosigmoid junction, a physiologic sphincter—if not an actual sphincter—seems to produce an area of high intraluminal pressure and a high frequency of phasic contractions. Very high pressure is thought to be an important factor in the pathogenesis of sigmoid colonic diverticula.

Transit

Luminal contents are propelled through the colon in response to a pressure gradient. Three patterns of colonic movement have been described, and there is marked regional variation among different portions of the colon (7–10). *Retrograde propulsion* is a pressure wave arising in the mid-transverse colon and moving orad. These annular contractions churn the contents and retard transit so that chyme is in contact with the cecum and ascending colon long enough to allow absorption. As ileal effluent continually enters the cecum, some of the column of liquid stool in the right colon is displaced, and it flows into the transverse colon.

Segmentation is the most common type of motor activity in the transverse and descending colon. Annular contractions create uniform segments that are nonpropulsive; both orad and aboral movements result. Segmental contractions form, relax, and reform in different locations following a pattern that appears to be random. *Mass movement* is a strong ring contraction moving aboral over long distances in the transverse and descending colon. It occurs only a few times daily and is most common after meals. Mass movements last only a few seconds.

The transit time for chyme to leave the stomach and arrive at the colon is about 12 hours. Transit through the normal large intestine occurs in 36 to 48 hours; about one-third of this interval is taken up in the right colon, another one-third in the left colon, and one-third in the rectosigmoid area. Movement of feces through the colon occurs at a net rate of about 1 cm per hour (7).

Physical activities such as changing posture, walking, and lifting are physiologically important stimuli to colonic transit. The rate of movement of colonic contents is affected by emotional states as well. A diet containing large elements of fiber is believed to hasten transit through the colon, and fat arriving in the right colon induces high-pressure contractions and rapid propulsion toward the left side.

Normal colonic movements are extremely variable, and the fecal stream does not move in an orderly fashion. Some ileal effluent will flow past feces remaining from earlier periods, particularly if feces enter the periphery of haustra, where they may lodge for 24 hours or longer. Mixing of bowel content in the colon may result in defecation of residue from a single meal in movements up to 3 to 4 days afterward (2).

Defecation

The urge to defecate is perceived when a small amount of feces or gas enters the rectum and stimulates receptors in the rectal wall or the levator ani muscles (7,9,11). The sensation may be temporarily suppressed by voluntarily contracting the sphincters and pelvic floor. The rectum has a great capacity to accommodate, and pressure diminishes slowly as the rectum expands. This mechanism allows the bolus to remain in the rectum, and it permits rectal contents to be sampled.

Sampling is a physiologic process that allows rectal contents to come into contact with the sensory epithelium of the upper anal canal to discriminate among flatus, liquid stool, and solid stool. Sampling results at least partly from a reflex relaxation of the internal sphincter. A short Valsalva maneuver contributes to sampling also.

When the rectum has filled beyond the maximum tolerable volume, the urge to defecate is impossible to deny. Maximum tolerable volume diminishes with aging (8).

Defecation is aided by assumption of a position with the thighs and hips flexed so that intra-abdominal pressure can be increased by a Valsalva maneuver. The internal and external anal sphincters relax, and the rectal contents are extruded by contraction of the colon and by increasing abdominal pressure. The pelvic floor relaxes, and the rectum looses its curves as feces are discharged from the anus. After defecation, sphincter tone returns, and the rectum normally remains empty until more feces arrive to trigger the cycle again.

The frequency of defecation is influenced by social customs and dietary habits. Among Western people the frequency of defecation varies from two or three times daily to once every 2 or 3 days. Dietary fiber and physical activity increase stool frequency. Inactivity is apt to result in infrequent passage of hard stools.

Continence

Mechanisms of anal continence are poorly understood and the subject of intensive research. The high-pressure zone created by contraction of the internal sphincter at rest and contraction of the external sphincters voluntarily is an important factor in fecal continence (9,11). If the puborectalis muscle is divided, incontinence invariably occurs (1). The anal canal is a slit at rest (Fig. 2.3), and the resistance to opening requires a Valsalva maneuver in most individuals.

The anorectal angle is a controversial factor in the maintenance of continence. Current research both supports and questions the importance of this angle, which is created by anterior pull of the puborectalis sling. Other mechanisms such as a proposed "flutter valve" effect possibly contribute as well.

The reservoir capacity of the rectum and its characteristic compliance probably plays a role. The vascular cushions known as hemorrhoids help fill the lumen and may assist in a small measure.

Colonic Gas

Most intestinal gas resides in the colon. The composition and volume vary greatly among normal people (2). Approximately 30 to 90% of intestinal gas is nitrogen arising from swallowed air; in some pathologic situations, nitrogen diffuses across the mucosa from blood to lumen because other gases are present in sufficient volume to lower the partial pressure of nitrogen.

Oxygen, carbon dioxide, hydrogen, methane, and trace gases such as hydrogen sulfide, indole, and skatole are also present in the colon. Carbon dioxide and hydrogen are generated by fermentation of ingested nonabsorbed carbohydrate in the right colon as described above. In people who are lactase deficient, milk provides a substrate.

About 25% of people produce methane by the action of colonic bacteria that use hydrogen to reduce carbon dioxide. Hydrogen is the other explosive gas in the colon and rectum, and it is found in every individual. The possible presence of these gases makes it unwise to do electrocautery procedures in the lumen of the colon and rectum in the absence of complete mechanical preparation. Polypectomy is not advised during flexible sigmoidoscopy because the preparation is inadequate to guard against explosion.

References

1. Goligher J. Surgery of the anus, rectum and colon. 4th ed. London: Baillière Tindall, 1984:1–29.
2. Schrock TR. Large intestine. In: Way LW, ed. Current surgical diagnosis and treatment. 8th ed. East Norwalk, CT: Appleton & Lange, 1988:586–630.
3. Schrock TR. Examination of the anorectum, rigid sigmoidoscopy, flexible sigmoidoscopy, and diseases of the anorectum. In: Sleisenger MH, Fordtran JS, eds. Gastrointestinal disease. Pathophysiology, diagnosis, management. 4th ed. Philadelphia: WB Saunders, 1988
4. Russell TR. Anorectum. In: Way LW, ed. Current surgical diagnosis and treatment. 4th ed. East Norwalk, CT: Appleton & Lange, 1988:631–648.
5. Wood BA. Anatomy of the anal sphincters and pelvic floor. In: Henry MM, Swash M, eds. Coloproctology and the pelvic floor. Pathophysiology and management. London: Butterworths, 1985:3–21.
6. Goldberg SM, Gordon PH, Nivatvongs S. Essentials of anorectal surgery. Philadelphia: JB Lippincott, 1980:1–33.
7. Pemberton JH, Phillips SF. Colonic absorption. In: Schrock TR, ed. Perspectives in colon and rectal surgery. St. Louis: Quality Medical Publishing, 1988;1:89–103.
8. Duthie H. Physiology. In: Goligher J. Surgery of the anus, rectum and colon. 4th ed. London: Bailliere Tindall, 1984:29–47.
9. Henry MM, Swash M. Faecal continence, defaecation and colorectal motility. A. Physiology of faecal continence and defaecation. In: Henry MM, Swash M, eds. Coloproctology and the pelvic floor. Pathophysiology and management. London: Butterworths, 1985:42–47.
10. Kumar D, Wingate DL. Colorectal motility. In: Henry MM, Swash M, eds. Coloproctology and the pelvic floor. Pathophysiology and management. London: Butterworths, 1985:47–61.
11. Whitehead WE, Schuster MM. Anorectal physiology and pathophysiology. Am J Gastroenterology 1987;82:487–497.

3

Indications and Contraindications of Flexible Sigmoidoscopy: Comparison with Rigid Sigmoidoscopy, Colonoscopy, and Barium Enema

Philip A. Christiansen, M.D.

INTRODUCTION

Overholt first reported the use of a flexible fiberoptic sigmoidoscope in 1968 (1). With the publication of Bohlman et al. in 1977 (2), who compared rigid sigmoidoscopy with a 60-cm flexible fiberoptic sigmoidoscope, the diagnostic superiority of the flexible sigmoidoscope emerged as the primary instrument of evaluation of the distal colon and rectum. This trend has become so pervasive that some gastroenterology and family medicine trainees receive little or no training in the use of the rigid instrument. The purpose of this chapter is to review the indications and contraindications of flexible sigmoidoscopy and to compare its use to rigid sigmoidoscopy, colonoscopy, and air contrast barium enema in certain clinical situations.

RIGID SIGMOIDOSCOPY

Rigid sigmoidoscopes are usually 25 cm long and 1.9 cm in outside diameter. They are usually illuminated distally by fiberoptics and have a magnification lens that closes off the proximal end. Longer or shorter instruments, or those of smaller or larger diameter, seldom are needed. Anoscopes are usually 10 cm in length and 2.5 cm in diameter with a beveled edge or, preferably, a "slotted" distal end with approximately 90 degrees of the side of the distal 5 cm opened. Both rigid sigmoidoscopes and anoscopes are inserted with an obturator in place. The power source for the sigmoidoscope is a simple transformer plugged into an electrical outlet. Except for the fiberoptic bundles and the lens, all parts are metallic and last for years without repairs. Accessory equipment includes long suction tubes, overbiting "alligator" forceps, and a cotton-ball-carrying single-tooth forcep. The cost of two or three instruments and accessory equipment is in the one-thousand dollar range (very inexpensive disposable instruments are also available). The cost of the rigid sigmoidoscopes and accessories compared to flexible equipment is modest (Table 3.1). The subsequent professional charges usually are approximately one-third to one-half those of flexible sigmoidoscopy charges. Because of expense it is common to have only one flexible sigmoidoscope, whereas one can easily afford two or three rigid instruments. Flexible sigmoidoscopes are more fragile. They require more frequent and more costly repairs. Cleansing and disinfecting flexible instruments is more time consuming and complex.

The best position for performing rigid sigmoidoscopy is in the inverted knee-chest position, preferably on a Ritter-type, tiltable table. This position (uncomfortable for the elderly) can be achieved on a flat table, as can the standard left lateral decubitus (Sims) position. Although the latter position is

Table 3.1.
Relative Advantages of Rigid and Flexible Sigmoidoscopy

Rigid Sigmoidoscopy	Flexible Sigmoidoscopy
Lower equipment cost	Better patient acceptance
Lower procedure charge	Three times greater polyp discovery
Less training	Three times greater cancer discovery
Easier, faster cleaning and disinfection	Diagnostic information more often answers
Shorter procedure time	clinical question
Easier unprepped exams	More adequate evaluation of sigmoid colon
Less air inflation need	
Deeper and larger biopsies	
Better anal inspection	
Fewer complications	

more comfortable for the patient it may be more time consuming and may be associated with a more limited depth of penetration when performing rigid sigmoidoscopy. Although flexible examinations can be done in either position, the Sims position is preferable because it is more comfortable for patient and physician and less intimidating to the patient.

Rigid sigmoidoscopy is probably more easily learned because of the short distance traversed and because of the rigidity and simplicity of the instrument. Nonetheless, the lack of a useful teaching head to monitor the trainee makes rigid sigmoidoscopy training more inexact. Detailed studies with documentation of training of physicians in rigid sigmoidoscopy have not been reported as they have been for flexible sigmoidoscopy.

For most clinical indications, rectosigmoid cleansing preparation is desirable for both rigid sigmoidoscopy and flexible sigmoidoscopy. Cleansing for rigid sigmoidoscopy is more easily achieved. Two enemas (commonly Phospho-soda) 1 to 2 hours prior to the examination usually result in a more adequate preparation in rigid sigmoidoscopy. It is general experience that substantially more patients have satisfactory flexible sigmoidoscopy examinations (cleanliness and/or distance passed) when a cathartic (e.g., magnesium citrate) is given the evening before the examination and enemas are taken immediately before the examination. In general, rigid sigmoidoscopy requires less cleansing and can be manipulated around stool more easily than flexible sigmoidoscopy.

The safety of rigid and flexible sigmoidoscopy is detailed in Chapter 10. Rigid sigmoidoscopy has a lower reported perforation rate. Rigid sigmoidoscopy can more easily control rectal bleeding (e.g., after biopsy) by using cotton swab pressure or silver nitrate sticks or with cautery.

Patient tolerance of both modes of sigmoidoscopy has been well studied (3). The reports that use the inverted knee-chest position for rigid sigmoidoscopy and the Sims position for flexible sigmoidoscopy found a preference for flexible sigmoidoscopy. The examinations possibly are about equal in patient discomfort, and the discomfort is highly operator/position dependent.

The crucial factors in comparing the use of rigid sigmoidoscopy with flexible sigmoidoscopy are the length of the lower colon inspected and the pathology detected. The average depth is 20 cm for rigid sigmoidoscopy and 52 cm for flexible sigmoidoscopy. Given a wide spectrum of indications for the examinations, flexible sigmoidoscopy uncovered neoplasm at a 3:1 ratio compared to rigid sigmoidoscopy. This finding is to be expected with the relative incidence of malignancy migrating proximately in reports of the last 10 years. Marks et al. (4) found that flexible sigmoidoscopy was 4.6 times more likely to find pathology that explained the patient's symptoms than was rigid sigmoidoscopy.

COLONOSCOPY

Colonoscopy, when compared to flexible sigmoidoscopy, requires more expensive equipment, much more training, and more monitoring of the patient for potential complications. Usually, sedation analgesia is also required. The procedure takes substantially longer than flexible sigmoidoscopy and clearly carries a greater risk. For colonoscopy, besides a more substantial history and physical, a complete blood count (CBC) and coagulation studies may be recommended. In general patients should avoid salicylates and other drugs that affect coagulative function for several days prior to (and following) polypectomy. The charges for colonoscopy are three to four times higher than flexible sigmoidoscopy.

Comparisons of clinical situations where flexible sigmoidoscopy should be eliminated and the physician should go directly to colonoscopy are reviewed below.

When compared with barium enema, colonoscopy has the major advantages of offering both biopsy and therapeutic techniques, for example, polypectomy, cautery, foreign body retrieval, and laser tumor ablation. Additionally, colonoscopy more accurately evaluates mucosal detail for inflammatory or polypoid lesions.

BARIUM ENEMA

It is generally considered that there is relative underuse of sigmoidoscopy compared to colon X-rays. It is a common clinical practice to obtain a barium enema without a sigmoidoscopy. Only in unusual circumstance is this sufficient. Conversely, there are a number of circumstances where only a sigmoidoscopy (especially flexible sigmoidoscopy) is necessary (e.g., screening).

It is troubling that for the colon X-ray some radiologists resist performing air contrast barium enemas (ACBE). It is estimated that over one-half of the colon contrast studies currently performed remain the full column or regular barium enema. The arguments that a regular barium enema is faster, less expensive, uses thinner barium (in part to better detect fistulas), and requires less training are not sufficient to use this method. Air contrast techniques can evaluate most patients' colon disease better, particularly abnormal mucosa patterns (e.g., ulcerative colitis, Crohn's disease, or polypoid lesions), and with appropriate effort equally visualize the terminal ileum. The superiority of air contrast versus full column barium enemas (FCBE) is documented in an excellent review by Geland and Ott (6). They found that the sensitivity ratio of ACBE:FCBE for all colon polyps was 87%:57%, and for colon polyps under 1 cm in diameter the ratio was approximately 71%:28%. Others find a similar improved detection of polyps of all sizes by ACBE as well as more accurate diagnosis of inflammatory bowel disease (6). The preparation for both is the same, and presumably the complication rate of approximately 1 in 5000 (0.02%) for perforation is similar.

When deciding whether to obtain a colon barium X-ray (with sigmoidoscopy) versus colonoscopy there are several considerations (see Chapter 16). The relative advantages of barium enema compared to colonoscopy are universal availability, lower cost, lower complication rate, uniform survey of the entire colon, and easier viewing of the terminal ileum. The barium enema takes less of both the patient's time and the facility's time (i.e., there is no recovery period). Patient preparation is similar, and patient preference (sedation/analgesia with colonoscopy) seems to be variable.

LOCAL EXPERTISE

A major consideration of which strategy to use that is seldom included in didactic sources is the local expertise and/or availability of various diagnostic techniques. Conventional medical literature frequently reports results of comparative diagnostic methods of organ systems or diseases from major institutions. The presumption is that these methods are equally available and are performed with equal expertise everywhere. This clinical situation obviously does not always pertain to the locale where the majority of patients are evaluated and treated. Even today many radiologists discourage, if not refuse to perform, air contrast barium enemas. On the other hand, an expert colonoscopist may not be available locally. Adjustment in patient management with reference to local expertise is clearly needed.

INDICATIONS

Routine Screening for Neoplasia

One of the most frequent indications for sigmoidoscopy is screening. Assuming that the rectal exam is negative, that the patient is not anemic, and that stool is negative for occult blood, the flexible sigmoidoscopy is the preferred examination. This conclusion is based on several series showing the 3:1 superiority of flexible sigmoidoscopy over rigid sigmoidoscopy for both polyps and cancer discovery. The American Cancer Society recommends routine sigmoidoscopy in persons over 50 years of age. This is to be followed in 1 year by repeat examination and every 3 to 5 years thereafter (7).

With the finding of any neoplasia at flexible sigmoidoscopy a subsequent colonoscopy is recommended. This allows checking for synchronous lesions and biopsy or removal of the original lesion. Subsequent management strategy is covered in Chapter 15. Because of their costs and risks, colonoscopy and barium enema are generally considered unsuitable as modes of routine surveillance. Nevertheless, initial reports of screening colonoscopy are emerging, and the ultimate role of screening colonoscopy awaits further study (8,9).

Screening of Patients with Increased Risks for Neoplasia

Patients who are asymptomatic but who have clinical histories putting them into high-risk groups generally should have colonoscopy rather than lesser examinations. Such patients include those with previous colon polyps, strong family histories of colon neoplasm (especially familial polyposis), previous colon cancer resections, and prolonged ulcerative colitis being followed under a specific surveillance protocol. Women with uterine or cervical cancer also have an increased risk for colon cancer.

Positive Occult Blood in Stools

Up to 50% of patients with occult blood in the stool have been found to have neoplasia somewhere in the colon. Therefore, appropriate evaluation must include the *entire* colon. Chapter 15 discusses the generally preferred next step—colonoscopy versus flexible sigmoidoscopy *plus* ACBE.

Minimal Red Rectal Bleeding

In patients with minimal rectal bleeding, sufficient studies are unavailable for a dogmatic recommendation. The source for most of this bleeding is anorectal (i.e., hemorrhoids or fissures). It is frequently advised (Chapter 11) that the standard (rigid) anoscope be used first before sigmoidoscopy of any type. Generally, however, rigid sigmoidoscopy or flexible sigmoidoscopy can be satisfactorily used as the initial examination. The anal canal usually can be seen better with a rigid instrument than with a fiberoptic one; because of its increased rigidity, it is less likely that the patient will expel the instrument. If the patient is less than 35 years old, has no additional risk factors, and has only minimal bleeding (especially on the toilet paper only), sigmoidoscopy probably is all that is needed. It may be wise to have patients subsequently check their stools for occult blood. If bleeding reoccurs on several occasions, a full colon evaluation is warranted.

Severe Red Rectal Bleeding

Most patients with this symptom will be managed in a hospital rather than in the physician's office. The choice of the examination will depend on the disease possibilities; the patient's age, past history and any other accompanying symptoms or physical findings will be taken into account. Of great importance is whether the blood has stopped or is contained at the time of the examination. Either rigid sigmoidoscopy or flexible sigmoidoscopy is an appropriate initial test. For example, proctitis, trauma, tumor, internal hemorrhoids, and ischemia (one-third of the time for the latter) can be diagnosed at rigid sigmoidoscopy. Electrocautery can be performed through the rigid instrument more easily and safely than through the flexible sigmoidoscope in the unprepped bowel. Full cleansing is needed to cauterize via flexible sigmoidoscopy. Rigid sigmoidoscopy offers easier viewing in the unprepped state, and suctioning of luminal contents is more adequately accomplished. If sigmoidoscopy reveals that the bleeding is originating upstream, colonoscopy after enemas or oral electrolyte solutions is generally recommended. The need for the latter examination should be proportional to the rate of bleeding. In massive rectal bleeding, emergency colonoscopy has found a specific cause of the bleeding in 70 to 85% of cases (10). In certain instances, such as arteriovenous malformations or polyps, the bleeding can be controlled by electrocautery. Barium enemas have little or no role in acute colon bleeding. Nuclear studies and angiography have been disappointing in their diagnostic usefulness. Generally they are indicated only after colonoscopy has been attempted. Exceptions to this approach would be patients bleeding so rapidly that they might benefit from vasoconstriction therapy or those with more suspicion for a small bowel source.

Acute and Chronic Diarrhea

Sigmoidoscopy is one of the most important and possibly one of the earliest tests that should be performed when evaluating patients with acute or chronic diarrhea. (See Chapter 13 for discussion of infectious diarrhea). With either rigid sigmoidoscopy or flexible sigmoidoscopy, immediate samples may be obtained for fecal leukocytes. This examination is an easy, low-cost screening procedure that is reasonably sensitive and specific for inflammatory diarrheal conditions. One also may obtain samples for culture or biopsy.

If a contagious disease, such as AIDS, gonorrhea, or pseudomembranous colitis, is suspected, rigid sigmoidoscopy is preferable to flexible sigmoidoscopy because of the ease of rapid sterilization of the rigid sigmoidoscope. Rigid sigmoidoscopy also has better suction, allowing a more careful mucosal inspection in the "dirty" or unprepped colon. For the patient without a high index of suspicion for infectious diarrhea, either rigid or flexible sigmoidoscopy may be used. Finally, the choice of the instrument used depends substantially on whether the clinically anticipated abnormality will be within 20 to 25 cm. All active ulcerative colitis, 50% of Crohn's colitis, most infectious diarrhea (if there are any mucosal changes), and 77% (versus 91% with flexible sigmoidoscopy) of pseudomembranous colitis are found with rigid sigmoidoscopy (11). With ischemic colitis, only 33% is seen on rigid sigmoidoscopy, but 80% is seen on rigid sigmoidoscopy (12). Diverticulitis frequently is seen on flexible sigmoidoscopy and is only rarely identifiable on rigid sigmoidoscopy.

Change in Bowel Habits and Abdominal Pain

One of the most frequent indications for colon evaluation is the onset of constipation, alternating constipation and diarrhea, or diarrhea (see above in this chapter for evaluation of acute and chronic diarrhea). If the patient is less than 35 years old and this is the first episode of mild symptoms without bleeding, diagnostic studies may be unnecessary. Often dietary and personal habit manipulation and medications will suffice. Otherwise, and in older patients, a full colon evaluation is warranted. The diagnostic choices in the latter circumstances are flexible sigmoidoscopy plus air contrast barium enema or colonoscopy. A similar prep is necessary for either choice. With protracted diarrhea as the symptom, colonoscopy initially is preferable because biopsies can be obtained at any colon level. Otherwise, flexible sigmoidoscopy followed by ACBE is probably a more practical choice. Randomized studies are needed to determine which approach is more cost effective. If terminal ileal disease is also suspected and the X-ray or colonoscopy fails to visualize that area, then a small bowel barium study should follow. Enteroclysis (if available) is preferred to a small bowel follow-through for disease of the small intestine at any level. The latter also applies for the perianal fistula or abscess patient being evaluated for Crohn's disease.

For patients with abdominal pain without change in their bowel habits, an even more careful history is necessary. Diagnostic studies should be oriented toward the organ or disease of suspected origin (i.e., gallbladder, ulcer, bowel obstruction, and so on) initially. Some of these include abdominal and/or pelvic ultrasound, abdominal computerized tomography (CT) upper endoscopy, endoscopic retrograde cholangiopancreatography (ERCP), upper GI, and/or small bowel X-rays. These may be appropriate before any colon studies are performed.

Lesions Seen on Barium Enema

It is still a common experience to find lesions on the barium enema with no prior sigmoidoscopy. Most such lesions will be polyps or nonobstructing cancers, and colonoscopy should be the next step to remove polyps and biopsy suspicious lesions. If the air contrast barium enema was of the highest quality and the lesion in question is rectal, either rigid or flexible sigmoidoscopy is appropriate. In this setting, the sigmoidoscopist should be fully prepared to remove any polyps if found.

If a localized lesion is in the sigmoid colon the differential diagnosis is usually diverticular disease versus a possible malignancy. Less likely are such lesions as segmental Crohn's, radiation colitis, or endometriosis. High-grade narrowing and/or rigidity may indicate the need for smaller diameter instruments (whether sigmoidoscope or pediatric colonoscope). Such lesions are commonly painful and may require sedation and an experienced endoscopist to traverse the narrowing.

MISCELLANEOUS CLINICAL CIRCUMSTANCES

Perianal Disease and Masses Found on Rectal Examination

In the presence of very active hemorrhoidal disease, fissures, abscesses, fistulas, or rectal stricture, the timing of the sigmoidoscopy may need to be delayed. Alternately, these may be indications for parenteral analgesia prior to performing sigmoidoscopy.

If lesions are felt on digital rectal examination, either rigid or flexible sigmoidoscopy may be used. Rigid instruments permit better evaluation of anal lesions (see Chapter 11), but flexible sigmoidoscopy is often adequate. Biopsy of anorectal lesions is also covered in Chapter 9. Biopsy of any anal lesion may need local analgesia because of somatic innervation. The method of or need for removal of anorectal lesions will depend on the exact location, size, and nature of the lesions. However, with any anorectal neoplasia, if luminal patency permits, a colonoscopy is recommended to evaluate the entire colon.

Acute Bowel Conditions

If the total clinical circumstances suggest impending perforation of the colon, one needs to weigh carefully whether to endoscope at all, and if so, which instrument to use. A plain abdominal film should be done initially. This will help diagnose conditions such as toxic dilation of inflammatory bowel disease or free air. An abdominal CT, probably without rectal contrast, may also clarify the differential diagnosis.

The principles of which sigmoidoscope to use are based on the need to evaluate without air inflation, the lack of ability to prep with enemas, and the likelihood of disease below 20 to 25 cm. Rigid sigmoidoscopy can detect approximately 33% of acute ischemic colitis, 77% percent of pseudomembranous colitis, and 95% of acute-stage ulcerative colitis patients. Virtually no diverticulitis is seen below 20 cm. It therefore is recommended that in nearly all acute conditions, short of perforation of the colon, judicious use of rigid sigmoidoscopy without bowel preparation should be employed initially. Total colon evaluation with colonoscopy or barium enema generally is contraindicated until the inflammatory process subsides.

In lesser-risk clinical situations (e.g., acute diverticulitis or pseudomembranous colitis) the flexible sigmoidoscopy may be used initially. If the diagnosis is not determined, subsequent flexible sigmoidoscopy/colonoscopy, with the need for better cleansing and air insufflation, would be dictated by specific diagnostic need versus the implied dangers.

Rectal Biopsy

When the purpose of the sigmoidoscopy procedure is to obtain rectal biopsy, the use of the rigid instrument and alligator forceps is clearly superior to the more limited (in size) specimens obtained via flexible sigmoidoscopy (this is particularly true for diseases requiring deep biopsies, such as lymphoma, Crohn's, and vasculitis. See Chapter 9).

Assessing the Clinical Course of Known Disease

The clinical course and/or response to treatment should be evaluated in patients with ulcerative colitis (excluding cancer/dysplasia surveillance); rectal Crohn's (especially with perianal fistula); solitary ulcer of the rectum; radiation proctitis; or pseudomembranous colitis. A rigid sigmoidoscopy provides (usually without enema) a less expensive, quick, not uncomfortable view of the rectum; in such circumstances a flexible sigmoidoscopy is unnecessary. An alternative is to do a limited flexible sigmoidoscopy at a reduced cost.

Sigmoid Volvulus

When the clinical history, physical examination, and plain films of the abdomen support the diagnosis of sigmoid volvulus, rigid sigmoidoscopy has successfully resolved the volvulus in 51 to 77% of cases. The data on flexible sigmoidoscopy and colonoscopy are preliminary but probably comparable (13, 14). Following resolution of the volvulus, a complete evaluation by colonoscopy or air contrast barium enema is warranted.

Decompression of Acute Nontoxic Megacolon (Ogilvie's Syndrome)

The etiology of this difficult and dangerous condition is unclear. Traditionally it is seen following trauma or surgery in elderly patients (typically after hysterectomy). In our experience it most often occurs in patients with multi-

Table 3.2.
Relative Contraindications of Flexible Sigmoidoscopy

1. Severe colitis, toxic dilation
2. Large abdominal aortic aneurysm
3. Unstable cardiopulmonary disease
4. Suspected or impending colonic perforation
5. Recent colonic anastomosis
6. Uncooperative patient

system failure; these patients often are on ventilators. Flexible sigmoidoscopy may be helpful to rule out a rectosigmoid obstructing lesion, but a significant degree of decompression generally cannot be achieved by flexible sigmoidoscopy. The colonoscope is usually successful in decompressing the colon. Colon dilation reoccurs in 35% unless a decompression tube is left (via colonoscopy) in the right or transverse colon.

CONTRAINDICATIONS TO FLEXIBLE SIGMOIDOSCOPY

In certain clinical circumstances procedures to evaluate the colon can be considered either relatively or absolutely contraindicated. Table 3.2 is a list of the relative contraindications for flexible sigmoidoscopy. In extreme clinical circumstances there may be absolute contraindications, which include acute peritonitis or free bowel perforation. As has been discussed earlier, with a relative contraindication, the diagnostic gain as applied to the specific patient must be weighed against the risk. The basis for the fine judgments involved in arriving at these decisions must be individualized. In some of these conditions a rigid sigmoidoscopy may be an appropriate substitute with its superior view in unprepped patients and with little or no air inflation needed.

Reference

1. Overholt BF. Clinical experience with the fibersigmoidoscope. Gastrointest Endosc 1968;15:27.
2. Bohlman TW, Katon RM, Lipshutz GR, et al. Fiberoptic pansigmoidoscopy. An evaluation and comparison with rigid sigmoidoscopy. Gastroenterology 1977;72:644–649.
3. Katon R et al., eds. Flexible sigmoidoscopy. Orlando, FL: Grune and Stratton, 1985:73–82.
4. Marks G, Boggs W, Castro AF, et al. Sigmoidoscopic examination with rigid and flexible fiberoptic sigmoidoscopes in the surgeon's office. A comparative perspective study of effectiveness in 1,012 cases. Dis Colon Rectum 1979;22:162–168.
5. Geland DW, Ott DJ. Single- vs. double-contrast gastrointestinal studies: Critical analysis of reported studies. Am J Radiol 1981;137:523–528.
6. Laufer J. The double-contrast enema: Myths and misconceptions. Gastrointest Radiol 1976;1:19–31.
7. American Cancer Society. Cancer of the colon and rectum. CA 1980;30:208–215.
8. Johnson D, Gurney M, Volpe R, Jones D, Van Ness M, Chobanian S, Alvarez J, Buck J, Kooyman G, Cattau E. A prospective study of the prevalence of colonic neoplasms in asymptomatic patients with an age-related risk. Am J Gastroenterol 1987;82:957 (abstract).
9. Lieberman D, Denberg T, Smith F. Screening for colon malignancy with colonoscopy in asymptomatic subjects. Gastrointest Endosc (abstract) 1989;35:174.
10. Caos A, Manier J, Benner K, et al. "Golytely" preparation for colonoscopy in acute lower gastrointestinal hemorrhage. Gastrointest Endosc (Abstract) 1983;29:157.
11. Tedesco FJ, Corless JK, Brownstein RE. Rectal sparing in antibiotic associated pseudomembranous colitis: A prospective study. Gastroenterology 1982;83:1259–1260.

12. Scowcroft CW, Sanowski RA, Kozarek RA. Colonoscopy in ischemic colitis. Gastrointest Endoscop 1981;27:156–161.
13. Sanner CJ, Saltzman DA. Detorsion of sigmoid volvulus by colonoscopy. Gastrointest Endosc 1977;23:212-213.
14. O'Connor JJ. Reduction of sigmoid volvulus by flexible sigmoidoscope. Arch Surg 1979;114:1092.

4

Flexible Sigmoidoscopy: Instruments and Associate Equipment

Melvin Schapiro, M.D.

The term "flexible sigmoidoscope" is, in many cases, a misnomer because the commonly used instruments are 60 to 77 cm in length and are capable of examining a variable distance of the colon proximal to the sigmoid. Though longer-length instruments, that is, true colonoscopes, may be used to perform flexible sigmoidoscopy, they are more cumbersome to use, run the risk of increased breakage of fiber bundles for the fiberoptic varieties, and are more costly to repair.

BASIC INSTRUMENT DESIGN

The basic instrument design (Figs. 4.1 and 4.2) includes a proximal or insertion tip that houses an image apparatus of either a lens system or electronic charged coupled device (CCD) chip. There is an exit point for light transmission and three-channel ports: one for air insufflation, one for water insufflation, and the other for passage of endoscopic accessories or for suction of intestinal contents. The tip is shielded by a small protective hood that helps prevent fecal soiling of the lens and mucosal irritation during intubation. It also allows for further safety during electrosurgical conditions. The insertion tube is of varying length. It usually contains the inlet valve for the accessory/suction channel near its proximal junction with the control head. An auxillary inlet for forceful water irrigation is also combined here on some models. The control, or instrument head, houses the viewing and magnifying eyepiece with focusing ring on fiberoptic instruments or the exit port for the electronic signal to a video processor for electronic instruments. This unit also contains two control knobs with locking levers for insertion tip deflection, up and down, or right and left, as well as buttons that when depressed effect suction and air/water insufflation. An umbilical cord connects the instrument to light, air, water, and suction sources.

The materials and junctions that cover the control head are waterproof in most models, thereby allowing for immersion during the cleaning and disinfection process (see Chapter 6). The waterproof insertion tube containing the

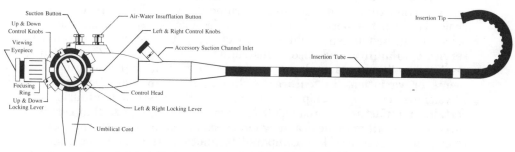

Figure 4.1. Component parts of flexible sigmoidoscope.

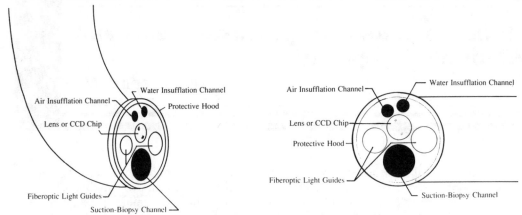

Figure 4.2. Component parts of insertion tip of flexible sigmoidoscope.

channels, noncoherent fiberoptic light source bundle, cables for tip angulation, and coherent fiberoptic image bundle or electronic signal conduits is covered by an inner metal mesh and an outer vinyl coat. This covering of the 10 cm of the insertion tube just proximal to the distal tip is more flexible, allowing for the acute angulation maneuvers. It is, as well, more vulnerable to trauma and may be a site of leakage or damage (see Chapter 6). In addition, the junction of the insertion tube with the control head is a frequent site of leakage arising from stress defects produced from excessive angulation. The question of whether the positional changes effected with video versus direct eyepiece visualization instruments will decrease the incidence of angulation-induced leakage at this junction is a theoretical possibility, particularly for learning situations where the tendency is for overangulation.

COMMERCIALLY AVAILABLE INSTRUMENTS

Tables 4.1 and 4.2 list the presently available instruments and their relative price range. For the most part, the less expensive instruments (Fig. 4.3) are constructed of less expensive material and usually lack an automatic water insufflation system for lens washing. These features, however, need not deter the individual who expects a low-volume experience because they have proved durable, they include satisfactory optics, and there is a minimal inconvenience for lens washing via an attached irrigation syringe.

One type of instrument contains only a single knob for tip control (up and down). This has been found to be difficult to use and is, at present, available from only one instrument manufacturer.

There are differences between models in accessory/suction channel diameter, insertion tube diameter, and instrument length. There is, in addition, a choice between fiberoptic and electronic video technology. Considerations when selecting an instrument include cost factors, quality of image, manufacturer service availability, and ease of instrument handling (feel). Controlled studies have not been carried out comparing different manufacturer's instruments or variations in features within or between manufacturer(s) lines. Physicians tend to develop a "feel" bias on the basis of familiarity with a certain manufacturer's product. It is important to recognize that certain features are overall more desirable when choosing an instrument than the "feel" of one manufacturer's line compared to another. It is probable that in the hands of the well-trained endoscopist, the clinical outcome of the examina-

Table 4.1.
Flexible Fiberoptic Sigmoidoscopes

Manufacturer Model	Field of View (degrees)	Depth of Field (mm/range)	Insertion Tube Diameter (cm)	Tip Deflection (degrees)		B/S Channel Diameter (mm)	Working Length (cm)	Air Insufflation	Water Insufflation	Immersible	Price (8-1-88)
				U/D	R/L						
Fujinon											
SIG-E4	105	4-120	13.0	180/180	160/160	3.2	77	Auto	Auto	Yes	6100
SIG-ET2	110	4-120	14.0	180/180	160/160	4.3	73	Auto	Auto	Yes	6100
Olympus											
CF-P20S	120	5-100	12.2	180/180	160/160	3.2	63	Auto	Auto	Yes	7300
OSF-2	100	3-100	12.2	180/180	160/160	3.2	60	Auto	Manual	Yes	3800/4195*
OSF-35-2	100	3-100	12.2	180/180	160/160	3.2	35	Auto	Manual	Yes	3800/4195*
Pentax											
FS-38H	120	3-100	12.8	180/180	160/160	3.8	70	Auto	Auto	Yes	7100
FS-34P	120	3-100	11.5	180/180	160/160	3.5	70	Auto	Auto	Yes	3950
Schott											
SC-5A	100	10-70	14.3	180/180	160/160	3.2	65	Auto	Auto	No	3375/3850*†
FPS-3	75	10-70	13.2	175/175	—	2.6	35	Manual	Manual	No	2295/2500*†
SC-36	90	10-70	13.4	170/180	140/140	2.6	35	Auto	Manual	No	2600/3100*†

*includes light source
†forceps accessory package not included

Table 4.2.
Flexible Electronic Video Sigmoidoscopes

Manufacturer Model	Field of View (degrees)	Depth of Field (mm/range)	Pixels	Insertion Tube Diameter End	Tube	B/S Channel Diameter (mm)	Working Length (cm)	Air Insufflation	Water Insufflation	Immersible	Price (8-1-88)
Fujinon											
EVS-E	125	4-100	100,000	13.5	13.3	3.7	77	Auto	Auto	Yes	6700
Olympus											
CF-V10S	140	5-100	32,000	15.4	13.8	3.2	63	Auto	Auto	Yes	7300
Pentax											
ES-3800	120	5-100	32,000	14.6	12.8	3.8	70	Auto	Auto	Yes	6800
Welch-Allyn											
VSDT-90	90	5-100	32,000	14.4	13.5	3.0	65	Auto	Auto	No	5500/8565*†

*includes processor and video monitor
†forceps accessory package not included

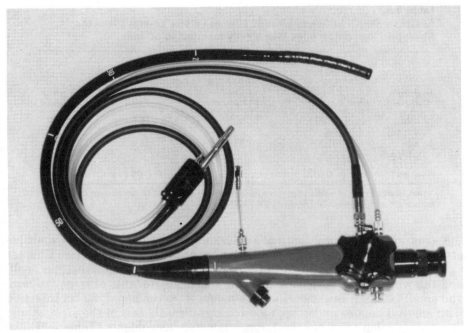

Figure 4.3. Olympus flexible fiberoptic sigmoidoscope Model OSF-2.

tions is affected very little, if at all, by the model variations once familiarity
with the instrument's characteristics have been acquired.

Instrument Length

Though, as mentioned previously, a limited left colonoscopic examination
may be carried out with short or long colonoscopes, for the purposes of this
discussion, flexible sigmoidoscopes are short (35 cm) or long (60 to 77 cm).
Though the former rarely examines beyond the sigmoid-descending colon
junction and best represents the term "flexible sigmoidoscope," the latter is
capable of examining a variable distance of the left colon and occasionally to
the splenic flexure. These longer instruments, which frequently examine at
least a portion of the descending colon, are the most popular and have come
to be called flexible sigmoidoscopes. The arguments for one length versus the
other surprisingly do not relate to cost factors, since the prices for short or
long flexible sigmoidoscopes are identical. Teaching and learning factors, at-
tainment of competency over a specific period of time or number of cases, and
concerns regarding pathology pickup are the important considerations in determining instrument length. These are discussed in detail in Chapter 5.

Insertion Tube Diameter

It has been shown that for upper GI endoscopy, the smaller diameter (thinner) instruments are better tolerated, particularly in the nonsedated patient.
This theoretical advantage of thinner instruments affording a more comfortable intubation has not been tested by randomized or double-scoping studies
for flexible sigmoidoscopy and may be associated with less desirable depths
of intubation. It has been demonstrated that the true anatomic depth of insertion is not necessarily related to the centimeters of insertion tube used for
intubation (1). Full 60-cm insertion, although usually allowing evaluation of
the entire sigmoid colon, will reach as far as the splenic flexure in less than
25% of the cases (2). This discrepancy is possibly related to the experience of

Table 4.3.
Anatomic Depth of Penetration of 16-mm versus 12-mm Diameter Fiberoptic Sigmoidoscopes When Fully Inserted to 60 mm

Instrument Diameter	At Least 75% of Sigmoid Colon	At Least Sigmoid Descending Colon Junction	At Least 50% of Descending Colon	Splenic Flexure
12 mm (N=37)	89%	59%	16%	8%
16 mm (N=58)	100%	81%	34%	22%
p values*	0.011	0.022	0.052	0.069

*From Hawes RH et al. Effect of instrument diameter on the depth of penetration of fiberoptic sigmoidoscopes. Gastrointest Endosc 1988; 34:28–31.

the examiner and to the patient's tolerance to the discomforts of multiple attempts at intubation during straightening of the sigmoid loop (see Chapter 8). It is, however, also related to the degree of sigmoid loop formation itself, and this varies from patient to patient. When instruments of large (16 mm) and small (12 mm) insertion tube diameters were compared, 60-cm insertion with small diameter endoscopes viewed significantly less of the sigmoid and descending colon than did the larger diameter instruments (Table 4.3). The greater flexibility and decreased stiffness of the insertion tube that is characteristic of thinner instruments may account for increased sigmoid loop formation (3). If flexibility and stiffness are important considerations for anatomic depth of insertion, and if certain thinner instruments cause discontinuation of intubation because of discomfort secondary to sigmoid loop formation, then, unlike upper GI endoscopes, thinner may not be better. Studies comparing depth of penetration with instruments of equal diameter but varying stiffness are needed.

Air-Water Insufflation

There is a small diameter channel through which air is insufflated automatically on each instrument except one (Table 4.1). This is facilitated by finger manipulation of the air button on the control section of the instrument. This channel, and its control button, is usually coupled to an automatic water irrigation function that cleans the lens of small amounts of debris or fecal residue when the button is fully depressed. Some of the lower-cost instruments provide the automatic air insufflation but have a separate port to which an irrigating syringe may be attached for manual water irrigation (Fig. 4.4). Though the syringe attachment for lens irrigation is more cumbersome to use, its manipulation is easily learned and may even provide a more forceful stream for cleaning of debris than with the automatic system. When a small syringe is attached at the beginning of the procedure it is ready for use immediately during the examination. The volume of fluid available from a small syringe, however, may not be enough during the course of certain examinations, and arrangements need to be made to refill the syringe or provide additional syringes for further irrigation. Attachment of a larger volume syringe throughout the examination interferes with hand function and unbalances the control section. The clinical facts of the matter are that water irrigation is not always required, particularly in well-prepared patients. This separation of the automatic air/water function is present only in the low-cost models and does not represent a desirable option but rather is a marketing means of providing an instrument capable of being used for accurate flexible sig-

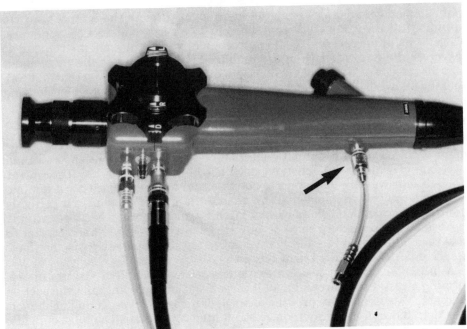

Figure 4.4.   Syringe attachment port for water irrigation. (arrow)

moidoscopy at a more attractive purchase price. If instrument purchase cost is a major consideration, the absence of this automatic lens irrigation is not a major drawback.

Channel Diameter

The instrument channel that provides a passageway for suction as well as passage of accessories such as biopsy forceps has a minimal diameter of 2.6 mm and at present a maximum of 4.3 mm, depending on the particular model. Instruments with the larger channel diameter have generally a thicker insertion tube. As discussed above, this may not be a disadvantage for intubation in most patients. It does allow the advantages of improved aspiration of retained semi-fluid fecal residue and ease of passage of biopsy forceps when the instrument is in a full-tip deflection position. If the colon lumen is narrow, intubation through and beyond may be possible only with instruments of smaller external diameter. These situations, however, are usually associated with indications for longer colonoscopes.

The placement of the channel inlet has, in most cases, been moved from a close proximity to the eyepiece position on the control head to an area near the junction of the control head and insertion tube. This feature allows a degree of safety from splashing and back spray toward the eyes when the channel is manipulated during direct visualization. This problem is of less concern with electronic video sigmoidoscopes, since hand-operating conditions occur at a considerable distance from the eyes. Nevertheless, with electronic instruments, the channel inlet has also been placed near the head-insertion tube junction, providing for a more standard feel between instrument types. The channel inlet consists of a cap with a rubber diaphragm. This is replaceable, since after multiple passages of accessories a leak will occur allowing for back-splashing of intestinal fluid as well as air release. An antisplatter device for the protection of endoscopic personel has been devised for attachment to the channel insertion port (4). In addition to this valve inlet, the main suction channel also exits the instrument through the control head via an umbilical cord that allows attachment to an external suction appliance. The exit point for external suction attachment varies. In some instruments it traverses the entire length of the umbilical cord, exiting at the attachment port for the power light source. In others, it is placed close to the control head, thereby allowing quick disconnection and mechanical cleaning when clogging occurs during the procedure.

Tip Deflection

Most instruments are capable of distal tip deflection of 180 degrees in the up or down position. Right/left deflection of 160 degrees is present in all but two, one of which—the Schott model FPS-3—has only one-way tip control. Though four-way tip deflection is not essential for the majority of examinations and may be supplemented by hand-torquing maneuvers, it is a highly desirable feature that allows ease of learning and performance. A potentially risky slide-by procedure may be obviated by a 110-degree knob-controlled side turn, allowing direct luminal visualization that may otherwise not have occurred with hand instrument torque.

A full 180-degree up or down tip deflection, for example, as occurs in performing a rectal turn-around maneuver, effects an acute angle on the suction channel. This angle may prevent passage of biopsy forceps through channels less than 3.5 mm and may require straightening of the tip angulation while the accessory is being passed.

Optics

Flexible sigmoidoscopes are available in either fiberoptic or electronic video formats. Though resolution studies comparing various manufacturer's fiberoptic bundles are not available, there are subjective differences between manufacturers' lines. Prominence of fiber bundle pattern, angle of view, and depth of field differences account for differences in optic image reproduction. Certainly, a high-quality fiber bundle will give a finer and more pleasing image. Wide-angle versus narrow-angle view, however, is usually a matter of individual preference, though a wider angle may allow for easier identification of luminal direction at bowel flexures. Greater depth of field is likewise helpful in this regard.

Electronic endoscopes have, for the most part, been shown to have improved image resolution when compared to fiberoptics, except when viewing at very close range (5,6,7). It is not likely, however, that at present the resolution differences between fiberoptic instruments or between fiberoptic and electronic images account for any clinical difference in pathology identification or success of intubation (4). The learning process for flexible sigmoidoscopy, using a video monitor rather than a fiberoptic teaching attachment, may be more favorable. In addition, assistant and patient participation in the procedure; ease of recording of images for quality control; and decrease in eye, hand, and body fatigue functions are among the advantages offered by video endoscopes (5). All of the manufacturers' electronic video systems, except for one (Welch-Allyn model 89006), however, are of considerable additional cost. This Welch-Allyn system, particularly designed for the primary care physician, is priced competitively and provides many of the advantages of electronic video endoscopy.

Power/Light Sources

A supply of light, generated from an external power source, is conducted through the umbilical cord and down the instrument via a noncoherent fiber bundle that exits in one or two coated areas on the distal tip regardless of

Table 4.4.
Light Sources for Fiberoptic Sigmoidoscopes

Manufacturer Model	Bulb	Watts	Flash	Air Pump	Price (8-1-88)
Fujinon					
FLX-2000	Xenon	300	Yes	Yes	5500
FIL-V	Halogen	150	No	Yes	950
FIL-150	Halogen	150	No	Yes	650
Olympus					
CLV-10	Xenon	300	Yes	Yes	6700
CLE-F10	Halogen	150	Yes	Yes	4700
CLE-10	Halogen	150	No	Yes	2400
CLK-3	Halogen	150	No	Yes	650/395*
Pentax					
LX-500A	Xenon	300	Yes	Yes	6500
LH-150PA	Halogen	150	No	Yes	650
LH-150A	Halogen	150	No	No	395
Schott					
1185-A	Halogen	150	No	Yes	475
1181	Halogen	80	No	No	325

*With OSF sigmoidoscopes

electronics or fiberoptic technology. These power/light sources vary in light intensity output, complexity, available options, and cost (Tables 4.4 and 4.5).

Simple low-cost halogen units offer satisfactory light for flexible sigmoidoscopy but are at a disadvantage for photography and combined use with a broader range of endoscopic instruments. Low-cost models are available without automatic air pumps but require external balloon attachments for air insufflation and are not recommended. Endoscopic photography of marginal quality is possible with the low-cost 150 W halogen units using "fast" film (see below section, Photography); however, instant hard copy and quality images require associated flash capability of the light source and/or preferably higher light output Xeon units. The broadest range of image documentation occurs with the expensive electronic video systems, though satisfactory video tape recordings, as well as still images, are possible by purchasing the necessary video accessories with the lower-cost Welch-Allyn primary care flexible sigmoidoscopy unit.

Accessory Equipment

The original purchase price usually includes a package of accessory equipment consisting of biopsy forceps, spare valves, channel-cleaning equipment, tubing, and carrying case. Some of these accessories, particularly the biopsy

Table 4.5.
Electronic Video Processors and Components for Electronic Sigmoidoscopes

Manufacturer Model	Bulb	Watts Video/Fiber	Processor Price	12 in. Monitor Price	Keyboard Price	Cart Price (8-1-88)
Fujinon						
EPX-301A	Xenon	300/300	13,500	930	Included	Included
Olympus						
CV-1	Xenon	300/300	13,700	900	Included	Included
Pentax						
EPM-3000	Xenon	300/300	13,500	975	Included	400
Welch-Allyn						
VP-2	Xenon	300/300	12,500	850	500	2600
VP-1	Xenon	300 (Video Only)	6,800/8,565*	850	500	—

*Includes sigmoidoscope and monitor

forceps, are, however, optional at additional cost for some lines. In addition, disposable cytology brushes and variations in types of biopsy forceps are available for optional purchase. Jumbo biopsy forceps, enabling larger tissue biopsies, are available but are not recommended. They require the larger channel diameter instruments, offer a greater risk at biopsy, and are not likely to contribute significantly to the clinical evaluation. Discovered lesions are usually an indication for total colonoscopy, for which the range of ancillary equipment and expertise is available. One type of biopsy forceps that combines electrosurgical coagulation current with the biopsy (hot biopsy) has value in combined biopsy-destruction of diminutive (less than 5 mm) polypoid lesions. These hot biopsy forceps, however, are contraindicated unless the colon is totally clean. Simple biopsy of these lesions to determine their histology may be safely accomplished without coagulation requirements. If adenomatous tissue is discovered, the indication again is for more formal colonoscopy (see Chapter 15). For these reasons, and considering the risks of electrical hazards in the incompletely prepared bowel (as is usual for sigmoidoscopy), ancillary electrosurgical equipment and their appropriate power sources are not recommended for purchase when the colon examination is limited to flexible sigmoidoscopy.

Assisting (Teaching) Attachment

This desirable but relatively expensive side arm coherent fiberoptic bundle attachment allows an endoscopy assistant to participate in the examination with direct visualization of the endoscopic field while assisting with manipulation of the instrument. Many physicians find that insertion/withdrawal assistance simplifies the procedure, particularly in the learning stages. Visualization by the assistant, particularly while passing the sigmoid-descending colon junction, is helpful in this regard and may be an additional safety factor. The use of such an attachment not only adds the increased expense of purchase of the attachment itself but generally requires a more expensive light source, since splitting of the image decreases light availability to each observer in proportion to the percent of image fiber bundle volume split. Additional value to the attachments, however, is for sharing of the live endoscopic image with other interested individuals without disrupting the normal flow of the endoscopic examination. Unless the video endoscopic system is employed, this attachment is essential for teaching flexible sigmoidoscopy.

Photography

Camera equipment, usually using 35 mm format but also using 110 mm format, is available. Photodocumentation of pathologic findings is an optional, but frequently desirable, feature. The 35 mm automatic camera with film speeds of ASA 400 or higher can give slides or prints of acceptable quality when used with low cost, low output light sources, but manipulation of the camera exposure system is required and is not recommended for the average photographer. The light sources with automatic flash or Xeon output will allow quality photography more simply obtained. Documentation of the total endoscopic examination on video tape, however, may offer certain clinical advantages. Video tape review for consultation or for comparative purposes may have occasional value. Flexible sigmoidoscopy performed by paramedical personnel with quality control through video tape review has been reported and may be an important screening technique of the future (8).

Instrument Selection

It is apparent now that multiple options are available when choosing a flexible sigmoidoscope. The selection will become easier when the considerations of costs, service, and features are made in that order.

Cost

Most readers of this text will not be purchasing a flexible sigmoidoscope as part of equipping a full spectrum endoscopic unit. In that circumstance the flexible sigmoidoscope cost is relatively minor compared to the total cost figure and will be part of the overall decision-making process (e.g., the electronic video versus fiberoptic systems and various manufacturer considerations). When the decision is made for flexible sigmoidoscopy as part of the office practice, considerations must be given to procedural volume. Most physicians soon find that once the technical aspects of the procedure have been mastered and the office staff has become competent in assisting, in scheduling, and in care and maintenance of the equipment, then the number of procedures performed rapidly increase on the basis of valid indications. The limiting factors seem to be the physician's time in developing expertise and in adding the procedures to a busy office schedule. Data is available to indicate that in trained hands, a 35-cm examination takes on the average 5 minutes, whereas adding a full 60-cm insertion consumes less than an additional 5 minutes. Considering overall setup time, cleaning, and so on, scheduling cases at 30-minute intervals seems appropriate (see Chapter 6). Indeed, a busy office that handles multiple sigmoidoscopy procedures usually requires multiple instruments. Before deciding on cost expenditures, it is a good idea to take a 1-month period of time and record all of the patients likely to undergo flexible sigmoidoscopy in the practice if the instrument and full expertise were available. Consideration should be given not only to suspicion of, or evaluation of, pathology but also to screening of well (average-risk) patients greater than the age of 50. If this volume is a significant one, offering multiple possible examinations on a daily basis, then it is cost effective to purchase equipment that offers most of the desirable features. The cost outlay soon becomes of less concern under the conditions where tax advantages contribute to and procedural reimbursements account for an appropriate profit margin. It is important at this point to consider in the calculations the procedural charges. Flexible sigmoidoscopy to be cost effective must maintain charges that will have a favorable impact on screening. Though the procedure with a 60- to 77-cm instrument will often examine farther than the sigmoid colon, it is not appropriate to charge for a short colonoscopic or left colon examination. Indeed, third-party carriers have for the most part limited reimbursement to flexible sigmoidoscopy or total colonoscopic charges. A reasonable acceptable guideline for physician charges for 60- to 77-cm flexible sigmoidoscopy is two times the usual charge for a rigid sigmoidoscopy examination and one and a half times the rigid charge for a 30-cm flexible examination. If the monthly volume estimation for procedures indicates only a casual or occasional experience, then the low-cost units may prove satisfactory and become cost effective at an earlier time. Another consideration for a lower-cost unit might be as a backup for the busy practice in which a second instrument and/or backup light source might be needed.

Service

Though each of the manufacturers provide a service for sales, follow-up, and repairs, there may be variation in this service in certain geographic areas. It is wise to meet with the sales representative and discuss the services offered. If one manufacturer seems deficient in this area, it is likely a good idea to look more favorably on the competition's lines. Though breakdown of the flexible sigmoidoscope is not a frequent occurrence, when it happens there may be a lag period for repairs. Rapid service, replacement instruments, and maintenance advice are valuable sales features. Sometimes instrument purchase is combined with course instruction for learning to do the procedure with video tapes, plastic models, and/or sales representative recommendations. Be cautioned that competency in endoscopic procedures cannot be gained without hands-on experience in live patients (9), and the learning experience should be undertaken with the instruction of a trained supervisor (see Chapter 17). More than one physician has given up the procedure after an initial enthusiasm was generated from an encounter with a plastic model. An expensive instrument purchase can occur before it is apparent that self-teaching in live patients proves time consuming and unpleasant for both the patients and the physician, as well as potentially dangerous. The learning, performance, and purchase of a flexible sigmoidoscopy system is a valuable and satisfactory occurrence when carried out according to these guidelines.

Features

The final instrument selection should now depend on the specific features offered within the cost structure of the instrument manufacturer selected. There is little practical reason for individuals to select 35-cm instruments, though limitation to 35-cm insertion in the early learning experience has merit. Institutions involved in training may have usefulness for the 35-cm instrument. When cost considerations indicate outlay for the more versatile instruments, then light sources for assistant attachments, these attachments, and photography capability should strongly be considered for additional purchase. In this regard, the electronic unit offering these features at a cost commensurate with more complete fiberoptic packages should be carefully considered.

References

1. Auslander MO, Schapiro M. The true depth of insertion of the 60-cm flexible sigmoidoscopy: Does it matter? Gastrointest Endosc 1983;29:192A.
2. Lehman GA, Buchner DM, Lappas JC. Anatomical extent of fiberoptic sigmoidoscopy. Gastroenterol 1983;84:803–808.
3. Hawes R et al. Effect of instrument diameter on the depth of penetration of fiberoptic sigmoidoscopes. Gastrointest Endosc 1988;34:28–31.
4. Laine L. A prospective trial of an anti-splatter device for the protection of endoscopic personnel from potentially AIDS-infective fluids. Gastroint Endosc 1988;34:470–471.
5. Schapiro M, Auslander MO, Schapiro MB. The electronic video endoscope: clinical experience with 1200 diagnostic and therapeutic cases in the community hospital. Gastrointest Endosc 1987;33:63–68.
6. Kayrim K et al. Video endoscopes in comparison with fiberscopes: A quantitative measurement of optical resolution. Endosc 1987;19:156–159.
7. Kayrim K et al. Optical performance of electronic imaging system for the colon. Gastroenterology 1989;96:776–782.
8. Schroy PC et al. Videoendoscopy by nurse-practitioners: A model for colorectal cancer screening. Gastrointest Endosc 1988;34:390–394.
9. Statement on role of short courses in endoscopic training. Gastrointest Endosc 1988;34:14S–15S (Supplement).

5

Choice of Length of Flexible Sigmoidoscopes: Longer Versus Shorter

Glen A. Lehman, M.D.

INTRODUCTION

The ideal length of a fiberoptic sigmoidoscope is not known. Most studies of fiberoptic sigmoidoscopy have used instruments of 30 to 35 cm in length (generally called *short*) and 60 to 65 cm in length (generally referred to as *long*). Recently, marketed 70- to 77-cm instruments are included in the latter group. Intermediate 45-cm length instruments have been tested (1) and colonoscopes (2) have been used for unsedated "fiberoptic sigmoidoscopy."

After initial experience with various length prototype instruments, Bohlman et al. (3) published their study comparing rigid sigmoidoscopy and 60-cm fiberoptic sigmoidoscopy. This instrument became the first commercially available fiberoptic sigmoidoscope and received wide acceptance. Subsequently, instruments with a variety of lengths and diameters have been marketed (Chapter 4). This chapter will review the pros and cons of sigmoidoscopes of various lengths.

ANATOMIC AREA VIEWED AT FIBEROPTIC SIGMOIDOSCOPY

Because the goal of fiberoptic sigmoidoscopy is generally to examine the rectum and sigmoid colon, studies of anatomic depth of penetration are appropriate to accomplish this goal. Several studies have reported depth of penetration with 60-cm instruments (3,4,5,6,7). Mucosal clip placement followed by barium enema and radiographically monitoring contrast media injection through the biopsy channel of the instrument are the most accurate methods to evaluate depth of penetration. Plain abdominal film, fluoroscopy, metal detectors, and barium enema without clips are acceptable estimates of anatomic area viewed, although 10 to 18% under- and overestimating depth of penetration respectively occurred in our series when only plain abdominal film was used (6) (compared to barium enema with clip). Endoscopist's determination of the depth of penetration by luminal appearance was not an acceptable estimate in the sigmoid and descending colon, since 39% overestimates and 20% underestimates occurred in our series. The splenic flexure and transverse colon were generally identified by the endoscopist if that distance was achieved.

Table 5.1 shows that when a 60-cm fiberoptic sigmoidoscope was fully penetrated, the sigmoid descending colon junction was visualized in 81% of examinations (i.e., complete sigmoidoscopy). At least half of the descending colon was viewed in 34%, and the splenic flexure was reached in 22%. If only 50- to 55-cm or 40- to 45-cm penetration with 60-cm scopes was achieved (as is commonly the case), viewing to the sigmoid descending junction was 68% and 27% respectively. Other series (3,4,5) largely confirm that a fully penetrated 60-cm instrument has an 80% probability of fully viewing the sigmoid colon. Depth of penetration studies are awaited for the 70- to 77-cm sigmoidoscopes.

Table 5.1.

Percentage of Examinations that Reached to Each Subdivision of the Colon Divided According to Depth of Insertion of Olympus 16-mm Diameter TCF-1S Fibersigmoidoscope

	Area Viewed				
	At Least 50% Sigmoid	At Least 75% Sigmoid	Sigmoid Descending Junction	At Least 50% Descending	At Least Splenic Flexure
Depth of insertion					
60-cm exam					
(58 patients)					
No. of patients	58	58	47	20	13
Percent of patients	100	100	81	34	22
50- to 55-cm exam					
(25 patients)					
No. of patients	25	23	17	5	4
Percent of patients	100	92	68	20	16
40- to 45-cm exam					
(15 patients)					
No. of patients	14	9	4	0	0
Percent of patients	93	60	27	0	0
30- to 35-cm exam					
(15 patients)					
No. of patients	9	5	2	2	1
Percent of patients	60	33	13	13	6

From Lehman GA, Buchner DM, Lappas JC. Anatomical extent of fiberoptic sigmoidoscopy. Gastroenterology 1983; 84:806. Used with permission.

No studies of depth of penetration with 30- to 35-cm sigmoidoscopes have been reported. Data from use of 60-cm instruments, with a stop at 30 to 35 cm to place a clip, is shown in Table 5.1. Such examinations gave complete sigmoid viewing to the sigmoid descending junction in only 13% of cases. Fifty percent of the sigmoid colon was viewed in 60% of patients. Such lesser anatomic area viewed has obvious implications to lesion detection.

PATHOLOGY DETECTED

The ultimate goal of fiberoptic sigmoidoscopy is to detect pathology. Winnan et al. (8) have analyzed the distribution of lesions in the sigmoid colon, especially in comparison to the centimeter level of fiberoptic sigmoidoscope penetration. Polypoid lesions were especially frequent in the rectum and distal sigmoid (35 cm and below). Three series (9,10,11) have specifically studied the same patients with both 30- to 35-cm and 60- to 65-cm instruments. Table 5.2 shows a comparison of those studies. Approximately 80% of the detected

Table 5.2.

Series Comparing Diagnostic Yield for Polypoid Lesions with Short and Long Fiberoptic Sigmoidoscopy in the Same Patients

First Author	Polypoid Lesions Found		
	Patient (N)	30–35 cm	60–65 cm
Zucker (Ref 10)	96	26	31
Sarles (Ref 11)	100	20	26
Dubow (Ref 9)	258	38	49
Totals	454	84*	106*

*$p < .001$ (two-tailed) McNemar's test

polyps are present in the first 35 cm, but an additional 20% (p<.001) yield was found with the 60-cm scopes. In reality, a portion of these latter patients would have been identified by the presence of a sentinel polyp within the first 35 cm.

The diagnostic yield for inflammatory bowel disease was similar with both instruments. Diverticular disease was seen three times more frequently with the 60-cm instruments (10,11). Similar studies are needed with 70- to 80-cm instruments.

The above two major factors, anatomic area viewed and pathology detected, strongly indicate that "longer is better." Multiple other less important factors favor shorter sigmoidoscopes.

DISCOMFORT

As would be expected, the further the endoscope is advanced into the colon, the more uncomfortable (painful) the examination becomes. Indeed, colonoscopy nearly always requires parenteral sedatives/analgesic medications to achieve cecal viewing. Discomfort experienced during screening examinations may discourage subjects from follow-up examinations. Dubow et al. (9) studied 25 asymptomatic, unsedated subjects with both 35-cm and 60-cm sigmoidoscopes. Subjects then graded discomfort on a 1 (mild) to 10 (severe) scale. The 60-cm examinations more frequently induced moderate (49% versus 21%) or severe (20% versus 8%) pain. Subjects with a preference (presumably just from a pain viewpoint) usually chose the 35-cm exam (72% versus 7%).

The above patient preference data are misleading. We questioned patients undergoing unsedated screening "fiberoptic sigmoidoscopy" with a 160-cm colonoscope (12). The instrument was advanced until mild-to-moderate pain occurred, stool was encountered, or luminal angulation was present that was difficult to traverse quickly. The mean depth of penetration was 68 cm, with a range of 20 to 140 cm. The mean discomfort score as judged by the subject (1 to 10 scale as above) was 4.6 and as judged by the examining physician was 3.6. Subjects were then asked if they would prefer a similar, equally uncomfortable examination or a less uncomfortable examination that had only a 75% chance of detecting distal colonic lesions. All patients favored another long examination. We therefore conclude that the average informed subject is willing to endure a more uncomfortable examination if the improved yield from the examination is explained.

DURATION OF EXAMINATION

Three studies (9,10,11) have directly compared the total time of fiberoptic sigmoidoscopy for 30- to 35-cm versus 60-cm examinations. The mean examination time for 30- to 35-cm examinations was 4.4 min versus 8.4 min for 60-cm examinations. Logically, less time is required to examine a smaller anatomic area. The total time for a patient's fiberoptic sigmoidoscopy examination is a combined time for preparation (patient room and instrument), the actual endoscopic examination, clean-up (room and instrument), and patient dressing and instruction. Little overall time is saved with a shorter endoscopic examination.

SAFETY

The major initiative for the development of short instruments, especially for the primary care physician with otherwise limited and or no endoscopic experience, was anticipated greater safety (13), i.e., fewer complications. Unfortunately, we are aware of no data that compare in a fair way the complication rates for short and long sigmoidoscopies, i.e., endoscopists with equal skill and patients with equal disease (screening versus symptomatic patients) (see Chapter 10). Logically, examinations with longer instruments would have higher complication rates because of greater sigmoid colon stretching, greater air distention during the longer examination, and manipulation of more potentially dangerous segments of colon with diverticulosis. It is unknown whether this anticipated increased risk is or is not significant.

Additionally, whether the added curable pathology detected by longer scopes will offset a higher complication rate is unknown. In general, the complication rates observed from use of 30- to 35-cm and 60- to 65-cm instruments have been acceptable (Chapter 10).

LOWER COST/CHARGES

Shorter sigmoidoscopes generally cost the same as longer models except for one manufacturer (see Chapter 4). Light source requirements remain the same. Sigmoidoscope manufacturers report that sales of shorter instruments have been very limited. Patient charges for shorter sigmoidoscopy examination should be less than for the 60-cm examination since such examinations detect less pathology and require less time.

SHORTER LEARNING/TEACHING TIME

Learning and teaching sigmoidoscopy such that the trainee achieves overall competence requires a significant commitment of time and effort (see Chapter 17). After attendance at a one-day seminar and practice on rubber models, Schapiro et al. (14) showed that seven to ten hands-on examinations under direct supervision were required for primary care physicians to achieve competence with 35-cm instruments. Hospital privileges could, therefore, be obtained relatively quickly. Hawes (Chapter 17) indicates that 20 to 30 examinations are generally required to become competent in 60-cm flexible sigmoidoscopy. After learning on a short instrument, the trainee may wish to graduate to a longer one. Unfortunately, it is not possible to trade in the short instrument; the physician or medical facility must simply buy a new longer one.

INSTRUMENTS GREATER THAN 65-CM LENGTH

Instruments used for unsedated flexible sigmoidoscopy that are longer than 65 cm have not received extensive testing (2,12,15,16,17). Unfortunately, some reports do not give the diagnostic yields above and below 60 to 65 cm. Colonoscopes are clearly more expensive than sigmoidoscopes and are more cumbersome to manipulate and clean. We tested whether trainees doing unsedated sigmoidoscopy could insert a 160-cm colonoscope within acceptable safety and time limits when observed by, but not assisted by, an instructor (16). Table 5.3 shows that trainees with prior experience in rigid sigmoidoscopy could insert the instrument to greater than 60 cm 32% of the time and greater than 80 cm 15% of the time. We interpret these data to mean that instruments less than 60 cm would underuse even trainee-level skills.

Rosenberg (2) reports viewing the splenic flexure or more proximally in 70% of 250 unsedated patients examined in an office setting with a 105-cm length instrument. Dervin (17) advanced a 105-cm sigmoidoscope to greater than 60 cm (mean 71 cm) in 30 of 49 patients. No polypoid lesions were found beyond 60 cm.

Table 5.3.
Percentage of Examinations Achieving or Exceeding Respective Distances in Depth of Penetration with 160-cm Colonoscope (Unsedated Exams)

	Distance (cm)						
	20	≥30	≥40	≥50	≥60	≥80	≥100
All examinations	78	65	60	46	20	9	1
Trainees with prior rigid sigmoidoscopy experience	89	77	72	59	32	15	2
Trainees with no prior rigid sigmoidoscopy experience	74	62	58	43	19	9	2
Experienced endoscopists	97	92	92	73	49	35	16

From Lehman GA, Hawes RH, Roth B, Hast J. A study of optimal length of flexible fiberoptic sigmoidoscopes for initial endoscopic training. Diseases of the Colon and Rectum 1986; 29:879–881. Used with permission.

We have also used 160-cm colonoscopes to perform greater than 500 screening fiberoptic sigmoidoscopy examinations in asymptomatic subjects (12). The mean depth of penetration was 68 cm. Examinations were ≥ 60 cm in 41%, ≥ 80 cm in 20%, and ≥ 100 cm in 7%. All examinations were done by experienced endoscopists. Polyps (hyperplastic or adenomas) were detected in 19.5% of examinations. One hundred and one of 106 polyps were detected at a distance of 60 cm or less. Only 3% of patients with polyps had a polyp detected at greater than 60 cm without a sentinel polyp found downstream. We interpret these data to indicate that longer than 60 cm is largely unnecessary for screening. Further studies of tolerance, yield, and safety using 75- to 100-cm instruments in symptomatic patients would be of interest.

Use of 160-cm colonoscopes by endoscopists with limited experience is to be discouraged. Such use tempts individuals to experiment with full colonoscopy and polypectomy. Unacceptable complication rates are predictable.

SUMMARY

The advantages and disadvantages of 30- to 35-cm versus 60- to 75-cm instruments are summarized in Table 5.4. I believe the advantages of the 60- to 65-cm instruments strongly outweigh the potential or real advantages of the 30- to 35-cm instruments. Physicians and hospitals purchasing sigmoidoscopes must agree, since sales of 30- to 35-cm instruments remain very limited. However, shorter instruments are not to be condemned and do remain as a good alternative for the physician or hospital who currently owns one, since diagnostic yields from 30- to 35-cm instruments clearly exceed those of rigid sigmoidoscopes (18).

Table 5.4.
Relative Advantages of "Short" and "Long" Flexible Sigmoidoscopes

30–35 cm	60–75 cm
Shorter learning time	Detects more pathology
Easier to manipulate	Greater anatomic depth of penetration
Less patient discomfort	
Lower instrument cost	
Shorter exam time	
Possible lower complication rate	

References

1. Lehman GA, Roth BJ, Hildebrand W. Prototype studies of a forty-five cm flexible sigmoido-scope. Ind Fam Resid J 1985;3(1):11–15.
2. Rosenberg I. Left-sided colonoscopy in the office. Dis Colon Rectum 1979;22:396–398.
3. Bohlman TW, Katon RM, Lipshultz GR, McCool MF, Smith FW, Melnyk CS. Fiberoptic pansigmoidoscopy, an evaluation and comparison with rigid sigmoidoscopy. Gastroenterol-ogy 1977;72:644–649.
4. Auslander MO, Schapiro M. The true depth of insertion of the 60 cm flexible fiberoptic sig-moidoscope. Gastrointestinal Endosc 1983;29:192A.
5. Ott DJ, Wu WC, Gelfand DW. Extent of colonic visualization with the fiberoptic sigmoido-scope. J Clin Gastroenterol 1982;4:337–341.
6. Lehman GA, Buchner DM, Lappas JC. Anatomical extent of fiberoptic sigmoidoscopy. Gas-troenterology 1983;84:806–808.
7. Leicester RJ, Hawley RR, Pollett WG, Nichols RJ. Flexible fiberoptic sigmoidoscopy as an outpatient procedure. Lancet 1982;1:34–35.
8. Winnan G, Gerci G, Panish J, Talbot TM, Overholt BF, McCallum RW. Superiority of the flexible to the rigid sigmoidoscope in routine proctosigmoidoscopy. N Engl J Med 1980;302:1011–1012.
9. Dubow RA, Katon RM, Benner KG, van Dijk CM, Koval G, Smith FW. Short (35-cm) versus long (60-cm) flexible sigmoidoscopy: a comparison of findings and tolerance in asymptomatic patients screened for colorectal neoplasia. Gastrointest Endosc 1985;31:305–308.
10. Zucker GM, Madura MJ, Chmiel JS, Olinger EJ. The advantages of the 30-cm flexible sig-moidoscope over the 60-cm flexible sigmoidoscope. Gastrointest Endosc 1984;30:59–64.
11. Sarles JE, Sanowski RA, Haynes WC, Bellapravalu S. The long and short of flexible sig-moidoscopy: Does it matter? Gastroenterology 1986;81:369–371.
12. O'Connor KW, Flynn J, Rex D, Hawes R, Crabb D, Lehman G. Fiberoptic sigmoidoscopy—Is longer better? Gastroenterology 1988;94:A328.
13. Winawer SJ, Cummins R, Baldwin MP, Ptak A. A new flexible sigmoidoscope for the gener-alist. Gastrointest Endosc 1982;28:233–236.
14. Schapiro M, Auslander MO, Getzug SJ, Klasky I. Flexible fiberoptic sigmoidoscopy training of non-endoscopic physicians in the community hospital. Gastrointest Endosc 1983;29:186A.
15. Foley DP, Dunne P, O'Brien M, Crowe J, O'Callaghan TW, Lennon JR. Left sided colonoscopy as screening procedure for colorectal neoplasia in asymptomatic volunteers ≥45 years. Gut 1987;28:A1367.
16. Lehman GA, Hawes RH, Roth B, Hast J. A study of optimal length of flexible fiberoptic sigmoidoscopes for initial endoscopic training. Diseases of the Colon and Rectum 1986;29:879–881.
17. Dervin JV. Feasibility of 105-cm flexible sigmoidoscopy in family practice. J Fam Pract 1986;23:341–344.
18. Grobe JL, Kozarek RA, Sanowski RA. Flexible versus rigid sigmoidoscopy: A comparison using an inexpensive 35 cm flexible proctosigmoidoscope. Am J Gastroent 1983;78:569–571.

6

Establishing the Flexible Sigmoidoscopy Area and Care and Maintenance of the Instrument

Melvin Schapiro, M.D.
John Trocino, R.N., G.I.A.

The introduction of the flexible sigmoidoscope has provided a superior examination than was previously available with a rigid instrument. The decision to perform flexible sigmoidoscopy in the office offers the physician a chance to provide a service to the patient in a cost-effective and convenient setting. The establishment of this technology, however, involves an initial significant monetary outlay (see Chapter 4), and special care and maintenance of the equipment is necessary. Arrangements should be made to provide a standard of care equivalent to flexible sigmoidoscopy performed at the hospital. Therefore, there are a number of factors that must be taken into consideration before beginning office flexible sigmoidoscopy. These include space requirements, personnel, procedural documentation, emergency precautions, economic considerations for equipment purchases, and care and maintenance of the instrument.

SPACE REQUIREMENTS

When a large volume of procedures (five or more) are performed on a typical day, it may be desirable to have a room designed and equipped specifically for performing sigmoidoscopy. However, it may not be physically or financially practical to incorporate this into the existing office space. Flexible sigmoidoscopy can, however, be easily adapted to the existing office because expansion of current floor space is rarely necessary. An examination room can be used for performing flexible sigmoidoscopy because this procedure is simply an extension of rigid sigmoidoscopy and does not involve the planning required for more elaborate endoscopic procedures. The typical examination room is approximately $10' \times 10'$. In general though, the room should be large enough to accommodate a portable cart that holds the endoscope, light source, suction apparatus, and accessory equipment. The doors should be large enough to allow passage of wheelchairs and guerneys, and ideally, the room should include a generous ventilation system.

Restroom facilities should be readily accessible to the patient. Although an adjoining restroom would be ideal, this may not be practical in an existing office. A restroom in close proximity to the examination room is usually suitable.

Desirable electrical features include wall outlets in varying locations throughout the examination room and overhead lighting that can be controlled with a dimmer switch. This allows for the appropriate lighting background when performing the procedure.

A small dressing area should be provided for the patient's privacy when changing both before and after the examination. The changing room should have hangers for the patient's clothes, a mirror, and tissues and moist wipes for use after the procedure.

An existing examination table may be all that is necessary for performing flexible sigmoidoscopy, since nearly all the examinations are performed with the patient in the left lateral decubitus position. A tilt table may provide an extra amount of comfort and may occasionally assist the physician in positioning for the procedure. If medication is given before the procedure, a guerney with siderails is needed so that there is a safe environment while the patient recovers from the medication. Consideration should be given toward obtaining a hydraulic guerney that can be adjusted easily to accommodate the endoscopist whether standing or sitting. A portable stool is essential, as the endoscopist will frequently find it more comfortable to sit while performing the procedure.

An endoscopy cabinet with lock should be incorporated into the plans, so that the endoscope and its accessories such as light source, forceps, cameras, and film may be secured at the end of the day. This cabinet need not be part of the examination room and indeed is often located in another section of the office. A central location used for the endoscope cabinet is an excellent area for cleaning the equipment after the procedure, as well as for storing and maintaining various pieces of equipment. More than one examination room in the office would require separate cleaning supplies in each room if an area is not dedicated specifically for performing cleaning and disinfection. A large stainless steel double sink should be provided, along with adequate counter space to support a disinfection tray. A pegboard can be used to hang endoscopic accessories after cleaning to ensure adequate drying. The care and maintenance of flexible endoscopes will be discussed later in this chapter. Adequate counter and cabinet space is important for procedural performance, as well as for storage of linens and supplies.

PERSONNEL

The training of appropriate personnel for assisting in office flexible sigmoidoscopy is important, but it is relatively simple. The office assistant should be trained not only in the proper handling and care of flexible instruments but also in assisting the physician with the instrument during the endoscopic procedure. Assistance in providing patient information, explanation of consents, and discharge instructions after the endoscopy are important functions of the assistant.

The decision concerning who will assist the physician with flexible sigmoidoscopy is an individual choice. Flexible sigmoidoscopy is not a procedure that requires an R.N. or L.P.N. An office assistant easily can be trained to assist with flexible sigmoidoscopy. Various institutions provide hands-on training courses for gastrointestinal (GI) assistants that are far more extensive than what is required for assisting with office flexible sigmoidoscopy (1). Although the overall training is provided by the physician, special arrangements can be made so that the office assistant can observe others assisting with the procedure, handling biopsy forceps and specimens, and cleaning, disinfecting, and maintaining the instrument in a hospital setting. This, along with the instructions provided by the instrument manufacturers on guidelines specific to their particular endoscope, is of exceptional value.

ENDOSCOPIC DOCUMENTATION

The patient's office chart should contain all information pertinent to the endoscopic examination. This includes vital signs if indicated, nursing notes,

Table 6.1.
Nursing Notes for Flexible Sigmoidoscopy

Name _____

Date _____

Allergies _____

Endoscopist _____

Instrument _____

Vital Signs Preop _____

Vital Signs Postop _____

_____

_____

IV _____

Medications _____

_____

_____

Time Started _____

Time Completed _____

Biopsies _____

Photographic Documentation _____

Nursing Notes _____

_____

_____

and the physicians' written, diagrammed, or checklist endoscopic recordings. An office that performs just a few procedures a day should have no difficulty in obtaining these reports through their current filing and dictation system. An example of nursing notes for flexible sigmoidoscopy is provided in Table 6.1.

EMERGENCY CONSIDERATIONS

Flexible sigmoidoscopy is a safe and effective procedure when performed by a trained endoscopist. However, one should be concerned with the potential for adverse reactions under varying circumstances.

In the unusual situation when medication is administered, one should be aware of the actions, side effects, and adverse reaction to these medications. Generally, the medication is given intravenously, and standard resuscitative equipment that includes oxygen, ambubag, and antagonists to the medication should be readily available. Table 6.2 lists the medications that may be used

Table 6.2.
Medications and Supplies

1. Meperidine (Demerol)
2. Midazolam (Versed) or Diazepam (Valium)
3. Naloxone (Narcan)
4. 0.9% NaCl
5. Atropine
6. Epinephrine (Adrenalin)
7. Diphenhydramine (Benadryl)
8. Nitroglycerine tablets (Nitrostat sublingual)
9. Oxygen
10. Ambubag
11. IV tubing and infusion setup
12. Biopsy specimen bottles
13. Suction traps
14. Culture specimen containers
15. Glass slides
16. Suppositories and enemas for bowel evacuation

for flexible sigmoidoscopy and the emergency medications that should be available.

All personnel should be trained in basic cardiopulmonary resuscitation. In the event of an emergency requiring extraordinary measures, arrangements should be made to readily summon paramedic personnel. It is helpful to rehearse an emergency routine with the office personnel. A call button located in the endoscopy area could serve to alert the office personnel to an emergency.

Flexible sigmoidoscopy is a relatively safe procedure, with an incidence of bleeding or perforation occurring in less than 1% of examinations. Therefore, safety concerns are not a deterrent, as long as personnel are aware of the complications that could occur and what to do should the occasion arise.

SCHEDULING

Scheduling for flexible sigmoidoscopy should include the time needed to set up and perform the procedure, to clean the room, and to disinfect the endoscope. With an experienced endoscopist and assistant this generally takes ½ hour. The patient and any accompanying individuals should be aware of the amount of time they will spend at the physician's office, as well as the bowel preparation required prior to the procedure. Patient information pamphlets, available without charge from the American Cancer Society, are quite useful. Though the simple administration of Fleet's enemas just prior to the procedure will suffice in many cases, the retention of stool just beyond the sigmoid-descending colon junction, particularly in constipated individuals, usually requires a more rigorous preparation. A clear liquid dinner the evening prior to the examination, coupled with 1 ounce of milk of magnesia or similar laxative at bedtime, followed by two Fleet's enemas 2 hours prior to the examination, provides satisfactory bowel preparation for most patients. If the examination is performed in the afternoon, a clear liquid breakfast may be allowed (see Chapter 7).

CARE AND MAINTENANCE

The rigid sigmoidoscope is simple to care for. Many models are made of stainless steel, so even if left out in the rain, they will not rust. In addition, the rigid sigmoidoscope's construction will withstand being dropped from a height of several feet without significant damage. Routine maintenance may be kept to a minimum. For example, the O-ring that seals the viewing window rarely requires replacement, and the lightbulbs are long-lasting and easily replaced. The rigid sigmoidoscope is easy to clean in any soap solution, and if standard disinfection is deemed inadequate, it may be autoclaved.

The flexible endoscope, on the other hand, is an entirely different instrument. It is constructed with a variety of different materials. These may wear out more easily or become damaged, resulting in costly repairs. Therefore, it is important to be familiar with the workings of the flexible sigmoidoscope, its care and maintenance, and ways to prevent unnecessary wear or damage.

THE ARRIVAL OF THE NEW ENDOSCOPE

The new flexible sigmoidoscope is shipped in a suitcase that has been neatly packed in a custom-built foam rubber bed. Remove the endoscope from the suitcase, but save the suitcase. This is needed if it becomes necessary to return the instrument to the manufacturer for repairs. The suitcase should not, however, be used for storing the instrument on a daily basis. In fact, the endoscope should be hung securely in a manner that allows the insertion tube to hang in a vertical position (Fig. 6.1). It should not be stored in a coiled position in drawers. This increases the chance of breakage of the fiber bundles, and the instrument may take on the shape in which it is stored.

THE COMPOSITION OF AN ENDOSCOPE

The insertion tube of the flexible endoscope has four layers of materials that house the internal working mechanisms (Fig. 6.2). The outer layer is a teflon-coated, petroleum-based product that is heat sealed around a middle two layers of wire mesh. These surround a coiled piece of brass. The four layers together provide a stiffness to the flexible endoscope while protecting

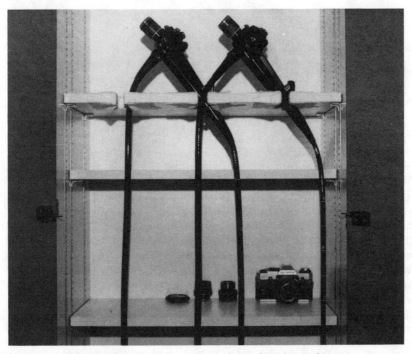

Figure 6.1. Flexible endoscopes in hanging cabinet.

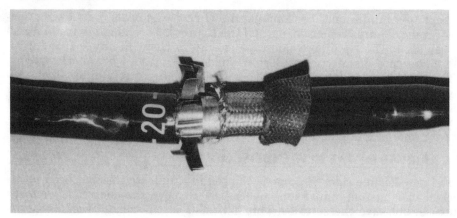

Figure 6.2. Internal layers of flexible endoscope.

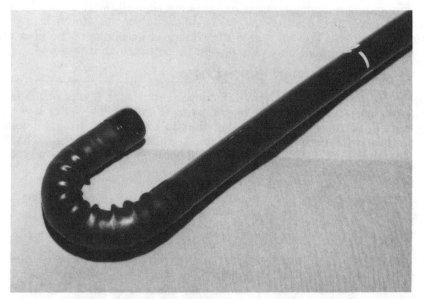

Figure 6.3. Angulated distal section of insertion tube.

the enclosed suction/biopsy channel, air/water channels, turning knob cables, and fiber bundles or electronic signal devices.

The distal end of the insertion tube is covered with a thin rubber membrane that allows the flexibility necessary for angulation and sharp turn-around views (Fig. 6.3). This portion of the endoscope frequently is subject to extreme bending and twisting. It must be carefully inspected for tears and perforations that could allow fluid to seep into the inner area during the cleaning and disinfection procedure. If leakage occurs, the result is severe damage, including corrosion of the enclosed inner working mechanisms.

The distal tip of the endoscope has several parts: an opening for the suction/biopsy channel, the termination of one or two light guides, and the air and water outlet (Fig. 6.4). The air and water ports are combined into one outlet on some models. The viewing lens, or electronic chip, is located on this distal tip. The lens is made of crystal glass and may crack if the tip strikes a

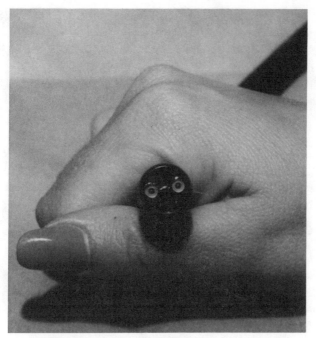

Figure 6.4.   Distal tip of flexible sigmoidoscope.

hard surface. The charged coupled device (CCD) chip likewise may dislodge from its appropriate alignment if the distal endoscope tip sustains blunt trauma.

The handle of the endoscope is made of lightweight steel or high-impact plastic, depending on the model. It is important to know whether the endoscope is waterproof. Some models are not, and the head of the instrument must not be immersed in fluids during cleaning. If water seeps into the internal control mechanisms and fiber bundles, the resulting damage usually is extensive and repair bills quite costly.

CLEANING

The following is a step-by-step procedure for basic cleaning and disinfection of a flexible sigmoidoscope with automatic air/water insufflation (2). A small but reliable suction machine is necessary not only for the performance of the endoscopic examination, but also for the effective cleaning and disinfection procedure. The suction collection bottle should be easily removable and the suction tubing disposable. Individual manufacturers will provide directions with slight variations that are specific to their models, particularly when air/water insufflation procedures are manually operated. It is important to remember at this point, however, that no matter how effective a particular disinfection solution has been shown to be, thorough mechanical cleaning of the endoscope and its component parts and accessories is the most important procedure (3). Indeed, disinfection procedures are frequently inadequate when mechanical cleaning is not appropriately applied. The following list shows the necessary cleaning equipment.

1. Three large plastic basins
2. Warm water
3. Low sudsing soap solution
4. Nonsterile 4×4 gauze pads, washcloths, and latex gloves

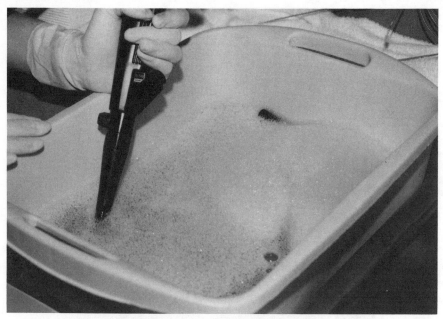

Figure 6.5.   Cleansing immersion.

5. Cotton-tipped applicators
6. 70% isopropyl alcohol
7. Cleaning brush (usually supplied with the endoscope)
8. Towels
9. 30-cc luer-tipped syringe
10. Gluteraldehyde or other appropriate disinfection solution

Step 1

After donning gloves, the bending portion of the endoscope is inspected for leaks. The turning knob locks should be left in the free position.

Step 2

Immediately after completion of the endoscopic procedure, the insertion tube should be immersed in a basin of warm, soapy water (Fig. 6.5). The air/water channels should be quick-dried by placing a finger over the disconnected inlet for the water bottle on the universal cord and then covering and depressing the air/water button until both channels are blowing bubbles in the water (Fig. 6.6). This allows any debris near the air/water ports to be removed, while preventing secretions from drying and blocking the ports.

Step 3

Gently wipe off the insertion tube with a clean washcloth.

Step 4

Suction 100 to 200 ml of soapy water through the suction/biopsy channel.

Step 5

Remove the distal hood and forceps valve. Wash these in the soapy water, rinse, and place them in the disinfectant solution.

Step 6

Some manufacturers' endoscopes allow for brushing the suction channel inside the insertion tube and universal cord by removing the suction valve.

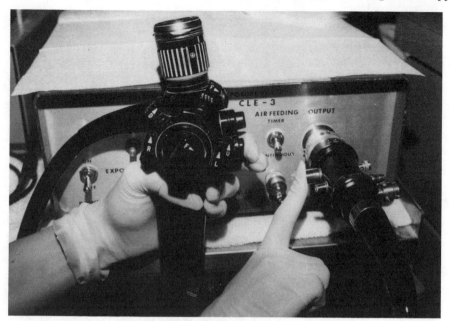

Figure 6.6.   Forcing air through instrument channel.

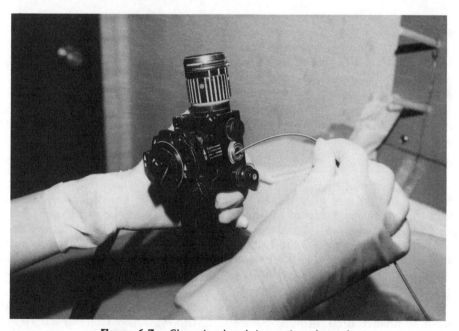

Figure 6.7.   Cleansing brush in suction channel.

In this case, if accessible, brush the entire length of both of these channels (Fig. 6.7).

Step 7

Use a cotton-tipped applicator to wipe debris from the biopsy channel inlet on the insertion tube and exit port on the instrument tip.

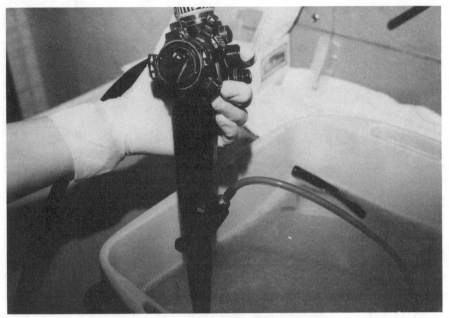

Figure 6.8.   Cleaning adapter on suction channel.

Step 8
Attach the channel-cleaning adapter to the biopsy channel opening and suction another 100 to 200 ml of soapy water through the instrument (Fig. 6.8).

Step 9
Immerse the insertion tube into a basin of clean, warm tap water. Suction another 300 to 400 ml of water through the distal tip, and wipe off any excess soap with a clean washcloth.

DISINFECTION
The two types of disinfectants that commonly have been used with endoscopic equipment are gluteraldehydes and iodophors. The iodophors tend to stain the white markings of the insertion tube a yellow-brown color. Gloves should be worn with all disinfectant solutions to prevent irritating the skin. In addition, disinfection should take place in a well-ventilated area to avoid inhalation of fumes. Table 6.3 lists the advantages and disadvantages of the various disinfectants and sterilants.

Step 1
Immerse the insertion tube into a pan of disinfectant solution. Unless leak tested to ensure airtightness, the head of the waterproof endoscope should not be immersed. (See the manufacturer's instructions for leak testing.)

Step 2
Attach a 30-cc luer-lock syringe to the channel-cleaning adapter, and insert the adapter onto the biopsy channel inlet port. Depress the suction button until disinfectant comes through the suction tubing at the universal cord. Attach a Kelly clamp to the suction tubing (Fig. 6.9). Remove the finger from the suction button and draw 20 to 30 cc of disinfectant solution into the syringe that is attached to the channel-cleaning adapter (Fig. 6.10). The disin-

Table 6.3.
Disinfectants and Sterilants

	Gluteraldehydes	
Advantages		*Disadvantages*
Rapid disinfection time		Skin sensitivity
High-level disinfection		Toxic vapors
Noncorrosive		
	Iodophors	
Advantages		*Disadvantages*
Rapid disinfection time		Medium-level disinfectant
Noncorrosive		Stains endoscope markings yellow
	Ethylene Oxide Gas	
Advantages		*Disadvantages*
Sterilizes instrument		Prolonged sterilization time
		Discolors fiber bundles
		Decreases life of endoscope

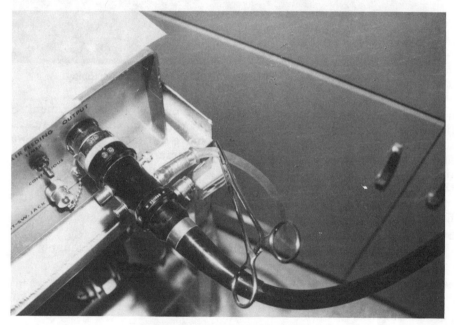

Figure 6.9.   Suction tubing clamp.

fectant is now trapped in both the suction channel of the insertion tube and the universal cord. Allow the endoscope to soak in the disinfectant solution for at least 10 minutes (3). In a busy unit, a minimum soak time of 2 minutes between cases has been used, but its effectiveness has not been documented (4). In contrast, however, overnight soaking in disinfectant solutions should not occur, as this tends to loosen the lens seal, with subsequent leakage into the insertion tube.

FINAL RINSE

Step 1

Remove the Kelly clamp from the suction tubing. Remove the syringe from the channel-cleaning adapter. Place the insertion tube of the endoscope in a basin of clean tap water with approximately 6 to 8 oz of 70% isopropyl alco-

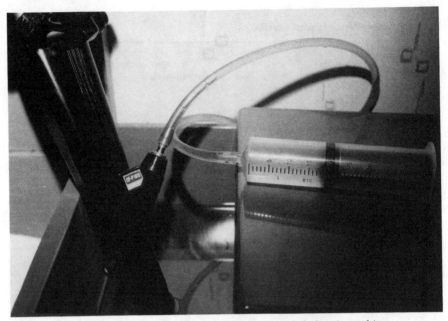

Figure 6.10.   Disinfection drawn into channel cleaning tubing.

hol. This aids in the dispersion of water and drying of the instrument. Suction 400 to 500 ml of water through the distal tip, and wipe off the insertion tube with a clean, dry 4×4 gauze pad. Remove the endoscope from the water and continue to suction the channel for a minimum of another minute. When the instrument is to be stored at the end of the day, it is important to dry thoroughly the suction channel. Pseudomonas organisms have been known to build up in instrument channels, especially if they have been stored without proper drying (5).

Step 2

Remove the channel-cleaning adapter, and dry the biopsy channel with a cotton-tipped applicator.

Step 3

Rinse the distal hood and forceps valve, and dry these with a 4×4 gauze pad or compressed air.

Step 4

With the endoscope connected to the light source, turn on the air/water pump, and with one finger covering the air/water inlet connection on the universal cord, depress the air/water button on the head of the endoscope. Any excess water in the air/water channel should be expelled through the distal tip of the endoscope. Continue depressing the air/water button until no more water is seen coming through these ports.

The head of the endoscope may be cleaned with a gauze pad dampened with 70% isopropyl alcohol. The distal tip and ocular lens also may be cleaned with 70% alcohol or lens cleaner.

The endoscope may now be stored in the instrument cabinet so that it hangs in a vertical position.

ENDOSCOPIC BIOPSY

Electrosurgical therapeutic measures such as polypectomy are rarely performed during a flexible sigmoidoscopic examination because of inadequate

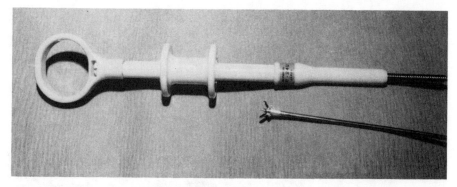

Figure 6.11.   Biopsy forceps.

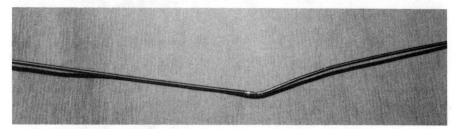

Figure 6.12.   Kink in biopsy forceps spring insertion.

bowel preparation and resultant risk of explosion. However, flexible sigmoidoscopes do allow passage of simple biopsy forceps that, in the absence of a bleeding disorder, are safe to use (see Chapter 9).

The biopsy forceps consist of a handle attached to a coiled metal sheath wrapped around a one-piece wire, which is in turn attached to forceps at the distal end (Fig. 6.11).

Inspection of the forceps should be made prior to the examination to make sure that they are in good working condition and that the jaws open and close smoothly. Occasionally, the jaws will not open, having become stuck with dried cleaning material. Placing them under hot running water usually will allow them to open and close. A drop of silicone lubricant placed on the hinges may also facilitate movement.

On gross inspection, the forceps shaft should not have any bends or kinks (Fig. 6.12). If present, they should be repaired or discarded, since the jaws may not perform smoothly and the portion where the kink is located can rub against the lining of the suction/biopsy channel and perforate it. The forceps also should be inspected for any sharp edges or burrs that may cause a tear in the suction/biopsy channel.

Make sure the forceps are in the closed position before inserting them into the biopsy channel. If not, the delicate jaws may break off. The same is true after a biopsy is taken.

CLEANING THE BIOPSY FORCEPS

The biopsy forceps should, at a minimum, be cleaned and disinfected in a similar manner as for the flexible endoscope. The coiled spring structure is a frequent site of contamination and must be meticulously cleaned prior to disinfection. Place the biopsy forceps in a basin of warm, soapy water. Using a washcloth, mechanically wash the coils of the forceps and the handle. A soft bristle brush, such as a toothbrush, should be used to clean the jaws of the

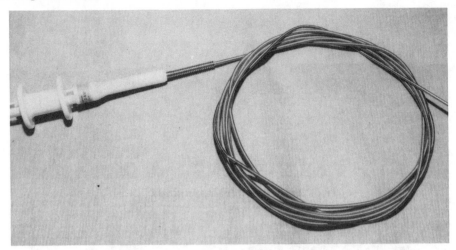

Figure 6.13. Inappropriate coiling of biopsy forceps.

forceps. Some forceps have a sharp metal spike between the jaws, and care must be exercised to prevent bending or breaking this.

Rinse the forceps in a basin of clean water and immerse them in the disinfectant solution. They should remain in the disinfectant for 10 minutes and then be removed for rinsing in another basin of clean tap water and 70% isopropyl alcohol. The forceps should also be hung to dry in a vertical position or placed in a forceps holder forming no more than a single loop. The forceps should not be coiled, as this tends to produce bends in the wire (Fig. 6.13). These heat stable forceps should be strongly considered for autoclaving (3).

If an ultrasonic cleaner is available, the forceps should be periodically cleaned in this. The small crooks and crevices of the biopsy forceps are not always accessible to standard mechanical cleaning, and ultrasonic cleaning increases the cleanliness and life of the forceps.

PREVENTION OF NOSOCOMIAL INFECTIONS

One of the reasons for endoscopic transmission of infections is that there is improper or poor mechanical cleaning of the endoscope prior to disinfection. The gastrointestinal assistant who performs this duty should be instructed as to the proper method of cleaning and disinfection of flexible endoscopes and the importance of this function. The assistant should be aware of the shelf life of the disinfectant solution to maintain its effectiveness.

In regard to acquired immune deficiency syndrome (AIDS), the human immunodeficiency virus (HIV) is relatively unstable and can be readily destroyed by several easily obtainable solutions (6). The problem is that not all of these products are safe to use on flexible endoscopes. Endoscope manufacturers currently recommend the use of gluteraldehydes as the safest solution for disinfection. These solutions are capable of destroying the HIV virus when a high-level disinfection is properly performed (6). Sterilization of flexible endoscopes and accessory equipment with ethylene oxide gas (ETO) may be carried out when known exposure to HIV or hepatitis virus occurs. One should be cautioned that this method of sterilization may reduce the life of the endoscope and typically extends the down time of the instrument for up to 24 to 48 hours. When ETO gas sterilization is not available, a prolonged 30-minute gluteraldehyde soak is an acceptable alternative to gas sterilization,

Table 6.4.
Flexible Sigmoidoscopy Report Form

Name _____

Address _____

_____

Social Security Number _____

Date of Birth _____   Sex: M   F

Phone Number _____

Referring M.D. _____

Appointment Date _____

Indication for Procedure _____

Instrument Used _____

Medications Used _____

Endoscopist _____   SPLENIC FLEXURE

Findings _____

_____

_____   DESCENDING COLON

_____

_____

Depth of Insertion _____   (cm)

Complications _____

_____   SIGMOID-DESCENDING JUNCTION

RECTUM

Impression _____

SIGMOID

ANUS

Plan/Recommendations _____

_____

_____
Signature

providing the endoscope is the type that is capable of being completely immersed in the disinfectant solution (7,8,9).

In addition to care and maintenance of the instrument, the potential for contamination of health care personnel must be considered. The Center for Disease Control (CDC) has recommended that health care personnel should consider all patients as potentially infected with HIV and/or other blood-borne

pathogens (6). These individuals should adhere to infection control procedures to minimize the risk of exposure. If circumstances indicate, the addition
of masks, goggles, and protective clothing should be used (3,8).

Disinfection of the examination room can be easily accomplished with any
phenolic solution or 10% bleach, by wiping down countertops, sinks, and various pieces of equipment. Any equipment that is disposable should be discarded in plastic bags and labeled infectious waste.

POSTEXAMINATION

On completion of the examination, the patient may want to use the restroom. The patient should be assisted into a sitting position, and, providing
they do not show any sign of postural hypotension and feel capable of walking, they should be assisted to the restroom.

Prior to discharge, the patient should receive instructions regarding diet,
activity, and what to expect following the examination. These instructions
preferably should be written, as verbal instructions may be easily forgotten
or misinterpreted. The patient's instructions should include the following:

1. *Diet:* Most patients will resume their regular diet.
2. *Activity:* Most patients will resume their regular activities unless they
   were given medication (sedation). In this case, the patient should be informed not to drive any vehicle or perform any activities requiring mental
   alertness until the following day. Also, no alcoholic beverages should be
   consumed for the following 24 hours.
3. *Information about the procedure:* The patient should be informed that some
   air remains in the colon after the examination, but that this is usually
   passed fairly quickly. Some minor abdominal cramping may be noted. The
   instrument may have irritated the colon and a few drops of blood may be
   seen. These are normal findings. The patient should be instructed to notify
   the physician immediately if severe pain, nausea, or difficulty breathing
   is experienced or if a large amount of blood is passed rectally.

RECORDING THE ENDOSCOPIC FINDINGS

An acceptable method for recording flexible sigmoidoscopic examinations is
the use of a checklist. This allows procedural information to be recorded easily and can be incorporated with the nursing notes. This information can then
be placed in the chart immediately following the examination, saving both
dictation and transcribing time. Table 6.4 shows an example of a flexible
sigmoidoscopy checklist.

The use of computers for recording endoscopic findings has been increasing
in popularity. Entry of the endoscopic findings into a computer database allows for endoscopic reports to be generated and for rapid retrieval of the information. Generation of recall letters is an added feature that is helpful for
notifying patients requiring follow-up flexible sigmoidoscopy (10).

References

1. Schapiro M. Kuritsky J. The gastroenterology assistant: A laboratory manual. Zepher Medical Enterprises, 5311 Aldea Avenue, Encino CA, 1989.
2. The Olympus Corporation. Instructions for care of sigmoid fiberscope. Olympus Corporation,
   4 Nevada Dr., Lake Success, NY, 1988.
3. Infection control during gastrointestinal endoscopy: Guidelines for clinical application. Gastrointest Endosc 34:375–405. (Supplement) 1988.

4. Schapiro, M. Gastrointestinal tract endoscopes: Cleaning and disinfection procedures. JAMA 1984;252:684.
5. Classen DC et al. Serious pseudomonas infections associated with endoscopic retrograde cholangiopancreatography. Amer J Med March 1988;84:590–596.
6. Bond W. Disinfecting and sterilizing of flexible fiberoptic endoscopes (FFE) and accessories. Endoscopy Review Jan/Feb 1987;4(1):55–58.
7. Classen M, Dancygier H, Gürtler L. Risk of transmitting HIV by endoscopes (letter) 1988;20:(3)128.
8. Dutta SK, Kowalewski EJ. Flexible sigmoidoscopy for primary care physicians. New York: Alan B. Liss, 1987:107–116.
9. Raufman JP, Straus EW. Gastrointestinal manifestations of AIDS: Endoscopic procedures in the AIDS patient: Risks, precautions, indications, and obligations. Gastro Clin North Amer 1988;17:495–506.
10. Kruss DM. The ASGE database: Computers in the endoscopy unit. Endoscopy Review 1987;4:64.

7

Patient Preparation for Flexible Sigmoidoscopy, Barium Enema and Colonoscopy

David C. Pound, M.D.

Patient preparation for colonic procedures includes preparing the patient psychologically and medically in addition to cleansing of the lumen. Because flexible sigmoidoscopy is often combined with barium enema (and at times colonoscopy), preparations for barium enema and colonoscopy also will be discussed.

PSYCHOLOGIC AND GENERAL MEDICAL PREPARATION

Psychologic preparation for the patient may vary greatly. Some patients may simply wish to get the examination completed promptly without detailed information, whereas others may desire precise details concerning the anticipated examination. Verbal instruction is important because it allows for interaction and often is perceived as more personal than a list of instructions. However, supplementing verbal instructions with written ones regarding the examination and the preparation serves as reinforcement. Providing a phone number where other potential preexamination questions may be addressed may also reassure the patient. A medical assistant may review many aspects of the preparation and the examination with the patient. The rationale, risks, benefits, and examination alternatives should be discussed (see Chapter 10). An assistant may do a portion of the latter instruction, but the sigmoidoscopist also should communicate directly with the patient. The examiner should be familiar with the patient's medical history, being mindful of the possible need for prophylactic antibiotics and adjustments in insulin or other medications (see Chapter 10). The examiner should also be aware of medications such as coumadin and aspirin or disorders that might interfere with coagulation. During the examination the patient should understand that he or she may experience discomfort from air insufflation or from instrument bowing. Patients should be advised to inform the examiner of excessive discomfort and be assured that the examiner will be attentive to their feedback. Showing the patient the instrument before the examination will sometimes help to relieve anxiety. Well-informed patients who have had their questions answered and their anxiety relieved will be more apt to consent to the examination, follow preparation instructions properly, and tolerate a complete examination.

FLEXIBLE SIGMOIDOSCOPY PREPARATION

Unprepped Flexible Sigmoidoscopy

Two common indications for flexible sigmoidoscopy in which an unprepped bowel may be preferred are inflammatory bowel disease and diarrhea of uncertain cause. In such conditions, a more accurate assessment of subtle inflammatory changes (granularity, erythema, friability) may be made in the unprepped state. Visualizing the unprepped bowel allows the examiner to see

83

the mucosa without any possible alterations due to the prep. Meisel et al. (1) demonstrated that both phospho-soda enemas and bisacodyl may cause sloughing of the surface epithelium in normal human rectal mucosa and may give a mild inflammation pattern by gross and histologic evaluation (see Chapter 9). If viewing in the unprepped state is inadequate, a 0.9% saline enema may be given without significant effect on the mucosa. Such changes are of no clinical significance when evaluating patients for polypoid lesions. Additionally, in the case of diarrhea of uncertain cause, the examiner may wish to obtain stool specimens for culture or ova and parasite analysis, which may be adversely altered by preparation. In active lower GI bleeding, some examiners advocate an unprepped examination, since blood itself serves as a laxative. However, generally some cleansing is necessary to view the lumen adequately.

Prepped Flexible Sigmoidoscopy

The purpose of bowel preparation is to provide the sigmoidoscopist with a feces-free lumen to permit optimal viewing of all of the luminal surface in the desired examination range.

Enemas

The enema is the traditional prepping agent for fiberoptic or rigid examinations. Common types of enemas used include phospho-soda, tap water, and saline. Soap enemas are usually avoided because of the potential risk of colitis (2,3).

All enemas promote bowel cleansing by softening the stool, stimulating mucous secretion, and stimulating defecation reflexes. The phospho-soda enema is also osmotically active. The commonly used Fleet phospho-soda enema is prepackaged in a disposable plastic bottle with a lubricated insertion tip and contains 19 g sodium biphosphate and 7 g sodium phosphate in 118 ml water diluent. The cost is approximately one dollar per enema.

Although most patients receive either one or two enemas before the examination, there are no randomized studies regarding the optimal number of enemas for sigmoidoscopy preparation. Weiss and Watkins (4) tabulated cleansing results after one versus two Fleet enemas in a nonrandomized nonblind study using a 35-cm flexible sigmoidoscope. Bowel preparation was considered adequate if the examination could be completed without fecal material obscuring visualization. In 54 subjects who took only one enema 1 hour before the examination, the prep was adequate in 87.1%. In the 55 subjects who took one enema 3 hours before the examination and a second enema 1 hour before the examination, the prep was adequate in 80% (p = 0.36). Some examiners instruct their patients to take the number of enemas necessary to provide a clear return (5). If the rectal effluent is clear after the first enema, it is unknown if a second enema will promote additional peristalsis and bring down additional stool that may obscure the bowel lumen during the examination. In cases where the rectal effluent is still not clear of stool after a second enema, a third or fourth enema may be required to provide sufficient preparation. Similar enema preparations may be used for either a 35-cm or a 60-cm examination.

Enemas may be taken at home or administered by the nursing staff. Administration by an assistant will require more personnel and room time but may facilitate proper enema administration and provide a better overall preparation. If enemas are self-administered, the patient should be instructed to deliver the enema in the left lateral decubitus position and to retain each enema until the urge to defecate is strong, usually within 5 to 10 minutes.

Diet Modifications

Dietary modifications such as clear liquids for the preceding evening meal and nothing by mouth after midnight before the examination are recommended by some examiners, whereas others do not specify any diet changes (see Table 7.1) Although we are aware of no controlled studies that address this issue, our clinical impression is that a clear liquid supper before the examination does facilitate the overall bowel cleansing.

Laxatives

Some examiners prefer patients to take laxatives in addition to enemas and dietary modifications (see Table 7.1). The inclusion of oral laxatives or suppositories as part of sigmoidoscopy preparation may be given on a more selective basis to patients who are chronically constipated, for example, or they may be incorporated as part of the routine preparation (see Table 7.2). Laxatives used in colon preparation include stimulants, saline and osmotic cathartics, wetting agents, and lubricants. Of these, stimulants and saline cathartics are the types most commonly used. Stimulant laxatives include bisacodyl, castor oil, and anthraquinones. Bisacodyl acts directly on colonic mucosa to induce motility in the colon through the parasympathetic nervous system.

Saline cathartics include magnesium salts and the sodium phosphates. These hypertonic solutions draw fluid into the lumen. Magnesium salts also can cause duodenal secretion of cholecystokinin, which may stimulate fluid secretions and motility (6). Osmotic cathartics such as lactulose, mannitol, and sorbitol are not recommended in colonic preparation because of their potential to form combustible gases.

As may be noted in Table 7.1, the percentage of the patients with inadequate preparation is relatively low and is similar among the different preparations used. However, a more extensive preparation including laxatives, dietary changes, and enemas may allow for a greater number of "excellent" as opposed to "adequate" preparations. The denotation of an "adequate prep"

Table 7.1.
Bowel Preparation and Results for Flexible Sigmoidoscopy

Enema Type	Number of Enemas Given	Instrument Length (cm)	Patients (enema no.) [instrument length]	Inadequate Preparation % (enema no.) [instrument length]	First Author*
Phospho-soda	1 or 2	35	55(1), 55(2)	12.9(1), 20.0(2)	Weiss (4)
Phospho-soda	"Until clear†"	35 & 65	227 [35 cm], 94 [65 cm]	2 [35 cm], 6 [65 cm]	Hocutt (5)
Phospho-soda	1	60	350	4.4	Vellacott (37)
Tap water	1 ‡	60	488	2	Crespi (38)
Saline	1 or 2	60	1012	3.2	Marks (39)
Phospho-soda	2	60	1015	5	McCallum (40)
Phospho-soda	2	60	5000	2	Traul (41)
Phospho-soda	2 §	65	116	2.6	Holt (42)
Phospho-soda	2 ‖	160	364	2.5	IUMC**

*First author and reference number.
†Enemas taken until the returns were clear 1 to 2 hours before the examination.
‡Two Dulcolax the day before the examination.
§Clear liquid supper the evening before the examination.
‖10 oz Magnesium Citrate at 4 PM and clear liquid supper the evening before the examination.
**IUMC = Indiana University Medical Center

Table 7.2.
Preparation for Flexible Sigmoidoscopy*

Exam Condition	Preparation
Unprepped	No prep desired due to exam indication (e.g., acute diarrhea, inflammatory bowel disease)
Unscheduled diagnostic exam	Two phospho-soda enemas immediately before the exam
Scheduled diagnostic exam	The day prior to the exam: Clear liquid supper 10 oz of magnesium citrate at 6:00 PM NPO after midnight except for meds The morning of the exam: Two phospho-soda enemas taken within 2 hours of the appointment

*This preparation is used at Indiana University Medical Center.

is in the eye of the examiner, and the definition varies between different studies. At Indiana University Medical Center we tallied the results of cleansing for examinations after preparation with a clear liquid supper, 10 oz (296 ml) of magnesium citrate at 4:00 PM the day before the examination and two phospho-soda enemas the morning of the examination. The preparation results in 364 patients were excellent in 67.6%, adequate in 22.8%, marginal in 7.1%, and poor in 2.5%. Randomized studies comparing the efficacies of enemas alone versus enemas plus dietary changes and/or laxatives are lacking and would be of interest. In our experience, the more extensive preparation is more likely to provide the best bowel cleansing.

Although a standardized preparation is desirable, individual modification may be necessary. Despite patient adherence to preparation and instructions, there will be occasions in which the bowel is inadequately cleansed. In such cases, additional cleansing and reexamination is generally appropriate. Occasionally, the suboptimal examination is accepted with description of examination findings and limitations.

From the patient's perspective the preparation should be convenient, inexpensive, and well tolerated. The examiner should consider the same factors but above all should choose the preparation based on its quality of cleansing. Our recommendations for fiberoptic sigmoidoscopy preparations are listed in Table 7.2.

Sedation

In general, parenteral sedatives or analgesics are not recommended or necessary for flexible sigmoidoscopy. To determine if oral sedation or analgesia is a good alternative, we performed a placebo-controlled randomized double blind study comparing diazepam 5 to 10 mg versus oxycodone hydrochloride 5 to 10 mg plus acetaminophen 325 to 650 mg (Percocet) as premedication for flexible sigmoidoscopy (7). We found no significant benefit toward lessening patient discomfort or improving the depth of examination penetration by giving oral diazepam (5 to 10 mg) or one or two Percocet tablets (DuPont Laboratories Manati, Puerto Rico) 30 to 60 minutes prior to the examination, compared with placebo (see Table 7.3). Sedatives or analgesics may be useful for particular patients who are very anxious, are mentally handicapped, or have painful anorectal or sigmoid disease.

In one randomized double-blind study, 1 mg of glucagon intravenously before fiberoptic sigmoidoscopy did not lessen patient discomfort or make the unsedated examination easier to perform (8).

Table 7.3.
Comparative Effects of Placebo, Valium, and Percocet on Different Sigmoidoscopic Parameters

Parameters	Valium		Placebo		Percocet
N	43		32		38
Mean total depth of penetration (cm)	50	←— NS* —→	48	←— NS —→	50
Mean effective depth of penetration (cm)	49	←— p<0.05 —→	43	←— NS —→	45
Total side effects frequency (%)	60	←— p<0.05 —→	19	←— p<0.05 —→	57
Total exam time (min)	15	←— NS —→	14	←— NS —→	14
Exam discomfort score as graded by patient	4.8	←— NS —→	4.4	←— NS —→	4.2
Exam discomfort score as graded by physician	3.5	←— NS —→	3.4	←— NS —→	3.7

*NS—not significant
(Gastrointestinal Endoscopy 1989;35:270, with permission.)

BARIUM ENEMA AND COLONOSCOPY PREPARATION

Flexible sigmoidoscopy and barium enema frequently are used in combination for evaluation of the colon. Because the preparation for this combination of examinations is often very similar or identical to that used for colonoscopy, this discussion will address the preparation for both examinations. Additionally, certain evaluation strategies call for patients to go directly to colonoscopy if a polyp is seen at flexible sigmoidoscopy (see Chapter 15). This may be done safely on the same day.

Performing sigmoidoscopy immediately prior to the barium enema is recommended because it avoids separate bowel preps and saves the patient time, expense, and discomfort (9). In the past, however, such examination sequencing was often discouraged (10). This delay was due to the concern that air inflation used during sigmoidoscopy would produce excessive gas and colonic irritation, which might interfere with the performance and interpretation of the barium enema study. Lappas et al. (11), however, demonstrated in a study of 295 patients that rigid or flexible sigmoidoscopy can be performed the same day as single- or double-contrast barium enema examinations without adversely affecting the quality or interpretation of the barium study (see Table 7.4).

Performing a good quality barium enema immediately after a suboptimal air-insufflated colonoscopy may be more difficult however. Phaosawasdi et al. (12) found that 14 of 15 patients were considered to have too much intestinal gas after air-insufflated incomplete colonoscopy to undergo barium enema adequately on the same day. On the contrary, all 15 patients having carbon dioxide insufflated suboptimal colonoscopy completed good quality barium enemas the same day. Additionally, carbon dioxide is nonexplosive and rapidly absorbed, produces less patient discomfort, and interferes minimally with colonic blood flow (13).

A clean colon is imperative for examination by sigmoidoscopy, barium enema, colonoscopy, or surgery. A well-prepped colon is one of the most important steps in the early diagnosis of colon cancer (14) and is also crucial in finding lesions such as angiodysplasias.

Table 7.4.
Quality of Double-Contrast Barium Enema Examinations

| | Rigid Sigmoidoscopy | | Fiberoptic Sigmoidoscopy | |
| | Prior Day | Same Day | Prior Day | Same Day |
Quality	(n = 50)	(n = 26)	(n = 58)	(n = 61)
Excellent	30 (60%)	14 (54%)	37 (64%)	35 (57%)
Good	16 (32%)	9 (34%)	17 (29%)	20 (33%)
Impaired	4 (8%)	3 (12%)	4 (7%)	6 (10%)

Modified from Radiology 1983; 149:655–658, with permission.

Prepping Agents

A smorgasbord of colon preparation agents and/or schedules exists. "Conventional preparation" generally includes a combination of 1 to 3 days of a low-residue or clear-liquid diet, laxatives, and cleansing enemas (15,16). The 2000-ml tap-water cleansing enema, as described by Miller, plays a key role in the standard preparation (17). More recently, whole gut irrigation with electrolyte solutions or polyethylene glycol electrolyte solutions (PEG-ELS) have been used.

Although the conventional methods usually have provided clean colons (15,14), they have suffered from the disadvantages of often being time consuming, inconvenient, and uncomfortable. Whole gut irrigation with electrolyte solutions provided for more rapid colon cleansing than the conventional preparation. However, substantial absorption of sodium, chloride, and water with resultant weight gain occurred in some patients prepped with whole gut irrigation, thereby contraindicating this method in patients who have impairment of salt and water excretion (18,19). Although osmotic cathartics such as lactulose, sorbitol, and mannitol do not have these side effects and are effective cleansing agents, reports of severe postural hypotension in the elderly (20) and colon explosion at the time of electrocautery secondary to the formation of explosive gas mixtures have diminished the use of this type of preparation (21,22,23). Davis et al. (24) reported the development of a gut irrigation solution, Golytely, in 1980, which was derived by substituting sodium sulfate for some of the sodium chloride in a balanced electrolyte solution and adding polyethylene glycol (PEG), a nonabsorbable and nonfermentable solute, to adjust osmolality. (Golytely is a registered trademark of Brain Tree Laboratories, Brain Tree, MA.) Subsequently, another PEG/ELS, Colyte, has also become available. (Colyte is a registered trademark of Reed and Carnrick, Piscataway, NJ.)

Physiologic Properties of PEG-ELS

Various physiologic and physical properties of PEG-ELS have been evaluated. Clinical studies of PEG-ELS have shown insignificant changes in measured hematologic and biochemical parameters (15). The potential explosion risk of colonic gas mixtures from bacterial fermentation has been eliminated by the substitution of PEG for Mannitol. Pre- and postprep end-expiratory breath H_2 and CH_4 levels in patients receiving PEG-ELS were well below known minimal explosive levels (15). Pockros and Foroozan (25) prospectively studied the changes of colonic mucosa in patients receiving either PEG-ELS lavage of a standard preparation (48 hr, clear liquid diet, 240 ml of magnesium citrate, and X-Prep senna derivative [Gray Pharmaceutical Company, Norwalk, CT]). Epithelial and goblet cells were normal in all of the PEG-ELS patients, and there was less edema in the lamina propria compared to the standard prep group in which there were changes in the structure of the surface epithelial cells and a marked decrease in goblet cells.

Efficacy of Barium Enema Preparations

The efficacy of PEG-ELS for barium enema preparations compared with standard techniques has been judged to be equally effective (26,27,28,29). Some investigators have noted an increase in residual colonic fluid from PEG-ELS (30,31), whereas others have not (28). The degree of residual fluid may be influenced by the amount of time between the PEG-ELS administration and the examination. PEG-ELS administered during the mid-day preceding the barium enema help reduce fluid retention in the colon (26). Although this may be helpful, such timing is inconvenient for patients with scheduled activities. Girard et al. (29) found that the administration of 20 mg of Dulcolax (Boehringer Ingelheim, Ltd. Ridgefield, CT) following PEG-ELS administration significantly improved the prep quality in their barium enema study.

Efficacy of Colonoscopy Preparations

For colonoscopy the preparation quality with PEG-ELS was considered more favorable in four studies than the quality using conventional methods (16,28,30,31). The timing of PEG-ELS administration for colonoscopy in respect to preparation quality is of less concern than with barium enema preparation, since retained fluid may be suctioned during the examination. Di-Palma et al. (32) noted no difference in the amount of colonic fluid retained or in colon cleansing with the addition of 10 mg of bisacodyl taken orally immediately after completion of PEG-ELS administration. Shaver et al. (33) demonstrated that the addition of simethicone to PEG-ELS preparation decreased the prevalence of colonic foam and residual stool in patients undergoing colonoscopy.

Patient Preparation Preference

Patient acceptance for the type of preparation varies. Some patients prefer the standard prep for barium enema and colonoscopy (26), whereas others choose the PEG-ELS (16,28,31). Patients over 60 years of age tolerated colon cleansing with either the standard prep or PEG-ELS well, as did their younger counterparts, with most patients in either age range having minimal discomfort (34). Brady et al. (35) demonstrated that patient acceptance was not improved by using either 10 mg or 20 mg of metoclopramide as premedication before PEG-ELS colonoscopy cleansing. Major factors for those patients who prefer PEG-ELS over the conventional prep include less dietary modifications, shorter preparation time, and personal dislike for enemas (Table 7.5).

Table 7.5.
Relative Advantages of Standard and Polyethylene Glycol-Electrolyte Solution Preparations for Barium Enema or Colonoscopy

Prep	Relative Advantages	Efficacy
Standard (Dietary modification, laxatives, enemas)	Less expensive	Adequate in 70 to 90% of exams
Polyethylene glycol-electrolyte solution (e.g., Golytely, Colyte)	Minimal sodium/H_2O absorption and secretion Minimal dietary modification Less time consuming No enemas	For barium enema: Similar to the standard prep For colonoscopy: Similar or superior to the standard prep

Table 7.6.
Colon Preparations for Barium Enema and Colonoscopy*

Prep	Methods for Barium Enema
Standard	*Days 3 and 2 before the exam:* Low residue diet *Day 1 before the exam:* Clear liquid diet† Drink at least one 8-oz glass of water each hour starting at 11:00 AM until 8:00 to 10:00 PM 2 oz of castor oil or four 5-mg bisacodyl tablets at noon 2½ oz of X-Prep or 10 oz of magnesium citrate at 4:00 PM *The morning of the exam:* A 2000-ml tap-water cleansing enema in the radiology department 30–60 min before the exam
PEG-ELS	No solid food for at least 4 hr before beginning the prep Oral: 240 ml (8 oz) every 10 min until 4 L are consumed or the rectal effluent is clear NG: 20–30 ml per min Begin the prep 14–24 hr before the exam 20 mg bisacodyl p.o. after the PEG-ELS

Prep	Methods for Colonoscopy
Standard	Same as barium enema
PEG-ELS	Same rate of administration as for barium enema Begin the prep 4–24 hr before the exam Simethicone 80 mg p.o. before and after the PEG-ELS; 20 mg bisacodyl p.o. after PEG-ELS

*These preparations are used at Indiana University Medical Center.
†Clear liquid diet: (Examples) Kool-Aid, Gatorade, carbonated beverages, coffee, tea, clear broth, bouillon, gelatin, apple juice, popsicles.

Patient's dislikes of PEG-ELS include its salty taste and the large volume to be ingested. The most frequent adverse reactions to the PEG-ELS are bloating, nausea, vomiting, and rectal irritation. The side effects generally disappear rapidly (36). The patient's preference of a colon preparation also may be influenced by its cost. None of the preps are very costly. Although prices vary according to location, the PEG-ELS prep is generally more expensive than the conventional one. Regardless of the colon prep used, the patient should be supplied with both verbal and written instructions for its usage. Patients receiving the conventional prep should understand what constitutes a clear-liquid diet. For patients using PEG-ELS, the manufacturers advise against adding additional ingredients or flavorings to the preparation. Refrigeration of these solutions before ingestion usually aids palatability. See Table 7.6 for examples of preparations used at the Indiana University Medical Center.

References

1. Meisel JL, Bergman D, Graney D et al. Human rectal mucosa: proctoscopic and morphological changes caused by laxatives. Gastroenterology 1977;729:1274–1279.
2. Lewis AE. Dangers inherent in soap enemas. Pacif Med Surg 1965;73:131–133.
3. Pike BF, Phillippi PJ, Lawson EH Jr. Soap colitis. N Engl J Med 1971;285:217–218.
4. Weiss B, Watkins S. Bowel preparation for flexible sigmoidoscopy. J Fam Pract 1985;21:285–287.

5. Hocutt JE Jr., Jaffe R, Owens G, Walters D. Flexible fiberoptic sigmoidoscopy in family medicine. Am Fam Physician 1984;29:131–138.

6. Harvey RF, Read AE. Mode of action of the saline purgatives. Am Heart J 1975;89:810–812.

7. Pound DC, Brown ED, Hawes RH, O'Connor KW, Lehman GA. Oral sedative/analgesic premedication for 60 cm fiberoptic sigmoidoscopy. Gastrointest Endo 1989;35:70–71.

8. Foster GE, Vellacott KD, Balfour TW, Hardcastle JD. Outpatient flexible fiberoptic sigmoidoscopy, diagnostic yield and the value of glucagon. Br J Surg 1981;68:463–464.

9. Rodney WM, Quan M, Gelb D. Friedman R. Barium enema after flexible sigmoidoscopy: is delay necessary? J Fam Pract 1984;19:323–326.

10. Thoeni RF. Questions and answers: timing of barium enema studies following sigmoidoscopy. JAMA 1979;241:941.

11. Lappas JC, Miller RE, Lehman GA, Eskridge JN, Morton JA. Postendoscopy barium enema examinations. Radiology 1983;149:655–658.

12. Phaosawasdi K, Cooley W, Wheeler J, Rice P. Carbon dioxide-insufflated colonoscopy: an ignored superior technique. Gastrointest Endosc 1986;32:330–333.

13. Brandt LJ, Boley SJ, Sammartano R. Carbon dioxide and room air insufflation of the colon: effects on colonic blood flow and intraluminal pressure in the dog. Gastrointest Endosc 1986;32:324–329.

14. Miller RE. The clean colon. Gastroenterology 1976;70:289–290.

15. DiPalma JA, Brady CE, Stewart DL, et al. Comparison of colon cleansing methods in preparation for colonoscopy. Gastroenterology 1984;86:856–860.

16. Present AJ, Ansson B, Burhenne HJ, et al. Evaluation of 12 colon-cleansing regimens with single-contrast barium enema. AJR 1982;139:855–859.

17. Miller RE. The cleansing enema. Radiology 1975;117:483–485.

18. Adler M, Quenon M, Even-Adin D, et al. Whole gut lavage for colonoscopy—a comparison between two solutions. Gastrointest Endosc 1984;30:65–67.

19. Burbige EJ, Bourke E, Tarder G. Effect of preparation for colonoscopy on fluid and electrolyte balance. Gastrointest Endosc 1978;24:286–287.

20. Gilmore IT, Ellis WR, Barrett GS, Dendover JEH, Parkins RA. A comparison of two methods of whole gut lavage for colonoscopy. Br J Surg 1981;68:388–389.

21. Bigard M, Gaucher P, Lassalle C. Fatal colonic explosion during colonoscopic polypectomy. Gastroenterology 1979;77:1307–1310.

22. Taylor EW, Bentley S, Young D, Keighley MRB. Bowel preparation and the safety of colonoscopic polypectomy. Gastroenterology 1981;81:1–4.

23. Bond JH, Levitt MD. Colonic gas explosion: is a fire extinguisher necessary? Gastroenterology 1979;77:1349–1350.

24. Davis GR, Santa Anna Ga, Morawski SG, Fordtran JS. Development of a lavage solution associated with minimal water and electrolyte absorption or secretion. Gastroenterology 1980;78:991–995.

25. Pockros PJ, Foroozan P. Golytely lavage versus a standard colonoscopy preparation: effect on normal colonic mucosa histology. Gastroenterology 1985;88:545–548.

26. Chan CH, Diner WC, Fontenot E, Davidson BD. Randomized single-blind clinical trial of a rapid colonic lavage solution (Golytely) vs. standard preparation for barium enema and colonoscopy. Gastrointest Radiol 1985;10:378–382.

27. Davis GR, Smith HJ. Double-contrast examination of the colon after preparation with Golytely (a balanced lavage solution). Gastrointest Radiol 1983;8:173–176.

28. Ernstoff JJ, Howard DA, Marshall JB, et al. A randomized blinded clinical trial of a rapid colonic lavage solution (Golytely) compared with standard preparation for colonoscopy and barium enema. Gastroenterology 1983;84:1512–1516.

29. Girard CM, Rugh KS, DiPalma JA, Brady CE, Pierson WP. Comparison of Golytely lavage with standard diet/cathartic preparation for double-contrast barium enema. AJR 1984;142:1147–1149.

30. Goldman J, Reichelderfer M. Evaluation of rapid colonoscopy preparation using a new gut lavage solution. Gastrointest Endosc 1982;28:9–11.

31. Thomas G, Brodzinsky S, Isenbert JI. Patient acceptance and effectiveness of a balanced lavage solution (Golytely) versus the standard preparation of colonoscopy. Gastroenterology 1982; 82:435–437.

32. DiPalma JA, Brady CE, Pierson WP. Golytely colon cleansing—Does bisacodyl improve cleansing? Clin Res 1984;32:839A (Abstract).

33. Shaver WA, Storms P, Peterson WL. Improvement of oral colonic lavage with supplemental simethicone. Dig Dis Sci 1988;33:185–188.
34. DiPalma JA, Brady CE, Pierson WP. Colon cleansing: acceptance by older patients. Am J Gastroenterol 1986;81:652–55.
35. Brady CE, DiPalma JA, Pierson WP. Golytely lavage—Is metoclopramide necessary? Am J Gastroenterol 1985;80:180–184.
36. Physician's desk reference. Oradell, NJ: Medical Economics Co., Inc., 1988.
37. Vellacott KD, Harcastle JD. An evaluation of flexible fiberoptic sigmoidoscopy. Br Med J 1981;283:1583–1585.
38. Crespi M, Casale V, Grassi A. Flexible sigmoidoscopy: a potential advance in cancer patrol. Gastrointest Endosc 1978;24:291–294.
39. Marks G, Boggs HW, Gastro AF, Gathright JB, Ray JE, Salvate E. Sigmoidoscopic examinations with rigid and flexible fiberoptic sigmoidoscopes in the surgeon's office. Dis Colon Rectum 1979;22:162–168.
40. McCallum RW, Meyer CT, Marignani P, Cane E, Contino C. Flexible sigmoidoscopy: Diagnostic yield in 1015 patients. Am J Gastroenterol 1984;79:433–437.
41. Traul DG, Davis CB, Pollock JC, Scudamore H. Flexible fiberoptic sigmoidoscopy—The Monroe clinic experience. Dis Colon Rectum 1983;26:161–166.
42. Holt RW, Wherry DC. Flexible fiberoptic sigmoidoscopy in a surgeon's office. Am J Surg 1980;139:708–710.

Techniques of the Flexible Sigmoidoscopic Examination

Jerome D. Waye, M.D.

8

This chapter deals with the practical technique of flexible sigmoidoscopy, an easy and relatively rapid procedure to visualize the mucosa of the rectum, sigmoid colon, and most or all of the descending colon. The ideal way to learn how to perform flexible sigmoidoscopy successfully and comfortably is for a preceptor first to demonstrate then to observe and teach each step of the procedure in several cases. There are many "tricks of the trade" that an experienced examiner can teach the beginner to speed the learning process; this may be accomplished in less than 10 examinations but usually requires approximately 15–25 examinations.

The material contained in this chapter is intended to appeal to everyone who performs flexible sigmoidoscopy. For those with experience, it will freshen the memory and it is hoped that it will provide new insights into some of the finer technical points. For those beginning with a preceptor, this chapter will reinforce the teaching process. For the person starting from scratch, it covers every important point in the technique and will hasten proficiency.

Although all modern instruments may be purchased "fully loaded" with four-way tip control and push-button capability for both water and air insufflation, these conveniences are associated with a higher price tag. This discussion assumes the use of a four-way tip control instrument, although similar maneuvers can be performed with a two-way deflection endoscope (the tip can be moved up and down in one plane), but the handling is somewhat more cumbersome than when using a more expensive instrument. The four-way tip control gives the operator the option of using either torque (rotatory twisting) of the endoscope shaft and/or various amounts of right/left tip deflection as desired, whereas with limited tip deflection capability, all the right/left maneuvering must be accomplished with torque.

The operator should always keep in mind that insertion of a tube into the rectum is invariably a traumatic psychologic event for the patient, no matter how skilled the examiner. During flexible sigmoidoscopy, patients always appreciate verbal communication with their physician. The conversation should not be condescending (e.g., "All right, dear, this will only take a minute") and is best directed toward an explanation of what you are doing and the sensation that may be experienced by the patient. Often the patient does not wish to respond verbally during the examination, and one should avoid asking questions such as "How are you doing?" or "Does that hurt?" It is far better to tell patients that there will be a sensation of fullness due to the air being pumped in and that they will experience a cramp when the instrument goes around a bend. During episodes of discomfort (although you are fairly sure it is due to a loop in the colon), you take measures both to deflate the colon and to straighten the scope.

It has been well established that the flexible sigmoidoscope allows a larger amount of colon mucosa to be seen than does the rigid sigmoidoscope, but total insertion of the instrument should not be the goal of the examination, which is usually performed for screening purposes in a well patient who does not have any symptoms of colorectal disease. These patients will require repeated examinations in their lifetime, and their perception of the examination, its thoroughness, professionalism, and comfort are major impressions that will determine the patient's willingness to undergo repeated examinations. There should be two goals during each examination, the first being that the examination is performed safely and comfortably for the patient and the second being that any significant pathology within reach of the instrument will be discovered. Techniques described in this chapter should help in attaining both of these goals.

Sedation should be avoided during the flexible sigmoidoscopic examination, since the use of drugs makes the examination much more complicated, with the need to give parenteral medication at least 1/2 hour before the examination or to perform venipuncture for intravenous dosage. In addition, sedated patients should not be permitted to drive for several hours after receiving medication, and they may require an area in which to rest before leaving the examining facility. Medications for flexible sigmoidoscopy should be employed only in rare and unusual circumstances but should never be a substitute for the necessary psychologic support of the patient before and during the flexible sigmoidoscopic examination.

SETUP OF THE ROOM

A standard patient examining table with the leg area extended may be used, or a flat table 6 feet long and 32 inches high will function well. There is no need for a tilt table or kneeling attachment. The light source may be on a portable cart, table, or shelf 30 to 40 inches above the floor. The "examiner's space" between the front edge of the light source and the edge of the examining table should be about 3 feet wide. A suction machine is essential and should be located near the light source. The light source should be positioned 3 feet from the center of the examining table. (Fig. 8.1)

PRACTICAL EQUIPMENT NEEDED

The following equipment is needed for flexible sigmoidoscopy (see also Chapter 4):

Three gloves
Lubricant
Soft paper towels (absorbent), 4 × 4 pads, or cloth towels
Sigmoidoscope
Light source
Biopsy forceps
Suction machine
Tubing from suction machine to endoscope
Sink for cleaning
Disinfectant and containers for soaking instruments

POSITION OF THE PATIENT

Flexible sigmoidoscopy may be performed with the patient in the left lateral (Fig. 8.1) or knee-chest position, but because of the awkwardness of the latter, both patients and physicians overwhelmingly prefer the ease and comfort of the left lateral position. The entire examination can be started and completed without requiring the patient to change positions. Alternatively, if the knee-chest position is preferred and an electrohydraulically controlled elevating examining table is available with a kneeling attachment, this position may be acceptable. With the patient in the left lateral position, facing

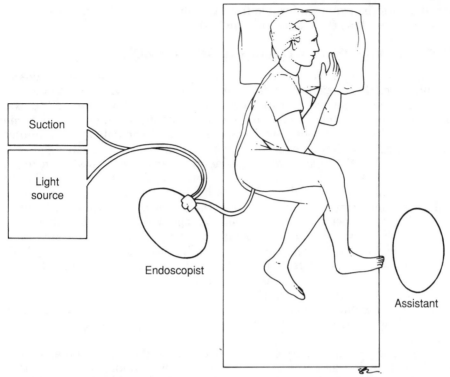

Figure 8.1. Patient position in relation to examiner, assistant, and light source.

away from the light source, the knees and hips are flexed at about 90-degree angles. The rectum should be approximately 4 inches from the edge of the examining table. An absorbent pad or paper towels may be tucked under the buttock to absorb any leakage of fluid from the rectum.

POSITION OF THE PHYSICIAN

The examiner will stand between the light source and the examining table, facing the back of the patient in the left lateral position. The doctor's left hip will be aligned with the patient's rectum. When the knee-chest position is used, the examiner stands directly behind the patient. During the examination, the umbilical cord of the instrument, containing the light transmitting fibers, air and water channels, suction, and so on, will be stretched comfortably between the light source and the examiner's hand. The umbilical cord will course across the examiner's waist instead of stretching across the examiner's back.

THE ASSISTANT

Although the presence of an assistant may not be required during purely diagnostic flexible sigmoidoscopy, the examination may be easier when an assistant can reassure the patient while providing more lubricant, absorbent sponges, and so on. If a biopsy is taken during the examination, the assistant will take care of the forceps, stabilize the instrument during the biopsy procedure, and handle the specimen, removing it from the forceps and placing it on a carrier before immersing the specimen in formalin. The assistant may stand across the examining table from the physician or, when the knee-chest position is used, at the examiner's right side.

ONE- OR TWO-PERSON EXAMINATION TECHNIQUE

There is no single "right way" to perform flexible fiberoptic sigmoidoscopic examinations. Some examiners feel more comfortable having an assistant hold the instrument near the rectum so that it will not fall out during the examination, whereas others prefer to have an assistant advance the instrument while the physician keeps both hands on the dial controls and manipulates up/down and right/left as needed to look behind folds of the rectosigmoid segments. On the other hand, with experience, many physicians learn to coordinate the shaft manipulations of torque (twisting the instrument to the right or left) advance and withdrawal while holding the instrument shaft in the right hand and controlling movements of the up/down dial with the left thumb.

Neophytes who perform flexible sigmoidoscopy will hold the instrument head in the left hand with the forefinger manipulating the buttons for air/water or suction and will use the right hand for manipulation of the control dials (i.e., up/down dial and right/left dial). With both hands on the instrument head, it is not possible to advance the instrument, and assistance from a second person will be necessary to complete the examination. The major function of an assistant in flexible sigmoidoscopy is to hold the instrument near the rectum so it will not fall out and to advance the instrument as requested by the examiner.

With a one-person technique, the shaft is held in the right hand and torqued to the right or left as necessary to swing the tip around colon folds with the amount of tip angulation controlled by the up/down wheel. The weight of the instrument is held in the left hand, and the left thumb hooks below the instrument head to move the large (up/down) dial backward and forward, producing up/down tip deflection (Fig. 8.2). Once the instrument tip is deflected either up or down, manipulation of the shaft in a clockwise rotatory torque will result in a movement of the tip in that direction (clockwise), in much the same fashion as would occur if the right/left knob were turned to the right. Therefore, the rotatory torquing capability of the right hand on the shaft of the instrument can be used effectively to turn the instrument tip to the right or left without requiring many manipulations of the right/left dial control mechanism. In similar fashion, the examiner who keeps the right hand on the shaft of the instrument for purposes of torque capability can also advance the shaft into the rectum or pull it out to reduce a sigmoid loop by pulling back the instrument while maintaining a clockwise twist on the shaft. Slight pressure in the direction of the rectum by the left hand holding the instrument head will prevent the shaft from falling out whenever the right hand is taken off the shaft to manipulate the right/left dial control.

Whenever the shaft of the instrument is held, a paper towel, gauze sponge, or cloth towel is used so that the gloved hand will not contact the instrument directly. The towel is useful because it prevents slippage of the lubricated instrument in the hand and protects the gloved hand from becoming soiled with fecal material, enema fluid, and debris. The towel should be changed frequently during the procedure so that it will not become soaked through and lose its effectiveness.

INTRODUCING THE FLEXIBLE SIGMOIDOSCOPE

With the patient positioned for sigmoidoscopy in either the left lateral or the knee-chest configuration, the perianal area should be inspected, usually

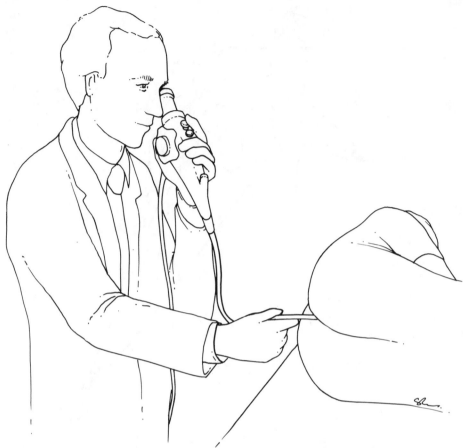

Figure 8.2. One-person examination technique. The right hand guides the flexible shaft for advancement, withdrawal, and/or torque, while the left hand holds the instrument head.

by spreading the buttock and looking as well as palpating with the index finger. A digital rectal examination is performed with a well-lubricated gloved finger. This will dilate the anal canal, will lubricate the passage for subsequent introduction of the flexible sigmoidoscope, and may detect pathology or the presence of stool. The anal canal, once entered with the finger, will easily accept the blunt end of the flexible sigmoidoscope, which may be difficult to introduce if the rectal examination was not performed. The examining glove may be replaced with a fresh glove prior to beginning the examination.

The instrument is held in the palm of the left hand (Fig. 8.3). The thumb extends below the head to rotate the large up/down wheel, providing tip deflection in one plane. The index finger is used to depress either the air/water button (located closest to the shaft) or the suction button (located closest to the eyepiece) when desired. The physician may or may not wear prescription eyeglasses when using the fiberoptic instrument because focusing the eyepiece before its introduction will adjust for diopter differences. When introducing the sigmoidoscope the distal tip is held in the right hand and placed in the rectum by grasping it like a screwdriver about 2 to 3 inches from the tip and advancing it directly into the anal canal. Alternatively, the distal

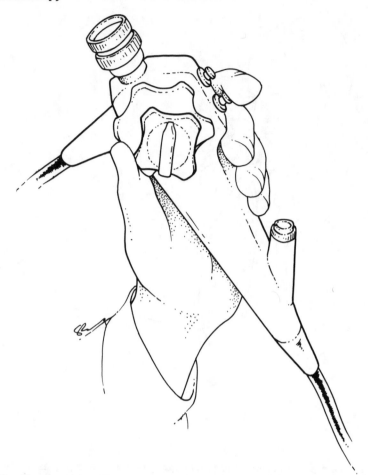

Figure 8.3. Hand position. The instrument head is held in the left hand with the thumb on the large up/down control wheel as the index finger depresses buttons for air/water or suction.

end may be held like a scalpel with the forefinger extended to the edge of the tip, guiding it into the rectum by flexing the forefinger and applying lateral pressure to the endoscope tip as it enters the anal canal.

LOOKING AT THE RECTUM

Once the tip has entered the rectum, a visual "red-out" is usually encountered, which indicates that vision is obscured because the lens is in contact with mucosa. Vision can be restored by insufflating air: The distention of the rectum will cause the mucosa to be pushed off the lens.

If a vascular pattern is not evident with air insufflation, first try moving the up/down dial control, then twist the shaft of the sigmoidoscope (apply torque) with the right hand. Torque may be counterclockwise or clockwise, and the twist (or torque) may be used in conjunction with tip deflection in the up/down direction. The beginner may be more comfortable having the instrument shaft held by an assistant so the examiner's right hand is free to manipulate the right/left dial control simultaneously with the movement of the left thumb on the up/down control. Sequential rotation of the four-way dial controls will enable the tip to travel through 360 degrees and the same maneuverability is possible with the use of rotatory torque on the instrument shaft while moving the up/down control knob with the left thumb. Although both methods will result in the same amount of tip deflection, the more advanced examiner will use rotatory torque, since control of shaft advance or withdrawal is another movement possibility when the right hand holds the instrument shaft. If none of the previous motions results in the visualization of the rectum's vascular pattern, try pulling back the instrument to move the tip away from mucosal contact. When the endoscope tip is against the mucosal wall, no vision is possible, and only a red image is seen (i.e., a "red-out"). When this happens, the tip control dials do not cause the anticipated degree of tip deflection and may not move the instrument tip at all. This principle can be demonstrated easily by holding the endoscope 20 cm from the tip and impacting it gently but firmly against a colleague's palm. Rotation of either or both control knobs results in movement of the bending section without tip deflection. Withdrawal of the tip off mucosal contact restores full tip movement.

LOCATING THE LUMEN

Air must be insufflated to distend the lumen for visualization. Although one should attempt to give as little air as possible for the procedure, the amount of air given is rarely a problem, since the patient will pass excess air through the anus or will inform you of discomfort due to air.

Once a vascular pattern is identified by the combination of air insufflation and tip motion movement, the lumen should be identified before advancing the shaft. The lumen in the rectum and sigmoid is never seen as a long tube because multiple folds, bends, and twists of the colon result in the ability to see only a short segment of bowel.

Because the colon is a cylindrical structure interrupted by multiple acute bends and twists, the lumen must be reidentified whenever each small segment is traversed. Several clues are available from the anatomic configuration of the colon to inform the endoscopist of the luminal direction. Many of these clues are self-evident but will be listed for completeness.

1. **Opposite Rule:** If movement of the dial controls or torque pushes the tip into the mucosa (as defined by a visual "red-out"), the lumen is usually in the opposite direction.
2. **Mucosal Contact Rule:** When movement of tip controls does not change the degree of redness during a "red-out," the tip is in contact with mucosa, and tip deflection capability will be restored by shaft withdrawal until the tip is seen to move away from the mucosa.
3. **Bright-Dark Clue:** There is no difficulty in seeing the lumen when the end of a cylindrical segment is entered parallel to the long axis of the cylinder. However, most often the tip of the sigmoidoscope enters each segment at an angle to its long axis, giving rise to the bright/dark phenomenon. Because of the tubular colon configuration, the wall closest to the scope will be brighter than the portion farther away; therefore the lumen will be toward the darker portion of the visual field. If tip deflection results in brightening of the visual image, the tip is moving closer to the colon wall, and the lumen is in the opposite direction.
4. **Lumen is Behind the Fold Rule:** In an area where tip deflection is adequate and where a segment of cylindrical large bowel is seen but the lumen is not evident, look for a curvilinear fold and lumen will be behind it. This clue can be reproduced by bending in half the cylindrical cardboard core of a paper towel roll. Looking through one end, it can be seen

that the sharp crease is on the inner portion of the bend, and the lumen is behind that crease. In addition, the sharpness of the bend can be estimated by the proximity of the two walls at the angle. With a gentle bend, the wall opposite the angle will be 10 mm or more away from the inner bend's sharp crease, whereas an acute angle is associated with the two walls touching.

5. **Lumen is Opposite the Ridge Rule:** In the colon, the mucosa and the submucosa lie on the circular muscle layer of the muscularis propria. When distended with air, the light reflections from the mucosa stretched over this muscular layer assume a curvilinear appearance as they are scattered over the ridges created by the circular muscle. Each of these curved light reflections is a portion of an arc, which, if extended, would become a circle around the bowel wall. The center of the circle is the middle of the lumen, and although a complete circle of light reflections is never present, the direction of the lumen can be estimated by constructing an imaginary circle using any arcuate reflection as part of the circle's edge.

DIRECTIONAL FORCES DURING INSERTION

The ease with which the flexible sigmoidoscope is passed depends to a great extent on identifying the lumen. Once located, the instrument tip may be deflected toward the lumen by either manipulating dial controls or using torque on the instrument shaft. In the one-person technique, the examiner's right hand on the shaft serves to rotate it as well as to insert or withdraw the instrument. Because of the multiple folds of the large bowel, pushing the shaft into the rectum may result in force vectors that tend to deflect the tip from advancing farther into the colon; in fact, advancing the instrument into the rectum occasionally may cause the tip to withdraw from its position, resulting in a paradoxical motion phenomenon. This is usually a sign that a loop is forming in the colon or an inverted "J" formation has occurred, and pushing on the shaft imparts a cephalad movement to the scope with the tip seeming to recede from its former position.

A LOOP IN THE COLON

Most discomfort during flexible sigmoidoscopy does not occur at the rectum, nor is it related to the amount of air insufflated; rather it is due to mesenteric traction. A large loop formed by the instrument causes patient discomfort, since this loop stretches the sigmoid mesocolon, creating painful traction on the root of the mesentery (Fig. 8.4). If the instrument could be passed without the formation of loops, very little discomfort would be encountered, as evidenced by the immediate cessation of pain with instrument withdrawal (Fig. 8.5). To ensure comfort, the withdrawal maneuver is used frequently during flexible sigmoidoscopy. As the loop is being reduced, there is a tendency for the tip to withdraw also; this usually can be prevented by twisting the shaft in a clockwise direction during withdrawal. This twist helps to keep the tip in place while the loop is removed because of the way the loop was originally formed. During introduction, as the shaft is advanced into the rectosigmoid while keeping the lumen in view, most of the tip deflection and torque on the instrument result in formation of a loop. Because of the anatomy of the colon, the loop that forms has a counterclockwise twist. If the instrument is pulled out without any torque, the tip will tend to slide back as the loop is withdrawn but will retain its position in the colon if clockwise torque is applied as the shaft is being withdrawn (Fig. 8.6). The amount that must be removed

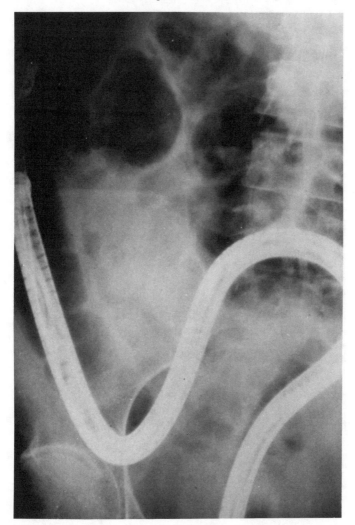

Figure 8.4. Loop in the sigmoid. This configuration takes much of the instrument length and may cause discomfort due to stretching of the mesentery.

to render a straight instrument configuration is related to the size of the loop and may vary from 10 to 40 cm. Occasionally, the tip will actually advance deeper into the colon as the loop is removed. The examiner can tell when the instrument is straight because the tip will begin to withdraw from its position. However, retreat of the tip also may indicate that the tip is sliding out along with loop removal before the endoscope is straight. The straightness of the instrument can be checked by jiggling the endoscope at the rectum, maintaining the clockwise twist, and observing the lumen through the instrument. When the instrument is straight, there will be a one-to-one transmission of the amount of shaft moved to and fro from the anus to the tip. The amount of tip motion over the mucosa can be estimated readily by the examiner. If the jiggle motion involves a 5-cm shaft excursion, a straight instrument will transmit that same amount of sliding movement to the endoscope tip, whereas in the presence of a loop, a smaller amount of tip motion

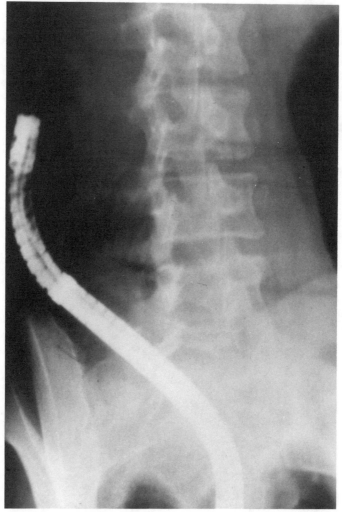

Figure 8.5. Loop removal. Withdrawal of the shaft in a clockwise fashion straightens the endoscope while the tip remains in the same position.

will be noted. Once the loop has been withdrawn, a slight clockwise torque on the shaft during the next insertion will assist in avoiding return of the loop.

PULLING BACK TO FIND THE LUMEN DURING INSERTION

The success in performance of flexible sigmoidoscopy is to insert the instrument to its full potential whenever possible, but the operator must always know the direction of the lumen. It is not acceptable to push the endoscope in blindly and hope that it advances into the sigmoid colon. Try to keep the lumen in view at all times from tip insertion in the rectum to full scope insertion by using the principles of lumen location previously described. If the lumen is lost, it can always be relocated by withdrawal of the shaft. One of the most difficult maneuvers for a beginner to learn is to pull back often during sigmoidoscopy to straighten the shaft and to locate the lumen. The

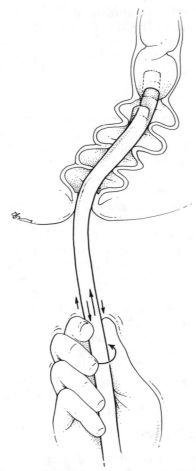

Figure 8.6. Loop withdrawal. Schematic representation of maneuvers for loop withdrawal in preceding X-rays. Torque the shaft clockwise and withdraw while jiggling. Once the loop has been removed, clockwise torque on the shaft during further insertion will tend to prevent loop reforming.

operator should keep the following points in mind when performing flexible sigmoidoscopy:

1. Pull back if the direction of lumen is not known.
2. Pull back if a "red-out" occurs, since that indicates the tip is against the mucosa.
3. Pull back to straighten the endoscope if the patient is having pain.
4. Pull back to straighten the endoscope if advancement is difficult.
5. Pull back to straighten the endoscope when the controls appear locked, since that is a sign that a loop is present.

VIEWING THE ENDOSCOPIC IMAGE

During the entire examination, keep your eye on the eyepiece or monitor screen. When using fiberoptic instruments, try to keep both eyes open during the examination and learn to suppress the vision in the eye that is not looking through the instrument, a technique used by microscopists to eliminate muscle strain of an eye that is voluntarily held closed while using monocular microscopes. Concentration on the visual field is important at every moment during the examination to prevent missing pathology in the colon. Attention to mucosal detail will also permit a full view of lumen at all times and allow for adjustments by torque, suction, insertion, and tip deflection.

DIAL CONTROL AND TORQUE

During insertion, the beginner turns the dial controls often to "steer" the endoscope toward the lumen. As confidence is gained and facility with shaft manipulation develops, it is possible to use rotatory torque on the shaft of the instrument to direct it left or right to maintain a luminal view. With tip deflection as a function of rotatory movements of the instrument shaft in combination with up/down deflection by the large control wheel, introduction of the endoscope will be easier, quicker, and better tolerated by the patient, since the right hand will advance and withdraw the instrument while torquing the tip around bends and folds, minimizing loop formation.

In the rectum and lower sigmoid, when most of the endoscope is external to the patient, grasping the shaft and torquing to the right or left does not affect the head of the instrument, which can be held in its normal position. Indeed, with video-sigmoidoscopes the instrument head can be held in any position while the examiner stands upright to view the monitor. However, with fiberoptic sigmoidoscopes as the instrument is advanced into the colon, the examiner must bend over to continue the examination, since the level of the eyepiece will become lower as the shaft is introduced farther into the colon. As more instrument is advanced, torque on the shaft is transmitted directly to the head of the endoscope so that performing a right torque moves the orientation of the head in a clockwise direction, requiring the examiner's head to move around as the shaft of the instrument is torqued.

PUSHING THROUGH THE LOOP

When the endoscope cannot be advanced because the patient has pain (almost invariably due to loop formation), but the total intubation distance has not been achieved, attempts at loop withdrawal should be made. If the instrument cannot be straightened (frequently a problem in the female patient who has had previous pelvic surgery), the scope may be reintroduced to the previous position and then further intubation attempted by "jiggling" the instrument with a 5 to 10 cm to-and-fro motion while keeping the tip deflected toward the lumen. This usually results in the tip moving more proximally, using the inherent springiness in the instrument. These small "jiggling" motions often help to advance the instrument, although a loop has formed by pleating the colon onto the shaft of the flexible sigmoidoscope.

WITHDRAWAL

Withdrawing the endoscope is the most important aspect of the procedure and is not intended merely to remove the tip from its most proximal position in the colon. The best views of the lumen are obtained during withdrawal. Air should be given to distend the lumen, and the tip should be moved in a 360-degree circle as it is being withdrawn. If the "accordioned" and pleated bowel on the endoscope shaft tends to unpleat, then the instrument should be pushed back in so that unvisualized segments of the colon will be seen. During withdrawal, slight motions to readvance the instrument are worthwhile to cause a small loop to form to stabilize the instrument and prevent the unpleating of the bowel. If the sigmoidoscope was withdrawn around an acute bend, the upper (inner) aspect of the bend may not be visualized, and the instrument should be readvanced beyond the bend and the tip deflected into the "blind" side of the angle so that full visualization can be obtained. There is no need to withdraw air continually during the withdrawal phase, since once the instrument is in the rectum, air may be aspirated.

When the tip of the instrument is in the rectum, retroflexion of the instrument should be performed so that the entire rectal ampulla may be seen from the inside (Fig. 8.7). This maneuver is accomplished fairly easily by inserting the instrument to approximately 15 cm from the anal verge and deflecting the right/left control maximally to the left and locking it in that position. The up/down control should be maximally flexed in an up direction and the instrument shaft gradually inserted while turning it counterclockwise. This will result in a "U"-turn maneuver in the rectum so that the instrument may be seen coming through the anus. Air insufflation will distend that area so that the dentate line can be seen as well as anal papillae, hemorrhoids, and perirectal pathology. On straightening of the instrument, prior to its removal, air may be aspirated.

TIPS TO AID IN SUCCESSFUL SIGMOIDOSCOPY

Endoscope Orientation Relative to the Patient

During the sigmoidoscopic examination it is extremely difficult to know the orientation of the visual field relative to any standard body position. Usually there are no clues as to which part of the visual field is the dependent portion, an observation that can be determined only if pooling of fluid is seen. If the pool is seen at the 12 o'clock position, then the examiner knows that the tip orientation is turned around, and therefore the lower part of the visual field is actually pointing toward the ceiling. There are no landmarks to inform the examiner as to the position of the mesenteric or antimesenteric border of the bowel or whether any given portion of the wall is anterior or posterior in relation to the body.

Cloudy Vision

Fluid or solid debris frequently become lodged on the lens during the examination. This results in a cloudy field that may be corrected by using the

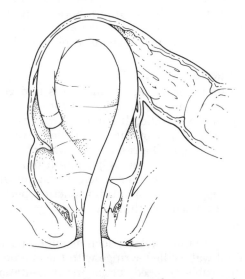

Figure 8.7.   "U"-turn in rectum affords a view of mucosa just inside the anal ring.

built-in lens washer, which, on most instruments, is activated by fully depressing the air/water button to squirt a fine water spray across the lens. A similar water spray is provided with the less expensive sigmoidoscope models but requires manual plunger compression of a water-filled syringe attached to the instrument head. A subsequent short burst of air usually results in a clear field.

Fluid in the Colon

If vision is obscured by fluid in the bowel, it may be aspirated through the suction/accessory channel by fully depressing the suction button. Suction may help to clear the field if water and air are not effective. The distal orifice of the accessory/suction channel is located at the 5 o'clock position on most sigmoidoscopes, making suction most efficient if that portion of the instrument tip is directed toward the pool of fluid to be aspirated. If the pool is at the 12 o'clock position, aspiration is best accomplished by elevating the tip toward the pool, directing the right lower portion of the visual field (because the 5 o'clock position is where the fluid will be suctioned) up into the fluid.

Suction of Mucosa onto the Tip

When the examiner attempts to aspirate fluid, mucosa often will be suctioned into the tip of the suction channel when the volume of fluid is small or if the tip is not directed into the fluid pool. This can be annoying and may be partially prevented by more careful tip deflection and avoidance of suction when the 5 o'clock portion of the visual field is close to the mucosa.

Releasing Suctioned Mucosa

When mucosa is suctioned into the suction orifice, a residual vacuum often will cause it to remain trapped in the end of the tiny channel even after the button is released. This may interfere with vision or may prevent another attempt at fluid aspiration. The "mucosal plug" can be dislodged by pulling the instrument back, but this may not be desirable. The plug also can be disengaged rapidly by injecting fluid or air through the suction/accessory port on the instrument head, breaking the vacuum.

Suction Artifacts

Mucosal suction artifacts appearing as red spots or little polypoid projections may be seen after the mucosa has been suctioned into the distal tip orifice. These must be distinguished from inherent pathology (colitis, inflammation, polyps, etc.). Although the reddened areas tend to persist for several minutes, the polypoid projections flatten out rapidly with air insufflation over 15 to 30 seconds.

Releasing Debris Suctioned onto Tip

When a foreign body (fiber, stool, or mucosa) is impacted on the tip by an aspiration attempt (depressing the suction button), it may obscure vision or prevent further aspiration of fluid. If small, it will be seen as an adherent object on the 5 o'clock position of the visual field, always maintaining its position relative to the image. Depressing the water button will not dislodge the object, which can be flushed out by placing a fluid- or air-filled syringe with an appropriate tapered adapter (such as an indwelling IV catheter) through the rubber-capped instrumentation/suction port on the scope head and injecting several cc down the channel.

Cleaning the Wall

When it is necessary to flush debris, such as adherent mucus or stool, from the colon wall, a 20-ml water-filled syringe with the appropriate adapter should be placed through the rubber-capped suction/instrumentation port, and a bolus of water should be given rapidly. Depressing the air/water button results in water being squirted across the lens for washing off debris adherent to the instrument tip but is not useful for washing the colon wall.

BIOPSY DURING SIGMOIDOSCOPY

Biopsies may be taken from any lesion seen during the examination or even from normal-appearing tissue when indicated (Chapter 9). It is difficult to do any serious damage with the small flexible forceps, which are capable of being passed through the suction/accessory channel of a sigmoidoscope. However, three points should be stressed:

1. Because the biopsy forceps enters the visual field through the same channel used for suction, the 5 o'clock portion of the endoscope tip always should be directed toward the lumen while the forceps are pushed through. This will prevent the forceps tip from being hidden and inadvertently pushed through the bowel wall as it exits from the instrument.

2. Suction is either markedly diminished or nonexistent (depending on the caliber of the channel in each brand of sigmoidoscope) when the biopsy forceps is in the channel.

3. The tissue retrieval is not a punch-type of biopsy where closure of the jaws severs the specimen from its bed; instead, the specimen is merely held within the forceps jaws and avulsed from its bed by forceps withdrawal. The piece of tissue held within the forceps is separated by being torn from surrounding mucosa that is stretched up to the flat face of the instrument.

HOW MUCH IS ENOUGH?

Almost all attempts at passage of the flexible sigmoidoscope will be successful to a distance of 25 cm. Because of looping in the colon, the entire length of the instrument may be inserted into the rectum, and the tip may not actually advance beyond the area of the mid-sigmoid colon. Usually, the formation of a large inverted "U"-loop causes significant patient discomfort from traction on the sigmoid mesocolon. However, in the elderly patient, a sensation of pain may not occur because of elasticity of these attachments. When stretch on the sigmoid mesocolon is associated with discomfort, maneuvers should be attempted to reduce the size of the loop. This can be accomplished by pulling back the instrument, usually with a clockwise torquing maneuver, so that the tip of the instrument will not withdraw in the same fashion as it was inserted. A slight rotatory torquing motion to the right frequently will keep the tip in its position related to that colon segment as the portion of instrument causing the loop is withdrawn from the rectum. During the rotatory torque and pull-back maneuver to reduce the loop, it is important for the endoscopist to be able to visualize the lumen at all times. This can be accomplished by moving the up/down control knob to keep the tip in the lumen. The technique of flexible sigmoidoscopy should not ever be considered a "blind technique," where the instrument is pushed in without the examiner's knowing the location of the lumen at all times.

The examination should be terminated if solid stool obstructs the lumen. Although this is unusual following two phosphate enemas, it may occur. If stool is present, the choices are to give another enema and continue the examination, to reschedule on another date, or just to terminate the examination if intubation and visualization were successful for at least 25 cm. There is no reason to continue the examination if a tumor obstruction is seen, an acute angulation of the colon is present, or severe diverticular disease impedes progress. If the instrument is inserted its total distance, the procedure may be terminated unless straightening maneuvers result in pleating the bowel so that the sigmoidoscope may be inserted farther into the colon. Patient discomfort is one of the most important parameters in the decision to stop the examination. Although it is desirable to pass the instrument to its full extent, this may not be accomplished successfully at all times in the unsedated patient. As experience is gained in the technique, patients will become more comfortable, and the capability of advancing the instrument farther into the colon during each examination will be increased.

Colorectal Biopsy

Christina M. Surawicz, M.D.

Colorectal biopsy is an important tool that increases the diagnostic ability of flexible sigmoidoscopy. This chapter reviews indications for biopsy, biopsy instruments, biopsy technique, and biopsy interpretation.

INDICATIONS FOR RECTAL BIOPSY

Rectal biopsy is helpful in further defining abnormal mucosa, polyps, or masses; in differentiating the etiology of colitis; in detecting dysplasia in chronic ulcerative colitis; and in detecting occult or submucosal disease in some systemic illnesses.

Diagnosis of Colitis

In patients with active or suspected colitis, it is best to perform sigmoidoscopy without a prior Fleet enema or Dulcolax suppository because these agents can injure the mucosa (1). If the unprepared examination is unsuccessful, a tap water enema can be given and sigmoidoscopy repeated.

In some situations, the gross appearance of the mucosa will be diagnostic, and biopsy may not be necessary. For example, sigmoidoscopy is often done in patients after abdominal aortic aneurysm surgery to look for ischemic changes. The dusky purplish color of ischemic mucosa is diagnostic in this setting, and biopsy is not necessary. Similarly, patients with antibiotic-associated diarrhea may have classical pseudomembranous colitis, and biopsy may not always be necessary for confirmation.

There are five indications for biopsy in colitis:

1. To confirm the presence of colitis;
2. To document either the extent or the severity of colitis;
3. To aid in differential diagnosis of colitis;
4. To follow the course of the disease in inflammatory bowel disease;
5. To detect dysplasia.

Each of these will be discussed (see Table 9.1).

Confirming the Presence of Colitis

Histology documents mucosal abnormalities and gives clues to the etiology of the colitis. In early inflammatory bowel disease, mucosal changes may be seen histologically when the mucosa looks normal grossly or when there is only induced friability ("positive wipe test").

Documenting the Extent and Severity of Colitis

This is important in ulcerative proctitis, where the inflammation does not extend above 10 to 12 cm from the anal verge. A biopsy showing normal mucosa above the 10- to 12-cm level is important because ulcerative proctitis may have a more benign course and prognosis compared to ulcerative colitis.

Biopsy may be an indication of severity of disease. The extent of inflammation and disruption of architecture usually correlate with disease as visualized endoscopically. However, severity of disease is best evaluated clinically, not by histology alone.

Table 9.1.
Indications for Colorectal Biopsy

Clinical Situation		Histology	Comments
1. Abnormal mucosa			
A. Colitis	Ulcerative colitis	Crypt distortion Diffuse chronic inflammation	Biopsy also detects dysplasia in CUC
	Crohn's	Granulomas; may have distorted crypts Focal chronic inflammation	
i. Differential diagnosis	Infectious (See Table 9.2)	Preservation of noraml architecture Acute inflammation	Culture (+) in only 40–60%
	Antibiotic associated pseudomembranous colitis	Typical pseudomembranes	Biopsy helpful in lingering cases C. difficile toxin will be (+) 90–95%
	Ischemic Postradiation	Superficial injury maximal Crypts "erased"; minimal inflammation	
ii. Detect dysplasia	Ulcerative colitis	Adenomatous change	Full colonoscopy and biopsy indicated at regular intervals after 7 years of disease
	Crohn's	Dysplasia can occur	Dysplasia may occur but screening not recommended currently
B. Polyps	Adenomatous	Villus, tubular or mixed tubulovillous	Neoplastic; malignant potential increases with size
	Hyperplastic	Serrated surface	No malignant potential
	Juvenile	Hamartomas	Rare in adults, no malignant potential, frequent in rectum
	Inflammatory	Inflammatory mass	No malignant potential
C. Mass	Adenocarcinoma Inflammatory polyps Other	Malignant cells	
D. Ulcers	Traumatic Infectious Ischemic IBD	Histology varies with etiology	Clinical setting helpful
2. Normal mucosa			
A. Detect occult disease	Crohn's	Granulomas occur in grossly normal mucosa	May be seen in 10% of biopsies of normal mucosa
	Collagenous colitis	Thickened subepithelial collagen layer	Chronic watery diarrhea
B. Detect submucosal disease	Hirschsprung's disease	Absence of neurons	Adequate submucosa necessary
	Amyloidosis	(+) Congo red stain with birefringence around submucosal blood vessels	Adequate submucosa necessary

Table 9.2.
Diffrential Diagnosis of Colitis

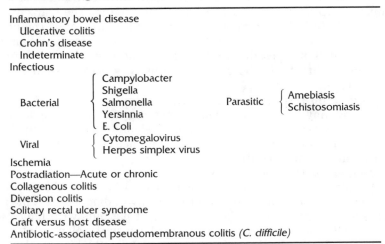

Inflammatory bowel disease
  Ulcerative colitis
  Crohn's disease
  Indeterminate
Infectious

| Bacterial | Campylobacter, Shigella, Salmonella, Yersinnia, E. Coli | Parasitic | Amebiasis, Schistosomiasis |

Viral — Cytomegalovirus, Herpes simplex virus

Ischemia
Postradiation—Acute or chronic
Collagenous colitis
Diversion colitis
Solitary rectal ulcer syndrome
Graft versus host disease
Antibiotic-associated pseudomembranous colitis *(C. difficile)*

Aiding in Differential Diagnosis of Colitis

Biopsy can distinguish IBD from other types of colitis (see Table 9.2). When a patient presents with acute bloody diarrhea, the clinician needs to know whether this is acute self-limited colitis, such as an infectious colitis, or whether it is the first episode of inflammatory bowel disease, such as ulcerative colitis. Stool cultures are positive in 40 to 60% of cases of infectious colitis; this is a good first step in evaluation. If the illness persists or is severe and warrants specific therapy, rectal biopsy should be done because rectal biopsies in inflammatory bowel disease have characteristic changes: distortion of architecture and chronic inflammation. Infectious colitis usually is characterized by preservation of normal architecture and acute inflammation (2,3). Sometimes biopsy gives a clue to an infecting organism: granulomas are seen in tuberculosis and in chlamydial and syphilitic proctitis. Viral inclusions can diagnose cytomegalovirus and herpes simplex virus type II colitis, which are usually seen in immunocompromised patients (4). Specific parasites such as E. histolytica, cryptosporidia and schistosomes can be seen in histological sections. Other forms of colitis include ischemic colitis and radiation colitis, which can be either acute or chronic.

Antibiotic pseudomembranous colitis will have diagnostic pseudomembranes, which are creamy yellow plaques adherent to the colonic wall. However, pseudomembranes can be seen in other diseases and thus are not specific for pseudomembranous colitis in patients without prior antibiotic ingestion. Ninety percent of patients with pseudomembranous colitis will have pseudomembranes visible within the reach of a flexible sigmoidoscope (5).

Homosexual men with proctitis or with acquired immune deficiency syndrome (AIDS) have frequent rectal symptoms. Biopsy is valuable in detecting infections such as cytomegalovirus, herpes simplex virus, and other infections, and it is a useful adjunct to culture in cases that are difficult to diagnose.

Biopsy is helpful in distinguishing between ulcerative colitis and Crohn's disease (6). Clinically, ulcerative colitis is characterized by rectal involvement with diffuse mucosal inflammation. Bloody diarrhea is the most frequent presenting symptom. In Crohn's disease, rectal involvement can occur but is not uniform as in ulcerative colitis, and inflammation is patchy or noncontiguous and may involve submucosa as well as mucosa. The classic endoscopic finding in Crohn's disease is linear ulceration in otherwise normal mucosa. Apthous ulcers may be an early finding. The transmural inflammation of Crohn's disease may result in fistula formation, a complication that is not seen in ulcerative colitis. In 10 to 20% of cases of inflammatory bowel disease, it is not possible to distinguish the two diseases clinically or histologically. With time, these diagnoses usually become clear in these cases of indeterminate colitis.

Following the Course of the Disease

Biopsy may be used to document healing of colitis or to document progression. In general, histologic information should be used to supplement clinical information in specific cases. There is no need for frequent rectal biopsies in most patients with colitis.

Detecting Dysplasia

Dysplasia occurs in some patients with ulcerative colitis after 7 years or more of disease, and biopsy is the only way to diagnose it. This gives an early clue to the presence of colon cancer. Most patients with long-standing ulcerative colitis are screened on a regular basis with colonoscopy and biopsies at standard intervals throughout the colon. Rectal biopsy alone is not sufficiently accurate to rule out the presence of dysplasia elsewhere in the colon.

Diagnosis of Polyps and Masses

In adults, polyps are either neoplastic or nonneoplastic. Neoplastic polyps are usually adenomas and are classified as tubular, villus, or tubulovillus. These have malignant potential, and for this reason they usually should be totally removed. Their gross appearance is a characteristic mulberry or reddened mucosa. If they are of sufficient size, a stalk or pedicle may form.

A biopsy can be done to determine the histology of the polyps. However, all adenomas should be removed (see Chapter 15), and polypectomy should be done only by an experienced colonoscopist using electrocautery after standard colonoscopy preparation. The colon preparation is necessary to reduce the bacterial load, thus decreasing the concentration of explosive gases that might be ignited by cautery. Total colonoscopy also allows detection of additional polyps that may be present proximally. The technique of polypectomy is well described elsewhere (7). For these reasons, the general recommendation is that polypectomy should not be done at the time of flexible sigmoidoscopy.

Hyperplastic polyps are the most common nonneoplastic polyps in adults, although inflammatory polyps, juvenile polyps, and other hamartomas can occur. These polyps do not have malignant potential. The presence of hyperplastic polyps in the rectosigmoid has generally not been considered to be correlated with adenomas elsewhere. Recent information (see Chapter 15) suggests a possible association between rectosigmoid hyperplastic polyps and adenomas elsewhere in the colon. Because the need for colonoscopy in patients with hyperplastic polyps is controversial, biopsy of newly discovered diminutive polyps at sigmoidoscopy is helpful in defining adenomas, which then clearly indicates a need for total colonoscopy. Alternatively, many physicians elect to bypass biopsy of such polyps at sigmoidoscopy and refer all patients with colon polyps regardless of size for total colonoscopy and polypectomy. Additional data are needed to define which of these approaches is optimal for patient care.

Colonic masses always should be biopsied for diagnosis. Occasionally, benign inflammatory conditions, such as solitary rectal ulcer present with a firm rectal mass that can be mistaken for carcinoma. Colonic ulcers are seen in Crohn's disease and other inflammatory diseases, and biopsy usually is indicated. Be careful not to biopsy the base of the ulcer, as perforation may result. Biopsy of normal mucosa is indicated in specific situations, such as searching for submucosal amyloid in systemic disease or looking for ganglion cells to exclude Hirschsprung's disease. In addition, some patients with Crohn's disease may have diagnostic granulomas in biopsies taken from grossly normal rectal mucosa. Finally, biopsy detects early inflammatory bowel disease or patchy, less common diseases such as collagenous colitis or microscopic colitis, which may elucidate the etiology of chronic diarrhea in some patients.

When Not to Biopsy

If flexible sigmoidoscopy is to be followed by a barium enema, biopsy generally should be deferred. Colonic perforations have occurred at a biopsy site when followed by high-pressure barium enema. This risk is almost certainly less with the superficial biopsies taken with the flexible sigmoidoscope than with the biopsy forceps used with a rigid sigmoidoscope. Biopsy of mass lesions protruding into the lumen is acceptable immediately prior to barium enema. Generally a 7-day interval is preferable between rigid sigmoidoscopy with deep rectal biopsy and subsequent barium enema.

Patients with uncorrectable coagulopathy should not be biopsied, nor should patients on anticoagulants. In addition, aspirin increases the risk of bleeding and should be discontinued if possible several days prior to and after biopsy.

In general, there is no need to biopsy benign anal disease such as hemorrhoids, anal papillae, or fissures. Uncomplicated diverticulosis should not be biopsied. Melanosis coli has a characteristic appearance, and biopsy usually is not necessary to confirm this. The black color of the mucosa is due to pigment in the lamina propria macrophages, associated with anthraquinone laxative ingestion.

BIOPSY INSTRUMENTS

There are three different types of instruments that can be used to biopsy the rectum (see Fig. 9.1): Standard forceps for rigid sigmoidoscopy, suction biopsy instruments, and forceps for flexible endoscopes.

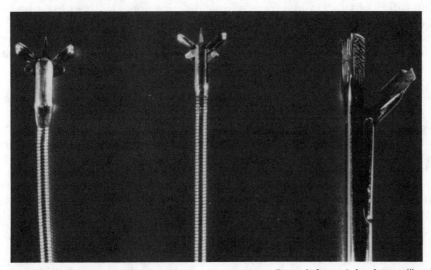

Figure 9.1. Photograph of three biopsy instruments. From left to right: Large "jumbo" biopsy forceps, standard biopsy forceps for flexible sigmoidoscopes, and straight forceps for rectal biopsy through a rigid sigmoidoscope. The flexible forceps have a central pin to aid in obtaining biopsies.

The standard proctosigmoidoscopic forceps, used through a rigid sigmoidoscope, can take large and deep biopsies and is especially useful when submucosal lesions are being evaluated. The major disadvantage of this instrument is the risk of bleeding (a significant hemorrhage occurs 1 in 400 times) and of perforation (rare but it can occur). These complications can occur because it is difficult to gauge the size of the biopsy. It is best to biopsy in the rectum within 10 cm of the anal verge, which is below the peritoneal reflection. After taking a biopsy, the author's practice is to pass a long cotton-tipped applicator through the sigmoidoscope and press the biopsy site for 1 minute. If the biopsy site continues to ooze, a silver nitrate stick can be used to cauterize the edges. Significant hemorrhage would require cautery with a hemostatic device such as a bicap or a heater probe. Rarely, a patient will require surgical intervention with a suture to stop the bleeding (see Chapter 10).

There are two suction instruments designed to take rectal samples without a sigmoidoscope (i.e., "blind" biopsies). They are the Quinton instrument, also known as the "Rubin tube," and the Crosby-Kugler capsule. Because they are small, these instruments often are used in children. They can be used to obtain biopsies from adults when a sigmoidoscopy is not necessary, such as diagnosing amyloidosis.

Flexible biopsy instruments are used with flexible sigmoidoscopes. These yield shallow biopsies, 2 to 4 mm in length, with little or no submucosa. The risk of bleeding and perforation thus is essentially nil. The major advantage, in addition to safety, is the ability to biopsy lesions above the rectum. The major disadvantage is the small size of the biopsy, which makes pathologic interpretation more difficult. Newer endoscopes with a larger channel up to 4.2 mm are a major advance because they allow for passage of a larger biopsy instrument ("jumbo forceps"), which takes biopsies over 4 mm in diameter. Because these biopsies are shallow, the risk of significant bleeding remains small. To the author's knowledge, colonic perforation has not been reported. These biopsies are adequate for evaluation of mucosal pathology, but they contain little submucosa and thus will not always detect submucosal disease.

The safety of this "jumbo forceps" has definite appeal. It can even be used through a rigid sigmoidoscope by sliding the biopsy forceps through a clear suction catheter to stiffen it.

The risk of biopsy parallels the depth of the biopsy; however, larger biopsies often yield more diagnostic information.

BIOPSY TECHNIQUE

Colorectal biopsy is painless because the mucosa has no pain receptors above the dentate line. It is best to take biopsies at least 7 cm above the anal verge to avoid inadvertently biopsying squamous epithelium (an "ouch" biopsy). Biopsies taken too low often contain confusing anal artifacts.

The closed biopsy forceps is passed through the suction channel of the instrument while the endoscopist watches the lumen to detect the forceps as it exits the endoscope tip. The forceps is then opened by the endoscopy assistant, and the endoscopist pushes the open forceps against the lesion or the mucosa. The assistant closes the forceps, and the biopsy forceps is tugged free and removed. Sometimes it is difficult to biopsy flat mucosa unless air is suctioned from the lumen. Biopsy instruments with a central pin are helpful to anchor the mucosa. Another solution is to biopsy the edge of a fold.

The biopsy should be removed gently from the cups of the opened forceps. The author uses the sharp point of a broken wooden cotton-tipped stick. It is advisable to orient the biopsy for better pathologic interpretation (8). The mucosa usually curls up, so it must be flattened with the side of a metal dissecting stick and placed on mounting medium mucosal side up. Mono-filament mesh, filter paper, or even cucumber slices can all be used. A well-oriented biopsy allows the histology technician to make nontangential sections that are easier to interpret because they lack confusing artifacts. The biopsy is then placed in fixative. The author uses a picric acid-based formula, Hollande's, because it decreases shrinkage artifacts. Formalin is more commonly used elsewhere.

It is important to label specimen containers if multiple biopsies have been taken from different areas. It is also important to provide the pathologist with adequate information for biopsy interpretation. Describe the clinical setting as well as the biopsy site and the specific questions to be answered.

BIOPSY INTERPRETATION

The normal mucosal biopsy (Fig. 9.2) contains surface epithelium, crypts, lamina propria, and some submucosa. The surface epithelium and crypts are composed of columnar absorptive cells and mucus-producing goblet cells. Normally, the crypts are closely packed and parallel. The lamina propria contains lymphocytes, plasma cells, occasional eosinophils, histiocytes, macrophages, and a rare neutrophil. The muscularis mucosa is below the crypt

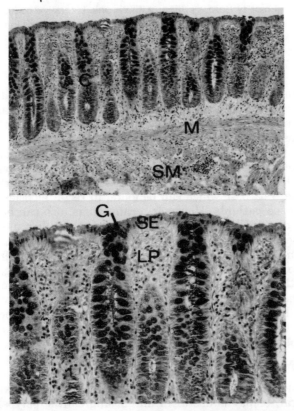

Figure 9.2. Normal rectal mucosa. The surface epithelium (SE) consists of columnar absorptive cells and darkly stained goblet cells (G, arrow). The crypts (C) are parallel and closely packed with lamina propria (LP) in between. Below is the muscularis mucosa (M) and submucosa (SM) with blood vessels. Top 90X, bottom 180X. All biopsies were stained with H + E, Alcian blue, and Saffron.

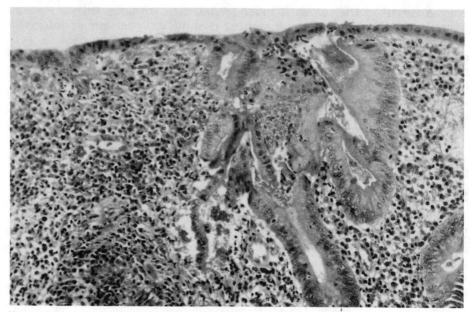

Figure 9.3.   Rectal biopsy from a patient with chronic ulcerative colitis shows crypt distortion and marked increase in acute and chronic inflammatory cells in the lamina propria (180X).

bases. The submucosa contains larger blood vessels. Acute self-limited colitis or infectious-type colitis usually is characterized by preservation of normal architecture and an increase in acute inflammatory cells in the lamina propria. In contrast, in chronic ulcerative colitis (Fig. 9.3) crypt architecture is distorted, and there is an increase in both acute and chronic inflammatory cells in the lamina propria. In Crohn's disease of the colon, crypt architecture may be normal, or it may be distorted. The histologic hallmark is the epithelioid granuloma (Fig. 9.4), which can be found in rectal biopsies from a quarter of Crohn's disease patients. However, granulomas also can be seen in infectious proctitis due to Chlamydia, syphilis, or, rarely, tuberculosis. Hyperplastic polyps (Fig. 9.5) consist of nonneoplastic epithelium with a serrated appearance to the mucosal surface. Dilated cystic crypts are frequent. These polyps have no malignant potential. Adenomatous polyps (Fig. 9.6) consist of neoplastic epithelium. The epithelial cells are hyperchromatic and increased in number. These polyps can be either tubular, villous, or both (i.e., tubulovillous). They have the potential to develop malignant adenocarcinoma. Adenocarcinoma (Fig. 9.7) is the most common colonic cancer and consists of clearly malignant cells.

CONCLUSION

Colorectal biopsy is an important diagnostic adjunct to flexible sigmoidoscopy. In general, biopsy is useful in diagnosing colitis, polyps, mass lesions, and ulcers. Biopsy of normal mucosa can help elucidate some cases of unexplained diarrhea. The new larger "jumbo" biopsy forceps provide adequate samples to diagnose most mucosal diseases. Submucosal lesions may require larger biopsies taken with a grasp forceps through a rigid sigmoidoscope.

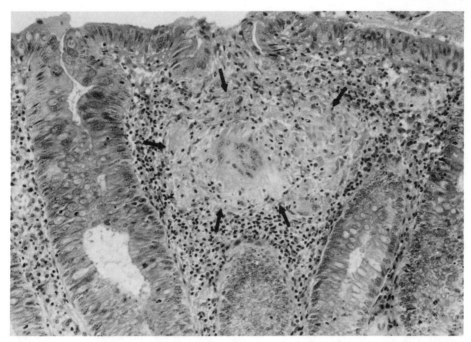

Figure 9.4. An epithelioid granuloma (arrows surrounding) in a rectal biopsy from a patient with Crohn's disease (180X).

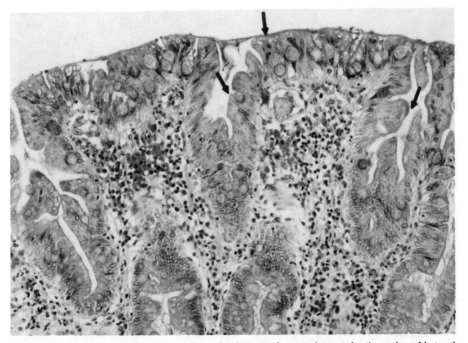

Figure 9.5. Hyperplastic epithelium in the biopsy from a hyperplastic polyp. Note the typical serrated appearance of the hyperplastic epithelium (arrow).

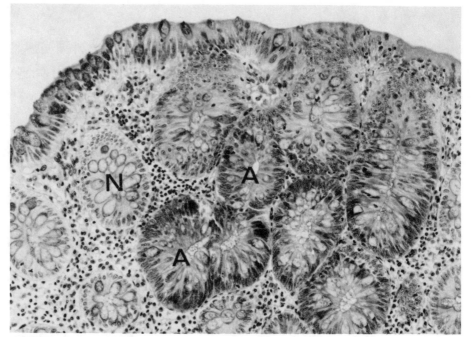

Figure 9.6. Adenomatous change (A) in biopsy of an adenomatous polyp. Contrast with the adjacent normal crypt (N).

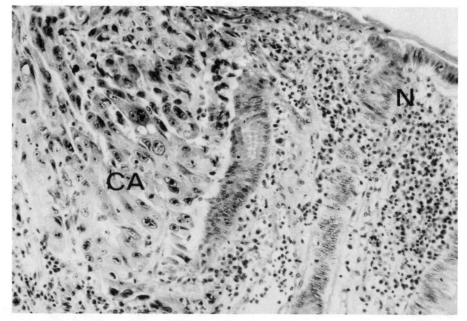

Figure 9.7. Adenocarcinoma (CA) of the colon. Adjacent nonmalignant mucosa for comparison (N).

References

1. Meisel JL, Bergman D, Graney D, et al. Human rectal mucosa: proctoscopic and morphological change caused by laxatives. Gastroenterology 1977;72:1274–1279.
2. Surawicz CM, Belic L. Rectal biopsy helps to distinguish acute self-limited colitis from idiopathic inflammatory bowel disease. Gastroenterology 1984;86:104–113.
3. Nostrant TT, Kumar NB, Appelman HD. Histopathology differentiates acute self-limited colitis from ulcerative colitis. Gastroenterology 1987;92:318–328.
4. Surawicz CM, Goodell SE, Quinn TC, et al. Spectrum of rectal biopsy abnormalities in homosexual men with intestinal symptoms. Gastroenterology 1986;91:651–659.
5. Tedesco FS, Corless JK, Brownstein RE. Rectal sparing in antibiotic associated pseudomembranous colitis: a prospective study. Gastroenterology 1982;83:1259–1260.
6. Yardley JH, Donowitz M. Colorectal biopsy in inflammatory bowel disease. In: Yardley JH, Morson BC, Abell MR, eds. The gastrointestinal tract. Baltimore: Williams & Wilkins, 1977.
7. Colonoscopic polypectomy, Chapter 10. In: Cotton PB, Williams CB. Practical gastrointestinal endoscopy, 2nd ed. Oxford, England: Blackwell Scientific Pub., 1982:142–154.
8. Shapiro M., Kuritsky J. The gastroenterology assistant: A laboratory manual. Zepher Medical Enterprises, 5311 Aldea Avenue, Encino, CA, 1988, pp. 63–68.

10

Complications and Informed Consent
K. W. O'Connor, M.D.

The endoscopist's goal should be to perform a safe, accurate, and expeditious examination of the distal colon with minimal discomfort. Although the balance between the knowledge to be gained by flexible sigmoidoscopy against the potential risk of a significant complication almost always justifies the examination, assessing the balance must be individualized and subject to change. Risk cannot always be anticipated before the procedure is started and it needs to be continuously reassessed as the procedure is being performed.

"Risk" should be viewed more broadly than just a major complication such as bleeding or perforation. A "safe" examination that the patient perceives as too painful, embarrassing, or frightening may be the last he or she will ever permit. Most patients have a preconceived idea of what undergoing sigmoidoscopy is like from jokes and anecdotes that stress the vulnerability and discomfort the patient can expect. Agreeing to have an instrument inserted into one's anus is an act of trust. Consequently, unpleasant surprises should be minimized. The patient should be told before the examination begins that he or she retains the right to terminate the procedure at any time during the procedure. Patients should also be told what to expect as the examination proceeds. Sensitivity to the patient's anxiety almost always results in the patient's reporting that the experience was not as intimidating as expected.

COMPLICATIONS

The more obvious potential complications of flexible sigmoidoscopy are bleeding, perforation, infection, and vagally mediated reactions. The limited published data on the frequency of complications indicate that major complications are rare. However, this reassuring information usually comes from "expert" series and from surveys that depend on voluntary reporting of mishaps. The natural tendency to resist disclosure of problems that reflect negatively on professional competence may skew data away from the true incidence and toward a somewhat biased sense of safety.

Lessons from Colonoscopy

The validity of using data from diagnostic colonoscopy by trained endoscopists to deduce the risk of flexible sigmoidoscopy for the inexperienced endoscopist must be adjusted by the facts that colonoscopy is a more difficult examination to complete than flexible sigmoidoscopy, but most complications occur within the rectosigmoid. In one very large series (1), 82% of the colonoscopy complications occurred in the rectum or sigmoid, and 96% were in the descending colon or distal to it. Additionally, most series citing complication rates for sigmoidoscopy and colonoscopy are based on data from experienced endoscopists. The low incidence of complications reported by fully trained endoscopists where a high degree of manual dexterity and experience is assumed should not lull the nonendoscopist into inattentiveness.

The Role of Experience

Complications are more likely to happen when the endoscopist has limited experience. In the survey by Geenen et al. (2) of colonoscopy complications, 85% occurred during the endoscopist's first 40 procedures. Fruhmorgen (1) reported on a survey assessing the complications in 23 hospitals where 35,892 colonoscopies were performed. There were 246 complications (or one major complication per 146 colonoscopies). Fifteen of the complications occurred during the first 10 procedures an endoscopist performed; 84 had occurred after the first 50 procedures; and 144 had occurred by the first 100 procedures, with a rapid decline in the frequency of complications thereafter, i.e., the complication rate was indirectly proportional to the experience of the examiner (1).

If flexible sigmoidoscopy is performed infrequently, dexterity and perhaps clinical judgment will deteriorate. Practice is necessary to maintain all physical skills; it is not practical to acquire the skill to perform flexible sigmoidoscopy unless the commitment also has been made to maintain and improve skills through regular use. Regular usage of the sigmoidoscope will be rewarded with more complete examinations that are more comfortable to the patient and accomplished in less time. The American College of Physicians Committee on Clinical Competence recommends that a minimum of 15 flexible sigmoidoscopic examinations be performed per year to maintain one's endoscopic skills with the 60-cm instrument; 5 per year may be sufficient with the 35-cm instrument (3). These recommendations are perhaps too conservative; 24 examinations per year (2 per month) would be a preferable minimal number.

Rigid Versus Flexible Instruments

There are no large series directly comparing the relative safety of the 25-cm rigid proctoscope with flexible sigmoidoscopes. If such data were known, it would have to be weighed against their differing diagnostic yields (and patient acceptability) to determine the "best" instrument. However, two large series indicate that the rigid proctoscope is a very safe instrument: a cancer detection center reported only five perforations in 103,645 screening rigid examinations performed in asymptomatic patients over age 45 (4) and the Mayo Clinic reported four perforations in 350,000 rigid examinations (5) (see Table 10.1).

Frequency of Major Complications

The colonoscopy data in Table 10.2 indicates that in expert hands perforations occur in about 1 in 575 cases; major bleeding (not defined) occurs in 1 in 4500 cases; and death due to colonoscopy (or flexible sigmoidoscopy) is decidedly rare in all series (less than 1 in 10,000). One might also conclude that perforations appear to happen less frequently in the 1980s than they did in the 1970s (0.18% versus 0.017%). The data are not available to determine whether these improved statistics reflect better endoscopic equipment, better

Table 10.1.
Rigid Proctosigmoidoscopy

Study	Date	N	Perforation	Bleed	Death
Marks (36)	1979	1,012	0	0	0
Jackman (5)	1974	350,000	4		
Gilbertsen (4)	1974	103,645	5	0	0
Totals		454,657	9 (0.00003%)		

Table 10.2.
Major Complications from Colonoscopy

Study	Year	N	Perforation	Bleed	Death
Roseman (41)	1973	627	5 (0.79%)	0	0
Wolf (42)	1973	2,000	0	0	0
Berci (32)	1974	3,850	7 (0.18%)	0	1 (0.03%)
Geenen (2)	1975	1,106	7 (0.63%)	0	0
Rogers (33)	1975	25,298	55 (0.22%)	12 (0.05%)	2 (0.008%)
Smith (34)	1975	6,290	5 (0.08%)	1[a]	1
Fruhmorgen (1)	1978	35,892	51 (0.14%)	3 (0.008%)	7 (0.02%)
Macrae (35)	1983	5,000	4 (0.08%)	1[b]	0
Totals		80,063	134 (0.17%)	17 (0.02%)	11 (0.01%)

[a]Mesenteric bleeding.
[b]Biopsy site.

training of endoscopists, or the general trend to report and publish "better" statistics.

Reported complication rates for flexible sigmoidoscopy are shown in Table 10.3. The composite perforation rate from these series was 1 in 8,000. There are insufficient data to separately calculate the complication rates for long versus short endoscopes, symptomatic versus asymptomatic subjects, and trainees versus experienced examiners. The overall major bleeding rate was 1 in 17,000 (the details on the number of patients receiving a biopsy or polypectomy are often not given). Bleeding is rare without biopsy or polypectomy and the bleeding rate will depend heavily on the number of such interventions. In the last 5 years, more than 10,000 sigmoidoscopic examinations have been performed at the Indiana University Medical Center, with more than half of the examinations performed by house officers learning flexible sigmoidoscopy under supervision. In this series there were two perforations (both required surgical closure), no major bleeding episodes, and no deaths. In no published series were any deaths directly attributed to flexible sigmoidoscopy; however, we recently performed a screening sigmoidoscopic examination on an asymptomatic 45-year-old man who died of an acute myocardial infarction within 30 days of his procedure. This apparently unlinked association demonstrates that coincidental or unsuspected diseases may affect complication frequencies.

Table 10.3.
Major Complications from Flexible Sigmoidoscopy

Study	Year	N[a]	Perforation	Bleed	Death
IUMC[b]	1989	11,112	2 (0.02%)[c]	0	0
Rodney (40)	1986	5,467	1	0	0
Sanowski (6)	1988	17,167	2 (0.02%)[c]	2[c]	0
McCallum (39)	1984	1,015	0	0	0
Traul (38)	1983	5,000	0	0[d]	0
Meyer (37)	1980	1,000	0	0	0
Marks (36)	1979	1,012	1 (0.1%)[c]	0	0
Totals		41,774	5 (.012%)	2 (.006%)	0

[a]The majority were performed with 60- rather than 35-cm scopes.
[b]Indiana University Medical Center, unpublished data 1983–1989. Procedures performed by residents, gastroenterology fellows, and staff.
[c]Unassociated with biopsies or polypectomy.
[d]8 bleeding episodes after polypectomy, 0 without polypectomy.

PERFORATION

Mechanisms

Perforation is the result of intraluminal pressure exceeding the tensile strength of the bowel wall. It can result from pushing too hard on the bowel wall with the instrument tip, from pushing an angled endoscope through a curve so that the bowed side of the instrument splits the bowel wall (away from the endoscope tip), or from pneumatic pressure (i.e., overdistention with air) (6).

Conditions that increase the probability of perforation are those that weaken the bowel wall or decrease its mobility: diverticular disease, severe colonic inflammation (infectious, ischemic, idiopathic) pelvic irradiation, prior pelvic infection or surgery, tight strictures, recent colonic anastomoses (less than 6 weeks old), and severe cachexia.

Pneumatic perforation is uncommon because excess air is usually refluxed through the ileocecal valve into the small bowel and expelled out the anus, or the patient expresses discomfort, indicating the need for the endoscopist to suction air from the bowel. However, the endoscopist's only clue to a competent ileocecal valve may be that the patient is unusually sensitive to air distention. Pushing too hard on the bowel wall with the tip of the instrument ("slide-by") is indicated by blanching of the small mucosal vessels and an increase in patient discomfort. When a large sigmoid loop (bow) occurs, the endoscope may exert excessive lateral pressure on the bowel wall while the tip of the endoscope is free within the lumen. This is probably the most common cause of sigmoid perforations (in the absence of polypectomy). Such a perforation may not be readily evident, as the perforation site is distal to the optical lens. The endoscopist needs to perceive that the amount of pressure needed to advance the instrument tip has increased and that the insertion of more instrument shaft is not associated with advancement of its tip. When this occurs the endoscope needs to be withdrawn, and straightening maneuvers should be used. Excessive distention, whether mechanical or pneumatic, is usually quite uncomfortable to the patient. Attention to the patient's comfort level provides a continuous "pressure indicator" that should influence decisions about continuing a difficult examination. Sedation is rarely necessary, but when it is used it may alter the patient's ability to warn the endoscopist that excessive pressure is being applied.

Perforation may be obvious, inapparent, or delayed. Free perforation of the bowel, in which the instrument enters the peritoneal cavity, should be readily apparent to the endoscopist. A tear may be manifest only by the sudden inability to maintain air distention of the bowel (due to the air leaking into the peritoneal cavity). Perforation may not be apparent for several hours or days after the procedure (the latter being limited to instances when cautery was used). Delayed perforation presents as persistent postprocedure pain, fever, or distention. With any of these findings, perforation should be looked for before overt peritoneal signs develop.

The mechanisms of perforation have some bearing on the size of the hole, the site of perforation, and the subsequent clinical presentation. Pneumatic perforation is most likely to take place in the cecum (even if the endoscope is in the sigmoid) or through a diverticulum. Perforations occur in the cecum because the bowel diameter is greatest there and the wall thinnest (tension in the bowel wall = distending pressure times the radius of the lumen divided by the thickness of the bowel wall). Diverticular perforations occur because the wall of the diverticulum lacks a muscular layer and is much thinner than adjacent bowel and because the diverticulum may be subjected to localized pressures or to wall tension that is far higher than the mean luminal pressure, e.g., when the scope tip is deflected into the mouth of a diverticulum while air is being insufflated (7,41). A serosal laceration, whether due to bowing of the instrument, bowel tethering by adhesions, or intraabdominal disease, may occur without an overt hole in the mucosa. Such a split in the bowel wall may produce pain alone or minimal pneumoperitoneum. Cecal, transverse, and sigmoid colon perforations are usually free perforations into the peritoneal cavity. On the other hand, virtually all rectal perforations and some descending and ascending colon perforations are confined, as these colon segments are totally or partially retroperitoneal.

Management of Perforation (Suspected or Confirmed)

If a perforation is suspected during the procedure, the examination should be terminated promptly, and luminal contents should be aspirated during instrument withdrawal. When perforation is not definite, the endoscopist should not be falsely reassured if the patient does not experience much pain shortly after the perforation because discomfort may be minimal if the hole is small, the colon is clean, the perforation is confined, or the patient is sedated. Similarly, shortly after the procedure, an air-filled bowel may be difficult to distinguish from free air, and bowel sounds may still be present, making it difficult to clinically confirm (or exclude) perforation by physical examination. If perforation is suspected, a radiologic acute abdomen series should be obtained promptly. If perforation either is still strongly suspected or is confirmed, a large-bore intravenous line needs to be established, broad spectrum antibiotics should be given, preoperative blood work should be sent to the laboratory, and a surgeon should be contacted. The patient should be told that a perforation is suspected (or has occurred) and that emergency surgery may be necessary. A family member or a friend of the patient should be notified to assist the patient in dealing with the complication. An enema using water-soluble contrast can confirm that a perforation has occurred and locate the site. Such diagnostic enemas should generally be reserved for situations in which the suspicion of perforation is high but perforation has not been confirmed by free peritoneal air, peritoneal irritation signs, or an obvious rent observed at endoscopy. However, a standard diagnostic barium enema is strongly discouraged when perforation is suspected because the enema may increase peritoneal soilage or may reopen a tiny perforation that may have already sealed itself.

If the perforation is obvious endoscopically or if the patient has peritoneal irritation on physical examination, urgent surgery is necessary. If enough air has entered the peritoneal cavity to cause respiratory compromise, percutaneous needle aspiration of free air may provide important temporary relief. On the other hand, if the pneumoperitoneum is small and peritoneal signs are absent on physical examination, conservative medical management with bowel rest, close observation with surgical consultation, and antibiotics have allowed spontaneous closure of small perforations (8). Benign pneumoperitoneum (without clinical signs of peritonitis) was observed following colonoscopy in 1 of 100 patients (8). How often this phenomenon occurs with flexible sigmoidoscopy is not known. Any degree of pneumoperitoneum must be followed closely and its significance interpreted in the context of the patient's overall medical condition. In any event, all perforation should be viewed as a potentially life-threatening complication in which the outcome is affected strongly by its prompt recognition and treatment.

BLEEDING

Major bleeding caused by sigmoidoscopy is quite uncommon. The amount of bleeding needed to count as a "complication" is not stated in most series, but procedure-induced bleeding usually is minor and self-limited. The cause of bleeding usually is mechanical abrasion (e.g., of inflamed mucosa, irritation, or laceration of hemorrhoids). Bleeding also can be caused by the traumatic insertion of an enema tip or by the end of the endoscope. Avulsion injuries often have a characteristic "gouged" appearance on the anterior wall of the rectum; they rarely require treatment but should serve as an indication of suboptimal insertion technique. In patients with friable rectal mucosa or with impaired coagulation, minor trauma can result in more significant bleeding. When the mucosa is usually friable, the endoscopist's decision to continue or terminate the procedure must balance the likelihood of detecting important diagnostic information against the possibility of causing more bleeding.

Patients who have undergone recent flexible sigmoidoscopy or colonoscopy during which a biopsy or polypectomy was performed may present with post-procedure bleeding hours or even days later. Management depends on the rate of bleeding: most bleeding stops spontaneously, but occasionally intervention is required to control it.

Treatment of Bleeding

Localized rectal bleeding that is not self-limited usually can be controlled with pressure, by chemical cautery with silver nitrate sticks, or by the injection of epinephrine into the site. Bleeding arising from the distal 5 cm of the rectum is virtually always within range of the gloved finger. After determining the location of the bleeding (its radial direction), direct finger pressure (with or without gauze packing) or pressure with a cotton pledget held firmly over the bleeding site for several minutes usually will control the bleeding. Alternatively, silver nitrate sticks applied to a bleeding site through an anoscope or a rigid sigmoidoscope, may control a persistent bleeding point regardless of whether it was caused by trauma, a biopsy, or polypectomy. For the more experienced endoscopist, cautery or the injection of epinephrine (1 ml of epinephrine at a concentration of 1/1,000 diluted with 9 ml of 0.9% saline) via a sclerosing catheter (a small-gauge needle-tipped catheter equivalent to that used for injecting esophageal varices) in a concentration of 1/10,000 in 0.5–1-ml increments up to 3–4 ml will control most bleeding from a discrete site (larger amounts injected into the rectum are likely to be absorbed with systemic effects). When the bleeding site is in the rectum and bleeding is brisk or the rectum is filled with blood clots, a rigid sigmoidoscope may be preferable to a flexible instrument because the flexible instrument's suction channel can be overwhelmed and clogged with clot.

If significant bleeding occurs, a large-bore intravenous line should be started; baseline coagulation, hemoglobin, and hematocrit studies should be obtained; and typing and cross-matching of blood should be requested. If the bleeding cannot be controlled easily by maneuvers such as applying pressure, an experienced endoscopist, surgeon, or invasive radiologist should be consulted. Depending on the probable site of bleeding, repeated endoscopy to cauterize or inject the bleeding point with vasoconstrictors, angiography with vasoconstrictor infusion, or surgery should be considered. If clinically significant bleeding has occured and been controlled, inpatient observation for rebleeding is still generally warranted.

CARDIOPULMONARY COMPLICATIONS

Major cardiopulmonary complications are rare during sigmoidoscopy and are uncommon during colonoscopy.

Vagal Complications

The most common cardiopulmonary problem encountered during flexible sigmoidoscopy is a vagally mediated reaction caused by air distention or mesenteric stretching of the bowel. Lightheadedness, nausea, and diaphoresis may occur with or without documentable bradycardia or hypotension. These symptoms may occur during the procedure or if the patient stands up too quickly after the procedure (orthostatic symptoms are much more common when the procedure is performed with the patient bent head-down in the position usually used for rigid sigmoidoscopy). Allowing the patient to recline for a few minutes or to sit after the examination before going to the bathroom usually is sufficient to allow these symptoms to pass. If prominent symptoms develop during the procedure, the procedure should be discontinued, and the patient should be encouraged to expel excessive gas. The patient should be kept flat or in Trendelenburg position with frequent pulse and blood pressure checks as would be appropriate for any vagal reaction. An electrocardiogram should be obtained if the patient is elderly or has suspected heart disease. Uncommonly, a patient with persistent symptoms may require intravenous fluid to restore blood pressure and reverse symptoms. The symptoms and objective evidence (e.g., heart rate, blood pressure, skin color, diaphoresis, emesis) should be recorded. Note of the reaction should be made on the procedure report because patients who are susceptible to vagal reactions may have these symptoms with subsequent examinations. The outpatient having an unexpected vagal reaction needs to be reassured and kept under observation until the symptoms have resolved. During future examinations, the procedure should be kept as short as possible with as little air distention as is feasible. Only rarely will it be necessary to administer an anticholinergic agent before the examination to prevent exaggerated vagal reactions.

Arrhythmias

Patients with known major arrhythmias may need electrocardiographic monitoring during flexible sigmoidoscopy, and patients with angina should have nitroglycerin available, but routine cardiac monitoring or oximetry during flexible sigmoidoscopy is not necessary. Monitoring of electrocardiographic changes during colonoscopy and during rigid and flexible sigmoidoscopy has shown that rhythm disturbances are very common but transient. Sinus tachycardia is the most common rhythm disturbance, followed by premature ventricular beats, but ST changes and bradycardia may also occur (9–11).

INFECTION

Bacteremia

Transient bacteremia is common, but its clinical significance is still unresolved; for example, the rates of bacteremia attributable to chewing hard candy and a digital rectal examination are 17 and 4%, respectively (12). Transient asymptomatic bacteremia has been reported after colonoscopy (13–15) and rigid proctoscopy (16, 17). How often it occurs during flexible sigmoidoscopy is not established, but when looked for rigorously during colonoscopy, it has been documented more than 25% of the time (13). The organisms cultured from the blood after rectal instrumentation are the usual colonic flora, but are not those that usually cause endocarditis. There are rare documented cases of endocarditis following colonoscopy or sigmoidoscopy (17–19). There have been no controlled trials showing that prophylactic antibiotics prevent endocarditis. Moreover, because of the number of subjects that would be required to show that antibiotics confer a statistical benefit, there probably never will be one.

Antibiotic Prophylaxis

Most cases of endocarditis would not be prevented by using antimicrobial prophylaxis because they occur in patients who do not have a recognizable predisposing cardiac lesion (20–22). This lack of data makes it difficult to determine which patients would be more likely to benefit from the antibiotic than have an adverse reaction to it.

Given how poor physician compliance has been in using prophylaxis for gastrointestinal procedures (23) and the low risk of causing endocarditis, it has been argued that antibiotic prophylaxis should be eliminated or considered optional for all patients except those with prosthetic valves (22). Precedent for this view has been established by the British Society for Antimicrobial Chemotherapy, which does not recommend antibiotic prophylaxis except for patients with prosthetic valves (24).

Who Should Be Treated?

The cardiac lesions for which the American Heart Association recommends prophylaxis are shown in Table 10.4. Mitral valve prolapse presents special problems because the lesion is so common. The recommendation of the American Heart Association is that only those patients with valvular insufficiency need to be treated. Interpretations of this recommendation range from all patients with mitral valve prolapse require antibiotic prophylaxis (25) to only those patients with mitral valve prolapse and a holosystolic murmur need treatment (22). Antibiotic regimens for gastrointestinal tract procedures are shown in Table 10.5. Although recommended by the American Heart Association the true risk of infective endocarditis following flexible sigmoidoscopy is unknown, the American Heart Association lists proctosigmoidoscopy (without biopsy) among the procedures that rarely, if ever, cause endocarditis (22).

The American Society for Gastrointestinal Endoscopy (ASGE) recommends antibiotic prophylaxis for patients with prosthetic heart valves, surgically constructed systemic-pulmonary shunts, and a history of a previously infected valve (26). Because firm data on the benefits and risks of antibiotic prophylaxis are so limited, there are differences of opinion between experts and independent professional organizations (18).

Patients with an Unknown Infection Risk

There are patients with a potential (but low) risk of acquiring a complication from the transient bacteremia that may occur during sigmoidoscopy: pa-

Table 10.4.
Cardiac Conditions That Require Endocarditis Prophylaxis According to the American Heart Association (22)

Prosthetic cardiac valves[a]
Most congenital cardiac malformations
Surgically constructed systemic-pulmonary shunts[a]
Rheumatic and other acquired valvular dysfunction
Idiopathic hypertrophic subaortic stenosis
Previous history of mitral valve prolapse with insufficiency
Lesions NOT requiring treatment
Isolated secundum atrial septal defect repaired without a patch 6 or more months earlier
Coronary artery bypass graft

[a]Require treatment according to the ASGE (26).

Table 10.5.
Antibiotic Regimens for Rigid or Flexible Sigmoidoscopy with Biopsy and Colonoscopy[a]

Standard
    Ampicillin, 2 g i.m. or i.v., plus gentamicin, 1.5 mg/kg body weight given i.v. or i.m. 1 hour before the procedure. One dose may be repeated in 8–12 hr.
For patients allergic to penicillin
    Vancomycin, 1 g i.v. over 1 hr, plus gentamicin, 1.5 mg/kg body weight given i.v. or i.m. 1 hr before the procedure. One dose may be repeated in 8–12 hr.
Oral regimen for low-risk patients (see text)
    Amoxicillin, 3 g orally, 1 hr before the procedure and 1.5 g 6 hr later.

[a]Antibiotics are not necessary for a diagnostic sigmoidoscopic examination without biopsy.

tients with atrial septal defects, syphilitic aortitis, and transvenous pacemakers (19). Patients with prosthetic joints or other orthopedic hardware, vascular grafts, or shunts and patients with ascites have a theoretically greater risk of acquiring a significant infection, but there are no firm guidelines on how to best manage these patients. The use of antibiotics in patients with an uncertain risk is not standardized and cannot be considered of proven benefit. Experts vary considerably in how and when they use prophylactic antibiotics (23), but antibiotic prophylaxis is not considered necessary for rigid or flexible sigmoidoscopy if a biopsy is not performed (19, 22, 27, 39).

Immunocompromised Patients

Immunocompromised patients (i.e., those receiving chemotherapy, transplant patients, and patients with AIDS) are clearly more vulnerable to any infectious agent than an immunocompetent patient. Additionally, they may at the same time be suffering from opportunistic infections. This means that an infected patient may also need to be protected from exposure to additional infection. Currently there are no universal recommendations on how best to protect the spectrum of immunocompromised patients. The use of antibiotic prophylaxis is left to the judgment of the primary physician. I use antibiotic prophylaxis (as in Table 10.5) for neutropenic patients with less than 1500 granulocytes.

Endoscopic Transmission of Disease

Although the transmission of an infection from one patient to another via flexible sigmoidoscopy has never been reported, a small cluster of cases of *Salmonella newport* was traced to an inadequately disinfected colonoscope that had been used to biopsy the index case (28). The potential for transmission should be considered when decisions are made about how the instruments are cleaned between cases and when a rigid (more easily sterilized or disposable) instrument should be used. Vigorous and thorough mechanical cleansing of the instrument with povidone-iodine and 2% gluteraldehyde will kill all known transmissible infectious agents, but gas sterilization is often performed after use in a patient with hepatitis B or AIDS. Because there are many more patients with unsuspected transmissible diseases (including cytomegalovirus, herpes, and AIDS) than patients who carry a specific diagnosis, precautions to prevent contamination of staff, equipment, and future patients should be routine.

Guidelines on Endoscope Disinfection

The joint guideline statement issued in 1988 by the American Society for Gastrointestinal Endoscopy, American College of Gastroenterology, and American Gastrointestinal Association recommends thorough mechanical cleaning of endoscopes immediately after use followed by the use of an EPA-registered liquid sterilant/disinfectant between each case (following the manufacturer's recommendations for achieving high-level disinfection) (see chapter 6). Most of these solutions are gluteraldehyde-based formulations that require at least 10 minutes of immersion. Forced air drying also is a necessary step to prevent proliferation of residual bacteria and fungi during storage overnight. Gas sterilization is another option following procedures on infected patients. Conversely, similar steps are appropriate prior to use of an instrument on the immunocompromised patient (26).

SPECIAL SITUATIONS

When to Consider Deferring the Examination

The endoscopist may wish to limit the examination or defer it in the patient who has a significant abdominal condition (e.g., a large aneurysm or a large hernia) that the sigmoidoscope might slide by (or into) as it moves within the bowel lumen (29). Flexible sigmoidoscopy is not contraindicated by pregnancy, but the clinical information to be gained by the examination should justify the increased discomfort and (infinitesimal) risk of complicating the pregnancy.

When to Consider Repeating the Examination

How often significant lesions are not seen or are misinterpreted by the endoscopist is unknown. A missed diagnosis is a disservice to the patient and an embarrassment to the endoscopist (with potential legal implications). When the view of the lumen is limited by stool, spasm, or marked angularity, the reported findings (especially if "normal") must be qualified. If the purpose of the examination was to rule out an obstructing lesion, a repeat examination may not be necessary, but a limited examination for a more specific clinical indication may need to be repeated (by the same or a more skilled endoscopist) to answer the clinical question definitively.

Documenting Complications

When a problem arises or the conditions of the examination are unusual, keep written records. For example, make note of an unusually pronounced vagal reaction, recording the blood pressure and heart rate and treatment given (if any). It should also be noted when sedation is used at the patient's insistence. If a complication occurs, tell the patient what happened, but avoid judgmental comments. Keep very detailed records of what occurred, when it happened, who was present, and what was done about it, because you may be asked to recreate precisely the chain of events years later if legal action is undertaken. The insurance carrier and hospital administrator should be made aware of any significant complications shortly after the event.

Keeping the Objective of a Screening Examination in Mind

For asymptomatic patients undergoing screening flexible sigmoidoscopy to detect polyps, the examination is elective and will usually be repeated at intervals. For that reason, extra effort should be taken to make the examination acceptable to the patient and the risk negligible. By way of contrast, when a symptomatic patient is being evaluated for lower gastrointestinal bleeding or a decrease in stool caliber, there is a high probability that a condition requiring therapeutic intervention will be detected by flexible sigmoidoscopy, and the risk of not identifying the source of the symptom may exceed the risk of performing a thorough examination even in a frail patient. Some common sense correlates of procedure-risk are the endoscopist's decisions as to when to defer the examination, quit, sedate the patient and continue, or refer the patient to another endoscopist. Despite the inconvenience in rescheduling patients, particularly when they have taken laxatives or enemas, the best decision is, at times, *not* to perform flexible sigmoidoscopy. For example, when a marginally cooperative patient is having a "bad" day, when the colon cleansing is inadequate despite repeated enemas, or when the endoscopy equipment is not working properly, it is easy to transform a routine procedure into one that is extremely difficult and needlessly more hazardous. Discretion is as important as finesse.

Excessive Patient Discomfort

Similarly, it is wiser to discontinue an uncomfortable examination before the patient gets extremely uncomfortable and decides never to submit to this again. Forward progress with the scope should stop when the patient experiences more discomfort than mild cramping or bloating that does not subside when the scope is withdrawn a few centimeters or when air is evacuated. The governing rationale should be that patients must not be made to feel that they are "victims" when they are undergoing an elective screening procedure. It is far wiser to stop centimeters short of the endpoint the endoscopist envisioned was obtainable and have the patient willing to undergo the procedure in the future than have the patient decide "never again." In most cases 10–15 minutes is a reasonable examination duration.

Sedation

Like all rules, there are exceptions to the generalization that sedation is not needed (and should not be used) for sigmoidoscopy. In most cases sedation should be used only by an experienced examiner since pain is the most important indicator the endoscopist has that excess force is being applied. When the patient experiences significant pain, the endoscopist must decide whether the pain is due to overdistention, scope pressure, pathology (which may be inapparent to the endoscopist) that decreases the mobility and distensibility of the colon, or a low pain threshold. When the clinical question that prompted the examination requires an answer and there are no better diagnostic alternatives available, sedating the patient and proceeding with an uncomfortable study may be the proper decision (e.g., when a patient's barium studies indicate a possible sigmoid mass). Sedation is not an acceptable substitute for inexperience or poor technique, but used judiciously, it can make an otherwise impossible examination possible. The vigor of the examination should be commensurate with the indication.

Referring the Patient for Sigmoidoscopy

In some situations the endoscopist's best decision may be to refer the patient to another endoscopist. Reasons for referral would include: a second opinion or the requirement for intervention that exceeds the endoscopist's realm of usual experience (i.e., cautery, polypectomy, biopsy, or greater expertise in maneuvering through a difficult sigmoid). Even the finest technician may wish to refer patients who are relatives or friends. Whatever the reason, referral may be preferable to undertaking an examination under suboptimal circumstances.

Documenting What Was Not Done

Although physicians are increasingly aware of the need to obtain informed consent and have become more conscientious in documenting what they do for patients, few are as sensitive to the need to document what is *not* done. When patients decline medical advice, the physician may need to prove that the recommendation was made so that the patient assumes the responsibility for receiving suboptimal care. Screening for colon cancer has been used as an example of this logic. The American Cancer Society recommends that everyone over age 50 should have a fecal occult blood test every year and flexible sigmoidoscopy every 3–5 years after two consecutive negative yearly examinations. It has been estimated that more than 50% of the 140,000 new cases of colon cancer being diagnosed each year could bring successful malpractice suits against their physicians for failure to screen for colon cancer (30). Physicians are encouraged to offer colon cancer screening to their patients and to document in the medical record the patient's response to such recommendations.

INFORMED CONSENT

When a patient consents to undergo a diagnostic procedure (whether for evaluation of symptoms or to screen for disease) the patient should know what information is sought, how it will be used, and that complications can occur during the procedure. Obtaining informed consent for flexible sigmoidoscopy means that patients agree to accept the possibility of a complication because they understand: the potential benefit from the procedure, which complications (adjusted to the age and medical problems of the individual patient) they would be most likely to experience, the low probability that a complication will occur, the consequences of *not* having the procedure done, and alternative ways of evaluating the condition. Most of these points can be covered in a brief discussion or paragraph. For example:

The procedure to be performed is flexible sigmoidoscopy. A flexible telescope is used to examine the lower colon for possible growths, inflammation, or bleeding. The wall of the bowel may be biopsied or cultures taken. Although the examination is generally very safe, possible complications of bleeding and making a hole (perforation) in the bowel occur in less than 1 in 100 persons but could require surgery. The reason for the procedure (and alternative tests such as x-rays and colonoscopy) has been explained to me, I have been encouraged to ask questions, and I have agreed to undergo the procedure (adapted from Ref. 31).

In obtaining a patient's consent, disclosure should vary with the age, intelligence, medical sophistication, and personality of the patient. When the patient and endoscopist discuss the procedure face to face this meeting becomes the basis for rapport during the procedure. The meeting also lets the endoscopist assess whether the patient has any special concerns about the procedure. It is desirable to have someone witness the discussion and be present while questions and answers about the procedure are taking place. Because the consent form should reflect the standards for disclosure in the endoscopist's state or country, it should be developed with legal advice.

Although there is no controversy over the primacy of consent, there is considerable debate over the role of consent forms. A consent form is not "required" for flexible sigmoidoscopy, but obtaining informed consent is. The legal basis for implied consent and verbal consent is less clear and varies among states. Many physicians use a written consent form defensively; however, the consent form cannot be used as a document to absolve the endoscopist from responsibility.

Written consent in many states is not routinely obtained for many procedures (e.g., intravenous lines, Pap smears and other office gynecological procedures, phlebotomy, and dental work, including extractions and root canal work). The risk of rectal bleeding and colonic perforation during sigmoidoscopy is less than the risk of a significant reaction to intravenous iodinated contrast (e.g., intravenous pyelogram, venography, and computed tomography). Written consent usually is not obtained for the latter procedures at many institutions. Ideally, the physician and patient view a consent form as documentation that a conversation about the procedure took place to their mutual satisfaction.

This discussion of potential procedure-related complications should not dissuade the endoscopist from performing flexible sigmoidoscopy. Knowledge of the dangers inherent in flexible sigmoidoscopy may temper enthusiasm for the procedure, but it is a necessary step, as caution precedes achieving skill and good clinical judgment. The endoscopist's goal is to obtain diagnostic information with minimal discomfort or risk to the patient. In reality, the best technique and attention to detail can approach that goal, but given human variability and enough examinations, complications become a statistical inevitability. Foreknowledge of the potential mechanisms of injury is preferable to learning about complications through experience and should help minimize them.

The attitude of patients and physicians about responsibility and risk has evolved greatly in the last decade and can be expected to continue to change. Texts on endoscopic technique published before 1985 generally covered the topic of informed consent in a few sentences; more recent texts devote chapters to the subject. This topic is not static, and endoscopists must assume the responsibility of staying current with their local legal standard of practice.

References

1. Fruhmorgen P, Demling L. Complications of diagnostic and therapeutic colonoscopy in the Federal Republic of Germany. Endoscopy 1979;2:146–150.
2. Geenen, JE, Schmitt MG, Wallace CW, Hogan WJ. Major complications of colonoscopy: Bleeding and perforation. Dig Dis Sci 1975;20:231–235.
3. American College of Physicians. Committee on Clinical Competence in the use of flexible sigmoidoscopy for screening purposes. Ann Intern Med 1987;107:589–591.
4. Gilbertsen VA. Proctosigmoidoscopy and polypectomy in reducing the incidence of rectal cancer. Cancer 1974;34:936–939.
5. Jackman RJ. Rigid tube proctosigmoidoscopy. In: Berry LH, ed. Gastrointestinal panendoscopy. Springfield, IL: Charles C Thomas, 1974:439–460.
6. Groveman HD, Sanowski RA, Klauber MR. Training primary care physicians in flexible sigmoidoscopy: Performance evaluation of 17, 167 procedures. West J Med 1988;148:221–4.
7. Kozarek RA, Earnest DL, Silverstein ME, Smith RG. Air-pressure-induced colon injury during diagnostic colonoscopy. Gastroenterology 1980;78:7–14.
8. Ecker MA, Goldstein M, Hoexter B, Hyman RA, Naidich JB, Stein HL. Benign pneumoperitoneum after fiberoptic colonoscopy. Gastroenterology 1977;73:226–230.
9. Fletcher GF, Earnest DL, Shuford WF, Wenger N. Electrocardiographic changes during routine sigmoidoscopy. Arch Intern Med 1968;122:483–486.
10. Alam M, Schuman BM, Duvernoy WFC, Madrago AC. Continuous electrocardiographic monitoring during colonoscopy. Gastrointest Endosc 1976;22:203–205.
11. Vawter M, Ruiz R, Alaama A, et al. Electrocardiographic monitoring during colonoscopy. Am J Gastroenterol 1975;63:155–157.
12. Botoman VA, Surawicz CA. Bacteremia with gastrointestinal endoscopic procedures. Gastrointest Endosc 1986;32:342–346.
13. Pelican G, Henteges D, Butt J, et al. Bacteremia during colonoscopy. Gastrointest Endosc 1976;23:33–36.
14. Rodriquez W, Levine JS. Enterococcal endocarditis following flexible sigmoidoscopy. West J Med 1984;140:951–953.
15. Murray JL. Enterococcal endocarditis after sigmoidoscopy [Letter]. West J Med 1984;141:689–690.
16. LeFrock JL, Ellis CA, Turchick JB, Weinstein L: Transient bacteremia associated with sigmoidoscopy. N Engl J Med 1973;289:467–469.
17. Rigilano J, Mahapatra R, Barnhill J, et al. Enterococcal endocarditis following sigmoidoscopy and mitral valve prolapse. Arch Intern Med 1984;144:850–851.

18. Shorvon PJ, Eykyn SJ, Cotton PB. Gastrointestinal instrumentation, bacteremia, and endocarditis. Gut 1983;24:1078–1093.

19. Durack, DT. Current issues in prevention of infective endocarditis. Am J Med 1985;78(suppl 6B):149–156.

20. Weinstein L, Rubin RH. Infective endocarditis—1973. Prog Cardiovasc Dis 1973;16:239–274.

21. Bayless R, Clarke C, Oakley C, Somerville W, Whitfield AGW. The teeth and infective endocarditis. Br Heart J 1983;50:506–512.

22. Kaye D. Prophylaxis for infective endocarditis: An update. Ann Intern Med 1986;104:419–423.

23. Meyer GW. Prophylaxis of infective endocarditis during gastrointestinal procedures: Report of a survey. Gastrointest Endosc 1979;25:1–2.

24. The antibiotic prophylaxis of infective endocarditis: Report of a working party of the British Society for antimicrobial chemotherapy. Lancet 1982;2:1323–1326.

25. Piecuch JH. Antibiotic prophylaxis for the dental patient with cardiovascular disease. J Conn State Dent Assoc 1984;58:83–84.

26. Statements and guidelines developed by the standards of training and practice committee of the ASGE. Gastrointest Endosc Suppl 1988;34:37S–40S.

27. Shulman S (Chairman), et al. Prevention of bacterial endocarditis. Circulation 1984;70:1123A–1127A.

28. Dwyer DM, Klein EG, Istre GR, et al. Salmonella newport infections transmitted by fiberoptic colonoscopy. Gastrointest Endosc 1987;33:84–87.

29. Gruber HE, Wiseman MH. Aortic thrombosis during sigmoidoscopy in Behcet's syndrome. Arch Intern Med 1983;143:343–345.

30. Plumeri PA, Rogers J. A lawyer's view of colon cancer in the 1980s. J Clin Gastroenterol 1988;10:229–231.

31. Katon RM, Keeffe EB, Melnyk CS. Flexible sigmoidoscopy. Orlando, FL: Grune & Stratton, 1985.

32. Berci G, Panish JF, Schapiro M, Corlin R. Complications of colonoscopy and polypectomy. Gastroenterology 1974;67:584–585.

33. Rogers BHG, Silvis SE, Nebel OT. Complications of flexible fiberoptic colonoscopy and polypectomy. Gastrointest Endosc 1975;22:73–76.

34. Smith LL, Nivatvongs S. Complications in colonoscopy. Dis Colon Rectum 1975;18:214–220.

35. Macrae FA, Tan KG, Williams CP. Toward safer colonoscopy: A report on the complications of 5,000 diagnostic or therapeutic colonoscopies. Gut 1983;24:376–383.

36. Marks G, Boggs HW, Castro AF, Gathright JB, Ray JE, Salvati E. Sigmoidoscopic examinations with rigid and flexible fiberoptic sigmoidscopes in the surgeon's office: A comparative prospective study of effectiveness in 1,012 cases. Dis Colon Rectum 1979;22:162–168.

37. Meyer CT, McBride W, Goldblatt RS, et al. Clinical experience with flexible sigmoidoscopy in asymptomatic and symptomatic patients. Yale J Biol Med 1980;53:345–352.

38. Traul DG, Davis CB, Pollock JC, Scudamore HH. Flexible fiberoptic sigmoidoscopy: The Monroe Clinic experience. A prospective study of 5000 examinations. Dis Colon Rectum 1983;26:161–166.

39. McCallum RW, Meyer CT, Marignani P, Cane E, Contino C. Diagnostic yield in 1015 patients. Am J Gastroenterol 1984;79:433–437.

40. Rodney WM, Albers G. Flexible sigmoidoscopy: primary care outcomes after two types of continuing medical education. Am J Gastroenterol 1986;81:133–138.

41. Roseman DM. Report from San Diego. Gastrointest Endosc 1973;20:36.

42. Wolf WI, Shinya H. A new approach to colonic polyps. Ann Surg 1973;178:367.

11

Diseases of the Anus, Rectum and Sigmoid Colon: The Proctologic Examination

Norman Sohn, M.D., F.A.C.S.

INTRODUCTION

Examination of the anus, rectum, and sigmoid colon is an integral part of a routine physical examination in patients over the age of 50 and is essential in the evaluation of patients with symptoms related to bowel disorders. The examination complements other essential components of the evaluation including flexible sigmoidoscopy, colonoscopy, or barium enema. The recent surge of interest in flexible endoscopic examinations and improved flexible instruments has diminished the intensity of interest in the traditional anorectal examination, which uses such proven mundane tools as inspection, palpation, anoscopy, and rigid proctosigmoidoscopy. Elegant high-tech devices, although sometimes inferior, are often favored over traditional tools. The combination of classical examination methods with flexible techniques achieves maximum results (1,2). This report will detail the evaluation of the anorectum, describe various anorectal disorders, and discuss other anorectal manifestations of systemic illnesses.

HISTORY

Historical factors that would cause the examiner to focus attention on the anus and rectum include rectal pain, rectal bleeding, rectal protrusion, a sensation of incomplete rectal evacuation, rectal discharge, and anal pruritus. The differential diagnosis of rectal bleeding, constipation, and diarrhea are not included in this paper.

Anorectal pain is almost always due to a disease process involving the lower 1 to 1½ inches of the rectum or the anus. Examination of more proximal areas of the colon with flexible instruments or barium enema examination rarely contributes any worthwhile information to the delineation of rectal pain. An analysis of the rectal pain pattern often reveals its etiology. Pain due to hemorrhoids is usually due to thrombosis or to the so-called "acute attack of piles," in which ulceration, thrombosis, or edema predominate. In the absence of thrombosis, edema, or ulceration, rectal pain should not be attributed to hemorrhoids.

Hemorrhoidal pain usually is maximum at the onset and then progressively improves. Pain due to an abscess typically worsens continuously until the abscess is drained either surgically or spontaneously. Anal fissure pain ordinarily occurs with or following a bowel movement, persists for several minutes to several hours, and then subsides, only to recur again at the time of the next defecation. These three conditions account for approximately 95% of causes of rectal pain in the nonhomosexual patient. In the homosexual patient other possibilities, include herpes, gonococcal proctitis, cytomegaloviral disease, and chlamydia.

Pain due to the levator syndrome, believed to be secondary to spasm of the levator muscles, usually is described as a high, vague sensation of pressure or a sensation of a foreign object in the rectum. This can awaken a patient from sleep, may be related to sexual orgasm, and may be associated with low back or coccygeal pain. Most cases are idiopathic in orgin. Other etiologies include low back disorders and prostatitis. In patients with rectal pain the examiner often makes the diagnosis on the basis of the history alone and confirms it with the physical examination.

Rectal protrusion can be due to internal or external hemorrhoids, to rectal prolapse, or, less commonly, to polyps. Rectal discharge can represent a low-grade form of anal incontinence or may be secondary to anal fistulas, large internal hemorrhoids, proctitis, or benign or malignant neoplasms. A sensation of incomplete evacuation can be due to large internal hemorrhoids, to intrarectal or complete rectal prolapse, to fecal impaction, or, infrequently, to benign or malignant neoplasms. Pruritus ani is discussed below.

The most common cause of rectal bleeding in adults is hemorrhoids. Other common anorectal causes include anal fissures and proctitis. Of utmost importance in the evaluation of patients with rectal bleeding is the possibility of benign or malignant neoplasms.

PHYSICAL EXAMINATION

Inspection

Simple inspection is a fundamental part of the rectal examination. Adequate lighting with a spotlight, headlight, or handheld light is necessary. The sacrococcygeal region is examined for pilonidal sinuses. These are characterized by small sinuses referred to as "pits." These occur in the midline or within 1 to 2 mm of the midline in the sacrococcygeal region. Protrusion of one ischiorectal space could be indicative of an underlying abscess. Inspection will also reveal the presence of external hemorrhoids, condyloma acuminata, or other benign or malignant neoplasms.

Painful hemorrhoids will be obvious on inspection with the eye-catching thrombosis, ulceration, or edema. Hemorrhoids classically occur in the right anterolateral, right posterolateral, and left lateral positions. Simple hemorrhoids located in the midline anteriorly or posteriorly are not common but usually represent "sentinel piles" occurring in relation to an anal fissure. In these circumstances the primary pathology is represented by the fissure, and the sentinel pile is merely secondary to it. Therapy, to be successful, must be directed to the fissure. Erythema or a visible bulge may suggest an underlying abscess.

Inspection of the rectum often is invaluable in evaluating patients complaining of protrusion. Protrusion most commonly is due to internal hemorrhoids. Its differential diagnosis includes rectal prolapse. It is very helpful to examine the patient immediately following a phosphate enema, with the patient instructed to strain as forcefully as possible during evacuation of the enema. This often will reveal hitherto concealed pathology. A variant of large internal hemorrhoids occurs in which all or most of the circumference of the rectum everts during defecation. This form of hemorrhoids is best diagnosed by inspection following evacuation of an enema and may be unappreciated by other examinations, including digital palpation or rigid or flexible endoscopic evaluations. The distinction between the longitudinal furrows of prolapsed hemorrhoids and the circumferential furrows of a rectal prolapse can also be appreciated.

Digital Examination

When digital examination is performed, the perirectal spaces are first palpated. The presence of tenderness or induration is determined. Gently spreading the buttocks in the midline, posteriorly or anteriorly, will unmask a fissure. This maneuver demonstrates most anal fissures. Even in the presence of pain, this maneuver can be performed with no added pain. The examining digit next is placed in the anal canal, and the presence of any tenderness and its location is noted.

The examining finger is then swept circumferentially, feeling for tumors or tenderness. The levator sling is appreciated best posteriorly and laterally, and any tenderness in it is noted. The examining finger is then inserted as high as possible, and the patient is asked to strain down. This may reveal hitherto unpalpated lesions. After the examining digit is removed, the examining glove is observed for any unusual contents, and a guaiac test is performed on any stool that is present (see Chapter 15). Sphincter tone is evaluated by noting the resistance of the sphincter on digital examination and by asking the patient to contract the sphincters during the examination. Bidigital examination or rectovaginal palpation of the rectovaginal septum bidigitally can be performed.

Anoscopy

Anoscopy is performed next. The author prefers a Hirschmann-type anoscope with a slanted tilt. Other styles are also useful. The standard Hirschmann anoscope is 10 cm long and 2.2 cm in diameter (Fig 11.1). A smaller instrument, measuring 8 cm in length and 1.7 cm in diameter, is useful when the patient has rectal pain. Other examiners may prefer other types of ano-

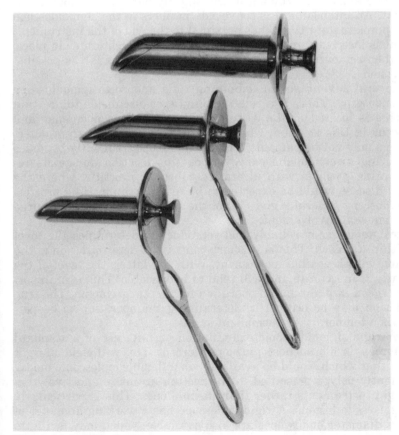

Figure 11.1. Hirschman anoscopes.

scopes. There are good models with a built-in light source. These are useful for diagnostic purposes, but the added length to accommodate the light source usually prevents the instrument from being used for therapeutic purposes. In particular, it is difficult to inject hemorrhoids or ligate them through these varieties of anoscopes.

Adequate lighting is essential. Overhead spotlights, headlights, handheld lights, or anoscopes with built-in light sources are all available.

The anoscope is placed in the anal canal with obturator in place. Pressure can be applied to the area of the dentate line, and this mild compression often will cause the internal hemorrhoids to distend. The anoscope, with the obturator in place, is rotated 90 degrees. The obturator is removed, and the area of the anorectum in view in the anoscope is inspected.

Rigid Protosigmoidoscopy

Much has been written about retroflexing flexible endoscopes to get a view of the distal rectum. However, anoscopy or rigid proctoscopy directly and most efficiently views this region. The mucosa can be seen readily, and subtle changes in the mucosa and its vascularity can be better appreciated than with a retroflexed sigmoidoscope. Proctitis that is limited to just a few centimeters of the rectum can be overlooked during a flexible endoscopic examination and is readily detected with anoscopy.

Anoscopy using a Hirschmann or other anoscope will evaluate up to 6 cm of the distal rectum. Rigid proctoscopy or sigmoidoscopy is performed next. The author prefers a 15-cm long rigid instrument. The diameter is either the standard 19-mm diameter instrument or the slightly narrower 15-mm diameter instrument. An intense light is conveyed via fibers in the sigmoidoscope up to a point approximately 1½ inches proximal to the end of the instrument. The instrument is inserted through the sphincters with the obturator in place. The latter is then removed, and the instrument is passed as far as possible under direct vision.

There are several advantages to combining rigid anoproctosigmoidoscopy with flexible endoscopy. There is a relative blind spot just inside the rectum posteriorly. This is located at the 4- to 6-cm level. Villous adenomas and carcinomas occur in this location, where they can be concealed from detection. Soft lesions may not be palpable. The flexible scope frequently bypasses that region during insertion and can overlook this location during its removal. In following patients with ulcerative colitis or proctitis, where the most advanced disease would be expected to be in the rectum, rigid proctoscopy or sigmoidoscopy generally gives all of the information that is required regarding the mucosal involvement.

Rigid proctosigmoidoscopy reliably and reproducibly determines the level of a lesion within its reach. This is in sharp contrast to determination of the level of a lesion with a flexible instrument. With the latter, the level of the lesion frequently is inaccurate and will tend to be variable. This is of importance to the surgeon in planning an operation for rectal carcinoma. The true level of the lesion may be critical in determining the operation to be performed vis-a-vis a temporary or permanent stoma.

Anoscopic or rigid sigmoidoscopic examination permits use of a standard rectal biopsy forceps or a bronchoscopic biopsy forceps. This will yield a larger specimen than that which would be available via a flexible endoscopic biopsy forceps. Frequently polyps presented in the rectum are more effectively excised using rigid instruments rather than flexible ones. This is particularly true with large sessile lesions. A rigid endoscope has a working diameter of 19 mm. Larger diameter endoscopes are also available, which may facilitate polypectomy. Of particular importance is the ability to achieve hemostasis using a rigid sigmoidoscope. This may not be possible with a flexible endoscope with a working channel of 3.5 mm diameter. This does not permit the rapid evacuation of blood from the rectal lumen that is possible with the rigid instrument. In addition, instruments designed to achieve hemostasis, such as rubber-band ligators or hemostatic staples, can be readily used through a rigid endoscope. These modalities are not available for use with a flexible endoscope. Biopsy of friable lesions such as Kaposi's sarcoma could be performed through a rigid instrument after first ligating the base of the lesion with a rubber band and taking the biopsy from the ligated portion. By no means can rigid anoscopy, proctoscopy, or sigmoidoscopy be expected to give the same information available from flexible endoscopy. However, the combination of the two maximizes the obtainable information.

PRIMARY PROCTOLOGIC DISORDERS—DIAGNOSIS AND MANAGEMENT

Hemorrhoids

Hemorrhoids are normal structures present in every human being. In the past they had been considered to be varicosities involving the lower rectum. More recent studies indicate that these are cushions of fibrovascular tissue that line the lower rectum (3). They probably contribute to continence by effecting a complete seal of the anus. Because hemorrhoids are ubiquitous, their treatment is indicated only when they cause symptoms.

There are probably many causes for the development of hemorrhoidal symptoms. Although various authors have incriminated every activity of daily living in the development of hemorrhoidal symptoms, the only consistent factors are constipation and pregnancy near term. Dramatic hemorrhoid complications, such as the acute attack in particular, have no consistent predisposing cause. The only rational effort that can possibly prevent the onset of hemorrhoidal symptoms is the prevention of constipation.

The usual symptoms are pain, bleeding, or protrusion. The availability of newer ambulatory modalities for treating certain types of hemorrhoids has aroused endoscopists' interest in them.

Hemorrhoids may be classified into five groups (4). The first group is *thrombosed hemorrhoids*. Thrombosed hemorrhoids can be painful. The pain that is present resolves rapidly over a period of a few days. The thrombus is then resorbed over a period of 3 to 8 weeks. When the thrombosed hemorrhoid is incapacitatingly painful it may be excised. Excision is preferred to incision and thrombectomy. However, deferring a decision for excision for a period of 24 hours usually obviates the need for this type of approach, as pain relief is to be expected. Reassurance and an explanation of the nature of the condition often is sufficient for the management of this condition.

The next type of hemorrhoid is the *acute attack of piles*. This shares some of the features of the thrombosed hemorrhoid. Multiple thrombi are present. The hemorrhoids are swollen and edematous, and necrotic areas may be visible. This is frequently a dramatic and exquisitely painful situation. Again, treatment directed toward this condition must take into account that this is likely to be a spontaneously resolving process. The pain subsides over a period of a few days, and the edema and thrombi are resorbed over a period of several weeks.

This condition is sometimes treated by immediate operative hemorrhoidectomy. It also can be treated as an ambulatory procedure consisting of rubber-band ligation of the internal hemorrhoid, partial excision of the external hemorrhoid, and extensive thrombectomy. Both of these approaches are intended to shorten the painful period or prevent recurrences. Both of these procedures carry a risk of fever and bacteremia. Formal operative hemorrhoidectomy during an acute attack carries a greater risk of postoperative complications, particularly stricture. As with thrombosed hemorrhoids, recurrences are possible but unpredictable. Prophylactic therapy to prevent recurrence, unless there have been multiple recurrences, is not indicated.

The third hemorrhoid group is *bleeding hemorrhoids*. They are the most common cause of rectal bleeding. Because hemorrhoids are unbiquitous, other possible etiologies must be excluded before rectal bleeding is attributed to them. It is rare to see the hemorrhoid actually bleeding. Bleeding hemorrhoids are usually internal hemorrhoids. Occasionally an external hemorrhoid in which a thrombus has eroded through the surface of the skin can cause rectal bleeding. However, most cases of rectal bleeding due to hemorrhoids are due to internal hemorrhoids.

Internal hemorrhoids form the fourth hemorrhoid group. Many authorities divide them into four grades. Grade I hemorrhoids do not protrude. Grade II hemorrhoids protrude and reduce spontaneously. Grade III hemorrhoids require manual reduction, and Grade IV hemorrhoids are irreducible. Thus, this popular hemorrhoid grading system only applies to one of five hemorrhoid groups.

Internal hemorrhoids are insensitive to pain and can be destroyed painlessly by many techniques. The simplest modality is that of injection sclerotherapy. In this technique, injections of a suitable agent, such as 5% quinine urea hydrochloride, are employed. One half milliliter is injected submucosally at the pedicle of each of the three hemorrhoids. Five percent phenol in peanut or other vegetable oil can be employed by injecting 3 to 10 cc at each hemorrhoid pedicle. Injection sclerotherapy causes a temporary cessation of hemorrhoidal bleeding. This effect can persist for up to several months. The potential for complications is minimal; rarely will there be bleeding at the injection site. This technique is excellent for patients who have rectal bleeding and who are anticoagulated. The injection of the phenol in oil, in some cases, can alleviate hemorrhoid protrusion. Complications from injecting phenol in oil, although more common than with quinine, are quite rare. The most important complication, precipitation of the acute hemorrhoidal attack, occurs in less than 1% (see Table 11.1).

Approximately 30 years ago, rubber-band ligation of internal hemorrhoids was introduced. This revolutionized hemorrhoid therapy by effectively eliminating hemorrhoids by a painless ambulatory procedure (5).

The technique involves placing a ¼-inch diameter elastic band around an internal hemorrhoid. The hemorrhoid is visualized through an anoscope. It is then grasped and squeezed with a clamp to ascertain that there is no pain sensibility. If there is pain, the rubber band can be placed in a location more proximal to the dentate line. A ligator is then used to place the rubber band around the hemorrhoid. Usually, one hemorrhoid is treated at a time. In some cases, multiple hemorrhoids can be ligated at once. Posttreatment pain is more common in the latter circumstance.

The main complications of this type of treatment are pain and late bleeding. Rare cases of sepsis and death have been reported following rubber-band ligation. Some of these unfortunate patients had rectal pain prior to the ligation, raising the possibility of a preexisting rectal abscess. Patients with rectal pain usually should not be ligated until the condition causing pain has subsided, with or without treatment.

Late bleeding, sometimes of great magnitude, can occur 4 to 14 days following treatment but has been seen as late as 30 days postoperatively. Accordingly, patients are cautioned to have medical care available to them if necessary for at least 2 weeks following a ligation treatment. This type of late bleeding can occur following any type of rectal surgery. Until proved otherwise, other techniques that destroy internal hemorrhoids probably are associated with the same risk.

As an outgrowth of the thermal methods used by endoscopists to treat gastrointestinal bleeding, similar methods have been used to treat hemorrhoids. Infrared photocoagulation and bipolar probe coagulation instruments have been introduced for the treatment of internal hemorrhoids (6,7,8). These techniques are designed to produce a burn on a hemorrhoid, which affects sclerosis and fixes the mucosa to the underlying submucosa and muscle. In selected cases they may be equally effective to rubber-band ligation, but for large protruding hemorrhoids, rubber-band ligation seems superior. Complications of late bleeding and rectal pain with bipolar and infrared coagulation treatments are similar to those with rubber-band ligation.

Recently, a device known as *Ultroid,* in which a low-voltage electrocoagulating current is applied to a hemorrhoid, has been introduced (9). This treatment modality has not yet offered significant advantages over rubber-band ligation and is probably less effective in eliminating them. Current comparative studies are in progress. Laser destruction of internal hemorrhoids also has been described (10).

All of these are ingenious ways of dealing with tissue that is not sensible to pain. Undoubtedly other modalities will be introduced in the future. Advantages of these newer modalities have not yet been demonstrated (11). A common feature is the high cost of equipment needed to perform these procedures. The rubber-band ligator is simple, inexpensive, and effective. Only when another modality can be shown to be safer, more efficacious, or less expensive should it be expected to replace rubber-band ligation.

External hemorrhoids compose the fifth hemorrhoid group. They are often associated with an internal hemorrhoid component. They produce cosmetic symptoms or make personal hygiene difficult. They are usually not the etiology of pruritus ani, and in the latter patient, hemorrhoid excision typically does not affect the anal pruritus. When the external hemorrhoid is associated with a significant internal component, rubber-band ligation of the latter may improve or eliminate external hemorrhoid symptoms. Those that fail to respond to removal of the internal component, or those in which there is no significant internal component, require hemorrhoidectomy.

Internal hemorrhoids associated with eversion of a significant portion of the circumference do not respond to simple therapy directed toward the internal hemorrhoids but do require excision, as do internal hemorrhoids that cannot be treated by local destruction. The results of operative hemorrhoidectomy have shown it to be a safe and effective procedure when suitably applied. The use of the contact YAG laser to perform operative hemorrhoidectomies seems to have resulted in diminished postoperative pain. The diminution in postoperative pain has transformed operative hemorrhoidectomy into an ambulatory procedure when performed by surgeons skilled with this technique (10).

Fissure-in-Ano

Anal fissures are small ulcers, usually located in the midline, more commonly posterior than anterior. The etiology is unknown but may be related to trauma from a hard stool or stretching of the rectum to accommodate a large-caliber stool. Once the fissure is established it is associated with an exaggerated response of the internal sphincter to distention and with thick-

Table 11.1.
Comparisons of the Advantages and Disadvantages of Various Hemorrhoidal Therapies

Technique	Hemorrhoid Type	Indication	Contraindications	Complications	Advantages	Disadvantages	Recurrences	Equipment Cost
Injection sclero-therapy	Internal	Bleeding Protrusion (where RBL is contra-indicated)	Rare	Rare	Simple Effective Ambulatory Minimal risks Can be used with antico-agulants	Effects are temporary	Common	$5
Rubber-band ligation (RBL)	Internal	Bleeding Protrusion	Inability to fol-low patient Anticoagulants	Pain 8% Acute attack 3% Late hemorrhage 0.2% Septicemia—rare	Ambulatory Minimal risks Inexpensive	Multiple visits	Depend on case selection	$150
Infrared coagula-tion (IRC)	Internal	Bleeding Protrusion ?	Anticoagulants	Pain 3% Late hemorrhage ?	Ambulatory Few risks Can sometimes be used where RBL is painful	Not as effec-tive as RBL for large hemor-rhoids	Frequent	$2000
Electrocoagulation (bipolar or direct current)	Internal	Bleeding Protrusion	Anticoagulants	Insufficient re-ported cases to compare to other techniques	Ambulatory Compares in efficacy RBL	New tech-nique—ad-vantage over prior techniques not yet demon-strated	Unknown but should be com-parable to RBL	$750-$4000

Procedure	Type	Indications	Contraindications	Complications	Advantages	Disadvantages	Recurrence	Cost
Laser (CO2, YAG, etc.)	Internal	Bleeding Protrusion	Anticoagulants	Insufficient reported cases to compare to other techniques	Ambulatory Compares in efficacy to RBL	Equipment expensive New technique—advantage over prior techniques not yet demonstrated	Unknown but should be comparable to RBL	$25,000-$100,000
Laser (CO2, YAG, etc.)	External Combined internal & external	Protrusion No response to prior therapy	Anticoagulants Age over 60–65 Incontinence	Pain despite Percocet 40% Pain requiring hospitalization 1% Late bleeding 1% Urinary retention 1% Fecal impaction 3%	Ambulatory Less postoperative pain Earlier return to work Accomplishes all that classical hemorrhoidectomy does	Equipment expensive	<1% require reoperation	$25,000-$100,000
Operative hemorrhoidectomy	External Combined internal & external	Protrusion No response to prior therapy	Anticoagulants Age over 60–65 Incontinence	Pain requiring injectable narcotics 95% Late bleeding 1% Urinary retention 10%	Hospital resources to care for possible complications	Increased risk of complications compared to ambulatory laser hemorrhoidectomy	<1% require reoperation	$25,000-$100,000

ening of the internal sphincter. Most fissures will respond to conservative therapy, which results in soft, formed stools, and to bland emollient suppositories. A role for corticosteroids in the treatment of anal fissures has never been documented. A fissure typically produces pain shortly following defecation. The pain persists for several minutes or hours and then subsides until the next defecation. Bleeding may be associated with this.

The pathologic triad seen with anal fissures consists of the ulcer with a sentinel pile external to it and an enlarged anal papilla at the level of the dentate line. The enlarged papilla has been termed a fibrous polyp or an anal polyp and is often confused with a true neoplasm. Specific etiologies for a fissure must be considered in its differential diagnosis, such as Crohn's disease, tuberculosis, syphilis, and herpes. The treatment when conservative management fails consists of an internal anal sphincterotomy or simple dilatation of the anal canal (12).

Abscesses and Fistulas

Abscesses and fistulas represent end points on a spectrum of perirectal infection. The abscess represents an acute stage of infection, and the fistula represents a chronic stage of infection. The pathogenesis of anorectal fistulous abscesses involves infection arising in the cryptoglandular epithelium lining the anal canal and penetrating to the intermuscular space. Scattered throughout the anal canal at the level of the dentate line are 8 to 12 anorectal glands. Normally the internal sphincter acts as a barrier to the passage of infection from the lumen through to the perirectal tissues. This barrier can be breached by the crypts into which the glands empty. The crypts penetrate through the internal sphincter. Once the internal sphincter barrier is breached the intermuscular abscess can then spread throughout the perirectal tissues.

Treatment of an anal fistula is surgical. The treatment is based on determining the origin of the fistula within the anal canal. Goodsall's rule relates the internal origin to the external orifice. It states that when the external orifice is in the anterior half of the rectum the fistula runs a radial course to the dentate line. When it is in the posterior half it runs a curved course to the posterior midline. Like many other rules, it is noted for its exceptions. However, the rule is a good guide in the search for the internal orifice of a fistula.

The classical operation for correction of an anal fistula consists of laying open the entire fistulous tract. A probe is placed in the external orifice and exits at the internal orifice, allowing the overlying tissues to be incised. This procedure can cause anal incontinence when a significant portion of the external sphincter must be divided. Under those circumstances a partial internal anal sphincterectomy, unroofing the intersphincteric abscess of origin, often is curative. Setons are heavy sutures or narrow drains that are placed through the course of a fistula. They are left in place for several weeks. These result in prolonged drainage, and by causing scarring and fixation of the sphincter mechanism, they diminish the possibility of incontinence (13,14).

The differential diagnosis of anal fistulas includes specific etiologies such as Crohn's disease, tuberculosis, fungal disorders, and hidradenitis suppurativa (Verneuil's disease). This disease is due to infection of apocrine sweat glands of the perineal region and is treated by simple excision of the affected tissue. Long-standing anal fistulas can become complicated by carcinoma.

Pruritus Ani

Pruritus ani can be a difficult condition to treat. Its treatment is largely empiric. Specific etiologies such as pinworm infection, Paget's disease, and syphilis must be excluded. The perianal skin may be totally normal, or it may be lichenified and hypertrophic. Fungal infection is often associated with pruritus ani (15,16). Antifungal therapy, topical corticosteroids, and attention to details of personal hygiene often are effective in resolving the problem.

Prolapse

Prolapse of the rectum is a complex condition. It more commonly affects females than males. Prolapse occurs at all ages, however, it more commonly affects the elderly. Anatomically it has been found to be associated with diminished anal sphincter function, with a long mesorectum, with a low culde-sac, and with a redundant sigmoid. Constipation or obstipation is a frequent accompaniment. The main point in differential diagnosis is to exclude it from mucosal prolapse or hemorrhoidal prolapse. The rectal mucosa in a true procidentia (prolapse) forms circumferential furrows, whereas the hemorrhoidal or mucosal prolapse has longitudinal furrows.

The treatment of rectal prolapse is controversial. An abdominal operation is preferred unless contraindicated. The authors prefers the modified Ripstein operation, in which Marlex mesh is used to anchor the rectum to the sacrum. This is over 95% effective and is a safe operation with a low mortality rate. In the poor-risk patient, the author prefers a Thiersch wire, in which a wire or other material is placed into the perianal tissues to prevent the prolapse.

An intrarectal or occult prolapse is one in which the prolapse is confined to the rectum and does not protrude through the anus. It can cause a sensation of incomplete evacuation of the rectum or a feeling of pressure in the rectum. It can be difficult to diagnose. Defecography in many hands has been found to be effective in demonstrating intrarectal prolapse (17). The author has found that a reliable way of diagnosing intrarectal prolapse is to ask the patient to strain while a large Hirschmann anoscope is in the anal canal. The mid and upper rectum can then be seen to intussuscept into the lower rectum or into the anoscope.

Correction of the partial intussusception can be difficult (18). Rubber-band ligation of the redundant portion of bowel has been reported to be effective, as has a Ripstein repair. However, the latter is associated with at least a 35% failure rate (19). The failures have discouraged widespread use of this approach for intrarectal prolapse.

Intrarectal prolapse can be associated with solitary rectal ulcer syndrome (20). One commonly sees a patch of ulceration or inflammation located anteriorly, usually at about the 6- to 8-cm level. The solitary ulcer can be diagnosed by observing the above ulceration in the presence of an intrarectal prolapse. This condition must be differentiated from nonspecific rectal ulcerations, particularly Crohn's disease.

Condyloma Acuminata

Condyloma or venereal warts are lesions usually caused by a sexually transmitted virus. Condyloma acuminata usually can be diagnosed from visual inspection. Some of these can be associated with Bowen's disease or squamous carcinoma. Therefore, biopsy is sometimes necessary. Anoscopy must be performed to search for intra-anal lesions. Most patients with condyloma acuminata have been exposed to anal intercourse. Most of those will have intrarectal lesions with or without perineal lesion. In patients in whom there is no history of anal intercourse, condylomata, when present, are usually perianal in location. A variant of cnodyloma acuminata is the Buschke-Löwenstein tumor, in which the condylomata are large and locally invasive lesions.

Treatment of condyloma acuminata primarily is with topical agents including podophyllum and bichloracetic acid. Those that fail to respond to that can be treated by electrocoagulation. Recently, laser photocoagulation using a contact YAG laser has been found to be very effective in eradicating these lesions and in minimizing, the potential for recurrences. Carbon dioxide laser has been used, but its results in rectal condyloma acuminata has been variable.

Proctitis

Nonspecific proctitis (also called ulcerative proctitis) is common. It can produce symptoms of bleeding or mucous discharge. The differential diagnosis includes specific etiologies and culture; parasite studies and biopsy must be obtained. Also the possibility of Crohn's disease with involvement of other portions of the intestinal tract must be considered. Nonspecific colitis, Crohn's colitis, or specific colitis also can produce bleeding, mucous discharge, or diarrhea (see Chapter 12).

Neoplasms

The anal canal and perianal region can be the site of benign or malignant neoplasms, including Bowen's disease or Bowenoid papulosis. Malignant lesions that occur include basal cell, squamous, and cloacogenic carcinoma; Kaposi's sarcoma; and Paget's disease. Leiomyomas, sarcomas, lymphomas, and carcinoids occur infrequently.

Lesions that have features equivocal for neoplasia either could be observed for a few days (to permit inflammatory changes to resolve) or could be biopsied promptly. The degree of suspicion that there is an underlying malignancy would dictate the approach. The anorectum is very vascular, and before embarking on obtaining biopsies in this region, the examiner must be capable of controlling bleeding with electrocautery or via suture ligation. Local anesthetics can be injected in or adjacent to the area in question prior to the biopsy.

Foreign Bodies

Foreign bodies can occur in the rectum. When a foreign body is lost in the rectum it frequently migrates to the midrectum. It usually is unable to negotiate the angle of the rectum at that position. It usually can be palpated by digital examination. Although there have been reports of successful extraction of rectal foreign bodies using sigmoidoscopes or flexible instruments, it is easier to introduce local anesthesia and a rectal retractor that permits the foreign object to be grasped and retrieved.

Local anesthesia can be induced using ½% lidocaine or bupivacaine to which hyaluronidase is added in a dose of 150 units per 10 to 15 ml of anesthetic solution. A 22-gauge 1-½-inch long needle, which is passed up to the hub in the right and left midlateral positions and in the anterior and posterior midline positions, is used to deposit 2.5 ml of the anesthetic solution. A continuous wheal is raised around the rectum with a 25- to 30-gauge needle. Complete anesthesia and total sphincter relaxation is thereby obtained.

THE ANORECTUM IN SYSTEMIC DISORDERS

The anorectum is also a site of involvement in systemic diseases that affect other organ systems. One of the most important is Crohn's disease. Crohn's disease anywhere in the gastrointestinal tract can be associated with rectal pathology. Anorectal pathology is reported in 25% of patients when the disease is limited to the ileum, and this increases to nearly 100% as the disease approaches the rectum.

The anorectal findings associated with Crohn's disease include skin tags, anal ulcers, anal fistulas, anorectal strictures, perianal lymphangioma, and perianal erythema (4). Skin tags are painless and protuberant and may be cyanotic. They have been termed elephant ears. Perianal ulcers are common. These can resemble the typical anal fissures, but unlike idiopathic anal fissures, those in Crohn's disease more commonly are not midline in position. Unlike the usual anal fissure, in Crohn's disease these typically are painless. Fistulas can resemble a typical anal fistula, but those that are complex, with distant orifices or chronic infection of the skin or subcutaneous tissue of the buttock, often are associated with Crohn's disease. Similarly, a rectovaginal fistula with no history of obstetrical or surgical trauma often is due to Crohn's disease. Other signs of Crohn's disease in the rectum include lymphangioma and perianal erythema without underlying pain or pruritus. These little bubbly type lesions can appear in the rectum and may be related to lymphatic obstruction in Crohn's disease. Most anorectal strictures are at the anal verge. In Crohn's disease these tend to be located 1 ½ to 4 cm inside the anal verge and are probably due to chronic ischiorectal abscess leading to stricture formation.

Another area of involvement of the rectum in systemic disease is AIDS (see Chapter 13). Herpes, cytomegaloviral infections, and chlamydia infections are common. In what is usually a late stage of AIDS, the patient can present with severely painful perianal and rectal ulcerating lesions. If the etiology is herpes, cytomegalovirus, or chlamydia, specific therapy can be directed toward them. In the absence of specific etiology, treatment is empiric and difficult.

Endometriosis rarely can cause a painful rectal condition and can be confused with an abscess (22). Rectal pain that varies with the menstrual cycle is characteristic.

Leukemia has been associated with perirectal infiltrates. Rectal pain in a patient with leukemia may be evaluated by limited biopsy (23). Incision and drainage usually is not necessary unless there is a frank abscess. Local radiation therapy is often beneficial. Granulocytopenic patients with or without associated malignancies, are particularly subject to acute rectal conditions (24).

The rectum is often the site for sexual abuse (25). Any child with suspicious rectal problems should be suspected as being the victim of rectal rape.

Primary and metastatic malignant melanoma, metastatic colon, breast and lung lesions to the anal canal and rectum have been described (26,27). Perianal hematomas have been found to be associated with aortic aneurysms (28).

References

1. Kelly SM, Sanowski RA, Foutch PG, Bellapravalu S, Haynes WC. A prospective comparison of anoscopy and fiberendoscopy in detecting anal lesions. J Clin Gastroenterol 1986;8:658–660.
2. Jaques PF, Fitch DD. Anal verge and low rectal bleeding. A diagnostic problem. J Clin Gastroenterol 1986;8:38–42.
3. Thomson WHF. The anatomy and nature of piles. In: Kaufman HD, ed. The haemorrhoid syndrome. Kent, England: Abacus Press, 1981:15–32.
4. Sohn N, Weinstein MA, Robbins RD. Anorectal disorders. Curr Probl Surg 1983;20:1–66.
5. Choi J, Freeman JB, Touchette J. Long-term follow-up of concomitant band ligation and sclerotherapy for internal hemorrhoids. Can J Surg 1985;28:523–524.
6. Ambrose NS, Hares MM, Alexander-Williams J, Keighley MR. Prospective randomised comparison of photocoagulation and rubber band ligation in treatment of haemorrhoids. Br Med J 1983;286:1389–1391.
7. Ambrose NS, Morris D, Alexander-Williams J, Keighley MR. A randomized trial of photo-

coagulation or injection sclerotherapy for the treatment of first- and second-degree hemorrhoids. Dis Colon Rectum 1985;28:238–240.

8. Griffith CD, Morris DL, Ellis I, Wherry DC, Hardcastle JD. Out-patient treatment of haemorrhoids with bipolar diathermy coagulation. Br J Surg 1987;74:827.

9. Norman DA, Newton R, Nicholas GV. Direct current electrotherapy of internal hemorrhoids: An effective, safe, and painless outpatient approach. Am J Gastro 1989;84:482–487.

10. Sankar MY, Joffe SN. Laser surgery in colic and anorectal lesions. Surg Clin of North Amer 1988 (Dec); 1447–1469.

11. Schapiro M. The gastroenterologist and the treatment of hemorrhoids: Is it about time? Am J Gastro 1989;84:493–495.

12. Weaver RM, Ambrose NS, Alexander-Williams J, Keighley MR. Manual dilation of the anus vs. lateral subcutaneous sphincterotomy in the treatment of chronic fissure-in-ano. Results of a prospective, randomized, clinical trial. Dis Colon Rectum 1987;30:420–423.

13. Held D, Khubchandani I, Sheets J, Stasik J, Rosen L, Riether R. Management of anorectal horseshoe abscess and fistula. Dis Colon Rectum 1986;29:793–797.

14. Christensen A, Nilas L, Christiansen J. Treatment of transsphincteric anal fistulas by the seton technique. Dis Colon Rectum 1986;7:454–455.

15. Allan A, Ambrose NS, Silverman S, Keighley MR. Physiological study of pruritus ani. Br J Surg 1987;74:576–579.

16. Dodi G, Pirone E, Bettin A, et al. The mycotic flora in proctological patients with and without pruritus ani. Br J Surg 1985;72:967–969.

17. Ekberg O, Nylander G, Fork FT. Defecography. Radiology 1985;155:45–48.

18. Berman IR, Manning DH, Dudley-Wright K. Anatomic specificity in the diagnosis and treatment of internal rectal prolapse. Dis Colon Rectum 1985;28:816–826.

19. Schoetz DJ, Veidenheimer MC. Rectal prolapse. A: Pathogenesis and clinical features. In: Henry MM, Swash M. Coloproctology and the pelvic floor. Pathophysiology and management. London, England: Butterworths, 1985:303–339.

20. Womack NR, Williams NS, Mist JH, Morrison JF. Anorectal function in the solitary rectal ulcer syndrome. Dis Colon Rectum 1987;30:319–323.

21. Wexner SD, Smithy WB, Milsom JW, Dailey TH. The surgical management of anorectal diseases in AIDS and pre-AIDS patients. Dis Colon Rectum 1986;29:719–723.

22. Gordon PH, Schottler JL, Balcos EG, Goldberg SM. Perianal endometrioma: report of five cases. Dis Colon Rectum 1976;19:260–265.

23. Boddie AW Jr, Bines SD. Management of acute rectal problems in leukemic patients. J Surg Oncol 1986;33:53–56.

24. Merrill JM, Brereton HD, Kent CH, Johnson RE. Anorectal disease in patients with non-haematological malignancy. Lancet 1976;1:1105–1107.

25. Hobbs CJ, Wynne JM. Buggery in childhood; a common syndrome of child abuse. Lancet 1986;2:792–796.

26. Dawson PM, Hershman MJ, Wood CB. Metastatic carcinoma of the breast in the anal canal. Postgrad Med J 1985;61:1081.

27. Kanhouwa S, Burns W, Matthews M, Chisholm R. Anaplastic carcinoma of the lung with metastasis to the anus: report of a case. Dis Colon Rectum 1975;18:42–48.

28. Antrum RM. Perianal haematoma: an unusual feature of a leaking aortic aneurysm. Br J Surg 1984;71:649.

The Use of Flexible Sigmoidoscopy in Special Clinical Situations

Francis J. Tedesco, M.D.

INTRODUCTION

This chapter will review the role of flexible sigmoidoscopy in a variety of predominantly noninfectious disease states. Differentiation of infectious from noninfectious disease is important and will be included here. This chapter, written by an internist-gastroenterologist, has some intentional overlap with Chapter 11, which presents a surgeon's experience. More detailed discussions of various infectious disease are found in Chapter 13.

In the evaluation of acute or chronic diarrhea (with or without bleeding), flexible sigmoidoscopy may detect mucosal inflammation, i.e., colitis. The rectum and sigmoid are a mirror of the entire colon in many types of colitides. Crohn's disease of the colon spares the rectum approximately 50% of the time, and the hemorrhagic colitis noted with *E. coli* serotype 0157:H7 involves the right side of the colon, but the majority of the other colitides involve the distal 60 cm of the large bowel.

ULCERATIVE COLITIS

This idiopathic inflammatory process predominately involves the mucosal layer of the bowel. One of the earliest features of colonic involvement by ulcerative colitis is mucosal edema, which is manifested at sigmoidoscopy by loss of vascular pattern. This is a nonspecific finding and may be secondary to enema or laxative bowel preparation as well as any inflammatory condition affecting the colon. Another early feature is the increase in mucosal blood flow, which can be manifested by diffuse erythema. This edematous, engorged mucosa is quite fragile and bleeds readily with minor trauma, i.e., friable mucosa. In addition to the edema, erythema, friability, and granularity with the accompanying disruption of the normal light reflex are all characteristic features of ulcerative colitis. These inflammatory changes are symmetric, uniform, and continuous, and the rectum is almost always involved (95% of cases). With progression of this inflammatory process, small superficial erosions and minute surface ulcerations occur on a background of severely inflamed mucosa. Large ulcers can also occur, but they also are always found on a background of inflamed mucosa. During the endoscopic examination, air insufflation should be kept to a minimum, and there is usually no need to proceed higher than the rectosigmoid area if severe inflammation is present. Biopsies can be obtained, which may help differentiate self-limited colitis from idiopathic inflammatory conditions of the large bowel. Cultures can be obtained, and treatment can be instituted based on clinical, sigmoidoscopic, culture, and stool examination results. Once the colitis is more quiescent, the full extent of the colonic involvement can be determined by barium enema examination or colonoscopy if the diagnosis remains uncertain. Full colon evaluation is generally contraindicated in severe colitis as toxic dilation may be precipitated. Ulcerative colitis and ulcerative proctitis are believed to be

149

familiar entities except that the latter is limited to the terminal 5–25 cm of colorectum.

CROHN'S COLITIS

Crohn's disease is another idiopathic inflammatory process that often has transmural colonic or small bowel involvement. Crohn's disease of the colon in contrast with ulcerative colitis spares the rectum and is visible via flexible sigmoidoscopy in only approximately 50% of the cases. One of the earliest features of Crohn's disease of the colon is aphthous-type ulcers. This ulcer is small, approximately 1–4 mm in diameter, with a surrounding narrow border of erythematous mucosa. These ulcers occur on a background of completely normal mucosa with normal vascular pattern. Progression of Crohn's colitis typically leads to large, often linear, ulcers surrounded by normal-appearing mucosa. In addition, surface nodules or bumps secondary to submucosal inflammation and edema give the characteristic cobblestone appearance noted in Crohn's disease. These features are usually seen in an asymmetric, discontinuous, or segmental distribution. Again, stool or exudate for culture as well as biopsies may be obtained, which may assist in differentiating the self-limited colitis from the idiopathic varieties.

INFECTIOUS COLITIS

This type of colitis accounts for approximately 30–40% of all newly diagnosed cases of acute bloody diarrhea. These are reviewed in detail in Chapter 13. There is no question that the most important diagnostic tool in defining the specific cause of infectious diarrhea remains the stool culture. What has evolved during the past decade is the belief that the direct observation of the rectosigmoid mucosa can lead the examiner to suspect a self-limited cause of the colitis or proctitis instead of considering the idiopathic inflammatory conditions such as ulcerative colitis or Crohn's colitis. To address this question, a prospective study of 29 patients in our institution presenting with mucoid bloody diarrhea was undertaken. All patients with a past history of ulcerative colitis, Crohn's colitis, Crohn's ileocolitis, or a history of bloody stools for greater than 6 weeks duration were excluded from this report. This study revealed that 11 of the 29 patients (38%) had infectious causes of the colitis (1). Further unpublished work from this group has expanded their study group to 37 patients. On sigmoidoscopic evaluation, the examiners felt that 17 patients had endoscopic features atypical for idiopathic inflammatory bowel disease, whereas 20 had features consistent with inflammatory bowel disease. The features considered suggestive for ulcerative colitis, Crohn's colitis, and infectious colitis are given in Table 12.1. When this group of evaluators at-

Table 12.1.
Endoscopic Features

Ulcerative colitis	Symmetric and continuous involvement
	Rectum almost always involved
	Diffuse erythema, edema, superficial ulcers involving entire mucosa, friability
Crohn's colitis	Asymptomatic and eccentric involvement
	Rectum involved in 50%
	Focal aphthous ulcers, cobblestoning of the mucosa, ulcers adjacent to normal mucosa
Infectious colitis	Patchy involvement
	Rectum usually involved
	Patchy, petechial hemorrhages, focal hyperemia, edema, and ulcerations

Table 12.2.
Atypical for Inflammatory Bowel Disease
(IBD)

Diagnosis	Number of Patients
Infectious colitis	12 (70%)
IBD	1 (6%)
Oral contraceptive colitis	1
Ischemic colitis	2
No diagnosis	1

Table 12.3.
Consistent with Inflammatory Bowel Disease
(IBD)

Diagnosis	Number of Patients
Infectious colitis	3 (15%)
IBD	13 (65%)
Oral contraceptive colitis	1
Ischemic colitis	2
No diagnosis	1

tempted to judge how accurate they were with their endoscopic evaluation, it appeared that in the 17 patients with features considered atypical for inflammatory bowel disease (Table 12.2) but more suggestive of infectious colitis, they were correct in 12 of 17 patients (70%), but there was a significant overlap. In the group of 20 patients with features consistent with idiopathic inflammatory bowel disease (Table 12.3), the observors were correct in 13 of 20 patients (60%), but again there was significant overlap. These findings reinforce the fact that the colon responds to a multitude of different insults in a defined and limited number of ways. Chapter 9 reviews the biopsy features that differentiate infectious colitis from noninfectious causes.

Campylobacter fetus is a short, thin, comma-shaped, motile, gram-negative rod, formerly placed in the genus Vibrio. It is felt that the organism is contracted most often from contaminated food or water and by the fecal-oral route in a nursing setting. *Campylobacter fetus* subspecies jejuni has been reported to cause a clinical syndrome with patients presenting with abdominal pain and diarrhea that may be bloody or mucopurulent (2,3). The sigmoidoscopic findings vary from mucosal edema, erythema, and friability to granularity with spontaneous bleeding. All findings are indistinguishable from ulcerative colitis. However, the involvement may be segmental and patchy with discrete ulcerations, which is more consistent with Crohn's disease.

Salmonellae are gram-negative, flagellated, nonencapsulated, nonsporulating, facultatively anaerobic bacilli that are transmitted to human beings almost solely by the ingestion of contaminated food or drink. *Salmonella* primarily involves the small bowel, but not infrequently salmonellosis of the large bowel has been reported (4,5,6). Patients present with abdominal cramps, fever, and bloody mucopurulent diarrhea. Sigmoidoscopic findings vary from mucosal edema with loss of vascular pattern to hyperemic granular mucosa with friability and petechial hemorrhages. Deep ulcerations also have been described. Again the visual similarity with both ulcerative and Crohn's colitis is obvious.

Shigella organisms are gram-negative rods that can be spread by human-to-human contact without interposition of a vehicle such as food or water. Besides direct fecal–oral transmission, the organism can be transmitted by contaminated water or food. Overcrowding and poor sanitary conditions enhance the dissemination of the organism. Shigellosis, commonly known as bacillary dysentery, primarily affects the large bowel. Patients present with crampy abdominal pain, tenesmus, fever, and mucoid bloody stools. Sigmoidoscopic findings range from mild edema, erythema, and granularity to significant hyperemia, friability, and multiple superficial ulcerations. This appearance can be confused with the findings in ulcerative colitis.

Yersinia enterocolitica is a nonlactose-fermenting, urease-positive, gram-negative rod. Although the clinical manifestations of yersiniosis are protean, *Yersinia enterocolitica* most commonly produces various gastrointestinal symptoms (7). *Yersinia enterocolitica* has been incriminated as the cause of acute enteritis with fever and diarrhea in children and terminal ileitis with mesenteric adenitis in adolescents and young adults. Recently, colonic infections have been reported, and patients present with fever, crampy abdominal pain, and watery diarrhea. Sigmoidoscopic features include diffuse granularity, erythema, edema, and friability, which mimic ulcerative colitis. However, some patients have patchy involvement or predominately right-sided involvement that includes terminal ileum, and this appearance mimics Crohn's ileocolitis.

Amebiasis is an acute or chronic disease caused by the organism *Entamoeba histolytica*. *Amebiasis* predominately affects the colon. Patients present with bloody diarrhea, abdominal crampy pain, tenesmus, and fever. Sigmoidoscopic findings vary from mucosal edema, granularity, and friability resembling ulcerative colitis to discrete ulcerations with undermined edges adjacent to relatively normal mucosa that resemble Crohn's colitis (8,9). With chronic involvement a fibrous reaction that involves the submucosa and serosa layer may occur; concentric narrowing also may occur.

ISCHEMIC COLITIS

Work by Scowcroft et al. (10) has better defined the usual anatomic distribution of ischemic colitis. The authors endoscopically observed that ischemia is a dynamic process with an acute, subacute, and chronic stage. The acute stage consists of an acute mucosal process of segmental distribution. Endoscopically one sees patchy areas of edematous and hyperemic mucosa alternating with areas of blanching mucosa. There is friability in the hyperemic area but much less so in the blanching area. Over the ensuing 24–72 hours there is coalescence of the erythematous area, the development of superficial ulcerations, and evidence of submucosal bleeding manifested by pinpoint petechiae or, less commonly, bluish submucosal blebs. Over the next few days, the ulcerative process involves more of the mucosal surface, tending to elongate into longitudinal or serpiginous ulcers somewhat similar to those seen in Crohn's colitis. This ischemic process usually progresses rapidly and goes on to complete healing in approximately 6 weeks. However, in some patients, because of the extent of mucosal and submucosal damage, changes of mucosal atrophy, loss of mucosal thickness, and submucosal replacement by granulation tissue lead to loss of haustrations and to stenosis or strictures.

This study also demonstrated that 12 of 15 patients (80%) could have been diagnosed with 60 cm flexible sigmoidoscopy, whereas only 5 of 15 (33%) could have been diagnosed with rigid sigmoidoscopy. This study demonstrates the dynamic nature of ischemic colitis, as well as the fact that a significant number of patients with ischemic colitis can be diagnosed and followed by flexible sigmoidoscopy. Clinically, it appears that during the initial phase in most such patients, clinical management can be guided by the clinical course and the endoscopic picture as revealed with flexible sigmoidoscopy. This approach seems to decrease the early need for more invasive studies such as total colonoscopy. If the patients have markedly severe abdominal pain, fever, marked leukocytosis, persistent bleeding, and/or peritoneal signs, more aggressive evaluation and intervention should be undertaken.

ANTIBIOTIC ASSOCIATED PSEUDOMEMBRANOUS COLITIS

Most studies on patients with antibiotic-associated pseudomembranous colitis (AAPMC) have shown that toxin-producing *Clostridium difficile* can be found in the stool. In addition to bacteriologic studies and tissue culture assays for toxin, endoscopic visualization of the colon has been advocated as a main means for diagnosing this condition. In patients receiving antibiotics who develop diarrhea, the majority will have normal sigmoidoscopy and negative clostridia studies (if performed). Many patients with *C. difficile* toxin in stools may have only nonspecific erythema or friability at sigmoidoscopy. In classic pseudomembranous colitis adherent yellow plaques are seen on a background of variably normal or nonspecifically abnormal mucosa with erythema or friability. The plaques may become confluent in more severe cases.

The optimal diagnostic instrument remains somewhat controversial. Seppala et al. (11), however, reported that these characteristic changes of AAPMC were observed in only 5 (31%) out of 16 patients by rigid sigmoidoscopy, whereas these changes were noted in 11 (85%) out of 13 patients in the colonic mucosa on whom colonoscopies were also performed. The authors emphasized that colonoscopy, instead of sigmoidoscopy, should be the method of choice in the early diagnosis of pseudomembranous colitis. A more recent prospective study (12) was performed to determine the incidence of rectal sparing in AAPMC. This prospective study of 22 patients with AAPMC demonstrated that the most distal location of the pseudomembranes was noted 0–25 cm from the anus in 17 patients, 25 to 60 cm from the anus in 3 patients, and greater than 60 cm from the anus in only 2 patients. The authors concluded that the pseudomembranes will be noted by the rigid sigmoidoscope in 77% of the patients and by the flexible sigmoidoscope in 91% of the patients. Colonoscopic examination beyond 60 cm from the anus was necessary for the diagnosis of AAPMC in 2 (9%) patients. This work strongly implies that flexible sigmoidoscopy is the diagnostic tool of choice when the colonic mucosa must be seen in patients with suspected AAPMC.

RADIATION COLITIS

In the clinical setting of recent pelvic irradiation and the onset of tenesmus, diarrhea, and a mucoid rectal discharge, the diagnosis of radiation injury must be considered. The use of flexible sigmoidoscopy may reveal dusky, edematous, and inflamed mucosa with loss of the normal vascular pattern. With reexamination in 24–96 hours, friability and mucosal ulcerations can be noted.

Patients with past history of pelvic radiation may present with constipation, diarrhea, a decrease in stool caliber, rectal pain, and/or rectal bleeding. Flexible sigmoidoscopy may reveal granular and friable mucosa with numerous telangiectasias. Focal ulceration may be seen especially on the anterior rectal wall in patients who have had implant radiation for gynecologic malignancies. At times firm stenotic areas are noted with or without adjacent ulcerations but usually with the telangiectasias being noted.

DIVERTICULITIS

Most persons with diverticulosis are essentially asymptomatic. Classically, diverticulitis presents as left lower quadrant abdominal pain, with or without fever and altered bowel movement pattern in an elderly patient. When the clinical impression and laboratory data suggest diverticulitis, the patient is usually treated medically initially, and further evaluation is delayed. After the acute episode and pain have improved, the physician will do a more complete evaluation to exclude other possibilities such as colitis, malignancy, or ischemic disease. In this instance, flexible sigmoidoscopy is a very reasonable next step. This examination should be gently performed with minimal bowel preparation and little or no air insufflation. In diverticulitis, the lumen may narrow abruptly. Usually adjacent diverticula without inflammation are present. With the narrowed segment, although the overlying mucosa is reddened, it remains intact, and the folds are symmetrical. Adherent exudate is occasionally seen. In malignant strictures, the mucosal folds are usually ulcerated or severely distorted. The stricture entrance is irregular and much firmer than noted in diverticular disease. If the narrowing cannot be traversed, the use of biopsies and brushing for cytology from within the segment may be quite useful. Full colon evaluation by barium enema or colonoscopy is recommended once the inflammation process has clinically resolved.

REDUCTION OF SIGMOID VOLVULUS

Volvulus of the sigmoid colon accounts for approximately 5% of all intestinal obstructions and 10% of all colonic obstructions. The treatment of sigmoid colon volvulus has included rigid sigmoidoscopy and rectal tube insertion, blind rectal tube insertion, barium enema, flexible sigmoidoscopy and/ or colonoscopy, and a variety of surgical procedures. Most recently the 60-cm flexible sigmoidoscope has been used because of the ease of examination and the increased therapeutic capability when compared with the rigid sigmoidoscope. With the 60-cm instrument being advanced under direct vision, a narrow area is usually noted at 30–35 cm from the anus. Mucosal folds leading to the narrowing usually show a twisted pattern. Gentle manipulation of the instrument tip through the narrowing will be greeted by a flood of stool and air with resultant decompression. Air is aspirated and the mucosa is carefully observed to ensure viability. Overdistention must be avoided. In many cases, decompression should be followed by the insertion of a long rectal tube.

In summary, in a variety of noninfectious and infectious diseases of the colon, FS may give valuable information that will aid in patient management. This information must be kept in perspective with the clinical condition of the patient and other colon diagnostic tools.

References

1. Tedesco FJ, Hardin RD, Harper RN, Edwards BH. Infectious colitis endoscopically simulating inflammatory bowel disease: a prospective evaluation. Gastrointest Endosc 1983;29:195–197.
2. Lambert ME, Schoefield PF, Ironside AG, et al. Campylobacter colitis. Br Med J 1979;1:857–859.
3. Willoughby CP, Piris J, Truelove SC. Campylobacter colitis. J Clin Pathol 1979;32:986–989.
4. Mandal BK, Mani V. Colonic involvement in salmonellosis. Lancet 1976;1:887–888.
5. Appelbaum PC, Scragg J, Schonland MM. Colonic involvement in salmonellosis. Lancet 1976;1:102.

 6. Saffouri B, Bartolomeco RS, Fuchs B. Colonic involvement in salmonellosis. Dig Dis Sci 1979;24(3):203–208.
 7. Vantrappen G, Agg HO, Ponette E, et al. Yersinia enteritis and enterocolitis: gastroenterological aspects. Gastroenterology 1977;72:220–227.
 8. Pittman FE, Henninger GR. Sigmoidoscopic and colonic mucosal biopsy findings in amebic colitis. Arch Pathol Lab Med 1974;97:155–158.
 9. Tucker PC, Webster PD, Kilpatrick ZM. Amebic colitis mistaken for inflammatory bowel disease. Arch Intern Med 1975;135:681–685.
10. Scowcroft CW, Sonowski RA, Kozarek RA. Colonoscopy in ischemic colitis. Gastrointest Endosc 1981;27:156–161.
11. Seppala K, Hjelt L, Sipponen P. Colonoscopy in the diagnosis of antibiotic-associated colitis—a prospective study. Scand J Gastroenterol 1981;16:465–468.
12. Tedesco FJ, Corless JK, Brownstein RE. Rectal sparing in antibiotic-associated pseudomembranous colitis: a prospective study. Gastroenterology 1982;83:1250–1260.

13

Infectious Diseases Encountered at Flexible Sigmoidoscopy

Sidney Niemark, M.D.

Acute infectious diarrhea is second only to upper respiratory tract infections as a cause of illness in our society. A causative agent can be determined in only 50% of cases. In most situations, the illness is mild, brief, and self-limited. In these cases, identifying the etiologic agent may not be important or even possible. Symptoms often resolve before complete evaluation can be undertaken. However, in certain situations, determining the etiology for an infectious diarrhea may be critical in preventing spread or selecting treatment. Homosexuals, immunosuppressed patients, infants in day-care centers, neonatal nurseries, and institutions caring for the mentally retarded may be at increased risk in disseminating infectious diarrheas. The very young and the very old are particularly susceptible to the devasting effects of prolonged diarrhea.

The definition of diarrhea differs (1). Clinically, diarrhea is a stool volume over 200 cc or stool weight over 200 g per day. Severe diarrheas can be defined as volumes over 1 L per day. From a practical standpoint, however, diarrhea is an increase in the number of stools passed associated with an increase in the fluid nature of the stool. Three mechanisms can result in an increased number of unformed stools. Increased gastrointestinal secretions, so-called secretory diarrheas, may be caused by bacterial enterotoxins that simulate adenylate cyclase. Enterotoxigenic *Escherichia coli* and *Vibrio cholerae* both produce such an enterotoxin. Decreased absorption of lumen contents also may occur with the production of certain bacteria enterotoxins, as well as with mucosal invasion, resulting in decreased absorptive capacity, and damage to the brush border enzymes, resulting in an osmotic diarrhea (2,3). Finally, increased gastrointestinal motility, which may occur with bacterial muscoal invasion or entertoxins production, may also cause diarrhea. Often, more than one mechanism is important in causing symptoms.

GENERAL CONSIDERATIONS IN EPIDEMIOLOGY, CLINICAL ASPECTS, DIAGNOSIS, AND TREATMENT

Epidemiology

Agents causing infectious diarrheas are spread by food, water, person-to-person contact, animal contacts, or other environmental contacts. Each agent often shows a characteristic mode of spread and may be dependent on a particular situation in the environment, such as a neonatal nursery. Inoculum size sufficient to produce infection also varies depending on the agent and possibly host susceptibility, as in infants or immune-suppressed patients. Rotovirus typically affects children under age 3. Seasonal variations also have been observed with rotovirus infections, which occur more frequently in cooler months.

Clinical Aspects

Clinical manifestations of infectious diarrheas often reflect the characteristics of the infecting agent. Symptoms occurring 1 to 4 hours after ingestion

157

of food and associated with nausea and vomiting in the absence of fever and other systemic signs imply ingestion of preformed toxin (food poisoning). Vomiting associated with diarrhea is also a characteristic of Norwalk and rotovirus infections. Fever and watery voluminous stool followed in 2 to 3 days by bloody, mucousy stools (dysentery) are often seen with *Shigella*. Dysenteric stools, however, are common with numerous other infections, including *Campylobacter* and enteroinvasive *E. coli* (4). Despite these features, in most patients a characteristic clinical picture is not present, and laboratory evaluation must be relied on to establish a diagnosis.

Diagnosis

The clinical situation often can categorize the etiology of the diarrhea: viral, bacterial, protozoan, or preformed toxin. A history of recent travel, antibiotic use, familial illness, and physical signs of toxicity and dehydration, such as orthostatic hypotension, tachycardia, poor skin turgor, or sunken fontanelles, should be elicited carefully. Patients with prolonged symptoms (greater than 1 week), voluminous stool volumes, marked systemic features, or in whom the possibility of an immune deficiency exists should undergo further evaluation to determine the etiologic agent.

Fecal leukocyte tests can be performed in the office. The presence of large numbers of leukocytes after methyline blue staining indicates an infectious or inflammatory etiology (5). Homosexuals should also have stools gram stained for the presence of intracellular diplococci, indicating gonococcal proctitis.

Stool cultures should be reserved for patients requiring hospitalization, patients with prolonged symptoms, or immunocompromised patients. Even careful, prompt culture technique may fail to detect a cause in 40 to 60% of infectious diarrheas.

Sigmoidoscopic evaluation may be invaluable in selected cases of acute diarrhea. Edema, friability, and punctate hemorrhages with exudate are common nonspecific findings in many types of infectious diarrhea. Necrotic ulcers may be seen in acute shigellosis, but discrete, flask-shaped ulcers are suggestive of amebiasis. The presence of raised plaque-like lesions are diagnostic of pseudomembranous colitis. Marked friability, discrete ulcers, pseudopolyps, and a cobblestone appearance to the mucosa all suggest inflammatory bowel disease. Large amounts of mucus in the absence of inflamed mucosa may be seen in "mucous colitis" or with a villous adenoma. Deeply pigmented mucosa (melanosis coli) suggests anthracene laxative abuse. Violaceous nodular mucosal lesions are typical of gastrointestinal Kaposi's sarcoma.

Rectal biopsy may help identify *Entamoeba histolytica,* ulcerative colitis, Crohn's colitis, or gastrointestinal Kaposi's but in general has a limited role in acute infectious colitis (6).

Treatment

In patients with acute diarrhea, intravascular volume status is of primary concern. Replacement of fluid and electrolytes is the mainstay treatment for all diarrheal illnesses. An oral solution recommended by the World Health Organization of 90 mEq/L of sodium, 20 mEq/L of potassium, and 20 g of glucose or other commercially available products such as Pedialyte (30 mEq/L sodium and 20 mEq/L potassium) or Gatorade (23 mEq/L sodium and 3 mEq/L potassium) can be used in milder diarrheal illnesses (7). Soft drinks, juices, and salted crackers are other alternatives in mild cases. When intravenous therapy is required, the fluid should approximate the electrolyte composition of diarrhea. Recommendations are sodium 120 to 140 mEq/L, potassium 20 to 40 mEq/L, chloride 40 to 50 mEq/L, and bicarbonate 40 to 50 mEq/

L. A simple formula is to add a 50-ml ampule of 7.5% bicarbonate and 20 to 40 mEq/L of potassium chloride to 1 L of half normal saline.

Hospitalization should be considered if any of the following exists:

1. Significant dehydration;
2. Intractable vomiting;
3. Extremes of age; or
4. Serious underlying disease.

Symptomatic relief using bismuth subsalicylate, loperamide, or diphenoxlate may be given to patients without dysenteric stools (8,9,10). Bismuth subsalicylate should be avoided in aspirin-sensitive patients (11). An 8-oz bottle taken over 3 to 4 hours will result in an equivalent salicylate level of eight ingested aspirins (11) and will help relieve abdominal cramping. Absorbent compounds such as Kaopectate will increase stool form, allowing better bowel control, but probably will do little to reduce fluid losses.

The role of antimicrobial agents will be reviewed under specific causes of infectious diarrheas.

TRAVELER'S DIARRHEA

Whether it is euphemistically called "Montezuma's revenge," "Delhi belly," "turista," or the "Aztec two-step," traveler's diarrhea, will affect almost half of all travelers visiting developing countries. Although traveler's diarrhea is a worldwide phenomenon, North Americans and Europeans appear to be at greatest risk when traveling to Latin America, Asia, or Africa (12,13,14,15).

The condition typically affects newcomers, with onset of symptoms 5 to 15 days after arrival, but ranges from 2 to 30 days. Onset is usually abrupt, with watery stools and abdominal cramps. Blood and mucus are generally absent. Nausea and vomiting, anorexia, and malaise accompany diarrhea in 10 to 20% of cases. A low-grade fever is present in one third of cases. Symptoms are usually self-limited, lasting 2 to 5 days. In 20% of cases, however, symptoms will last greater than 10 days (16).

Etiology

The etiology of turista has emerged only in the last few years. Infrequently, *Giardia, Salmonella, Shigella,* and ameba have been linked to turista. Viral studies also have failed to show a clear association. Studies by Kean (17) implicated *E. coli* in one-third of cases of traveler's diarrhea. An outbreak among British troops in Aden further identified *E. coli* in 54% of cases of traveler's diarrhea (18). Subsequent studies have demonstrated enterotoxigenic *E. coli* in 33 to 72% of cases of traveler's diarrhea (19,20). *Salmonella, Shigella,* or *Vibrio* was present in only 1 to 20% and rotavirus or *Campylobacter* was present in only 2 to 20% of cases (21,22).

E. coli produces both a heat-stable and a heat-labile enterotoxin. Immunologic evidence linking enterotoxigenic *E. coli* as a major cause of traveler's diarrhea is supported by demonstrating a rise in serum antitoxin to the heat-labile enterotoxin (20,23).

Therapy and Prevention

The efficiency of antimicrobial prophylaxis has been demonstrated in several studies (24,25,26). However, the emergence of multiple drug-resistant *E. coli,* the possibility of superinfection, and the risk of drug side effects such as photosensitivity still remain unsolved problems. Bismuth subsalicylate may help prevent symptoms. Tablets appear to be as effective as the liquid preparation. Patients taking bismuth preparation should be warned of passage of black stools and occurrence of black tongue.

Preventive measures should include careful attention to food and beverage preparation. Bismuth subsalicylate 60 ml or two tablets four times daily will decrease the incidence of diarrhea by 60% as will several antibiotic regimens. The problem with widespread use of antibiotics as prophylaxis is the common occurrence of side effects, including photosensitivity, Stevens-Johnson syndrome, rash, and antibiotic-associated infections. In addition, widespread prophylaxis enhances the reservoir of resistant organisms. Current recommendations include sensible dietary practices. Bismuth subsalicylate or antimotility agents such as loperamide or diphenoxylate should be taken with the first onset of symptoms. When fever, abdominal pain, or bloody diarrhea occur, antibiotics should be initiated. A 3- to 5-day course can reduce the severity and duration of symptoms. The best-studied regimen is trimethoprim-sulfamethoxazole (27) twice daily. Doxycycline 100 mg twice daily, norfloxacin 400 mg twice daily, or ciprofloxacin 500 mg twice daily are also effective in reducing symptoms (28,29). If diarrhea persists, evaluation for other causes, such as antibiotic-associated colitis, should be undertaken. Doxycycline, trimethoprim-sulfamethoxazole, or bicozamycin may also be effective in avoiding symptoms and may shorten the course of diarrheal illness once symptoms develop (27,28,30).

Pathogenesis

There are at least four different mechanisms by which *E. coli* produces symptoms. (a) With enteropathic *E. coli* the mode of action is unknown. It may produce diarrhea by affecting intracellular enzyme systems. (b) Enterotoxigenic *E. coli* produces a heat-stable toxin and a heat-labile toxin. The heat-labile toxin is cytotonic and is similar to the toxin produced by *V. cholera*. The toxin blocks adenylcyclase and results in reduced water reabsorption. Two general types of toxins exist. Cytotonic toxins interfere with intracellular enzyme systems and affect fluid secretion and absorption. These produce noninflammatory diarrhea typified by *V. cholera* and *E. coli*. Cytotoxic toxins produce injury to the surface mucosa, resulting in an inflammatory reaction that produces net fluid secretion. *Shigella, Campylobacter, Clostridium difficile, Yersinia* and *Clostridium perfringens* all produce such inflammatory diarrheas. (c) Enteroinvasive *E. coli* penetrates the colonic epithelium, producing an inflammatory diarrhea and dysenteric stools. Dysenteric stools may also be a result of enterohemorrhagic *E. coli* (31,32,33), a strain producing a shigella-like toxin. (d) Enteroadherent *E. coli* adheres to mucosal surfaces with penetration. Damage to the brush border and microvilli results.

SHIGELLA

The term "dysentery" was used by Hippocrates to indicate a condition characterized by the passage of small volumes of stool containing blood and mucus and often associated with urgency and tenesmus. Shiga established the cause of bacillary disentery in 1897. Four major serologic groups of *Shigella*, determined by cell-wall-specific antigens, are now identified. There are at least 50 serologic subtypes within these groups (34). Group A consists of *S. dysenteriae*, a species not generally encountered within the United States. Group B includes *S. flexneri*, a commonly identified subgroup in the United States. Group C includes *S. boydii*, which also is rarely isolated in the United States. Group D contains an isolated serotype, *S. sonnei*. This subtype is the most common agent associated with shigellosis in the United States (34).

Epidemiology

Shigellae have no natural intermediate host. Most cases are the result of person-to-person transmission via oral-fecal spread. Contaminated water and food sources of infection are well documented and may be a significant source of outbreaks, particularly in developing countries. Shigellae are remarkably efficient in producing symptoms with an inoculum as small as 200 organisms producing disease (35). At high risk are closed populations such as day-care centers, homes caring for the retarded, and prisons.

Pathogenesis

Bacillary dysentery is the most communicable bacterial diarrheal illness. The low dose of organisms required to produce infection explains the easy person-to-person spread and high secondary attack rate. Shigellae produce disease by invading intestinal mucosa. Infection is superficial, only rarely penetrating beyond the mucosa. This accounts for the rarity of bacteremia (34,36).

Shigellae produce an enterotoxin that probably plays a role in the local mucosal destruction and watery diarrhea that occurs in the first few days of infection.

After ingestion, bacteria transiently multiply in the small bowel, often producing cramps and watery diarrhea. Tenesmus and dysentery occur in the later stages of disease and correlate with diffuse colonic involvement. The incubation period ranges between 36 and 72 hours. Fever, abdominal cramps, and watery diarrhea usually occur within 48 hours, and subsequently bloody mucous stools develop.

Diagnosis

The presence of fever and diarrhea, particularly associated with mucus and blood, strongly suggests shigellosis. Definitive diagnosis however requires isolation of shigellae from stool. Sigmoidoscopic examination reveals diffuse erythema, multiple shallow 3-mm to 5-mm ulcerations, friability, and loss of transverse folds. The yield on stool cultures depends on minimizing inoculation time, as other microorganisms present give rise to acids that inactivate *Shigella*.

Prognosis

Shigellosis is usually a self-limited disease with fever lasting 3 to 5 days and dysentery resolving within 7 to 10 days. Shigellae may be recovered from the stool as long as 4 to 6 weeks after dysentery has subsided. Persistence beyond 3 months is rare.

Mortality is less than 1% in the United States and generally is related to complications from dehydration, shock, or severe electrolyte imbalance. Complications such as iritis, conjunctivitis, hemolytic uremic syndrome, or bowel perforations are rare. Arthritis is an unusual late complication that usually affects large weight-bearing joints.

Immunity following infection is species-specific but incomplete, and reinfections with the same strain may occur. There is no evidence of heterologous immunity.

Therapy

Prompt attention to fluid and electrolyte balance is important. Antidiarrheal agents that inhibit gastrointestinal motility are contraindicated (37,38). Because shigellosis is usually self-limited, antibiotic therapy is usually unnecessary. In addition, emergence of strains resistant to tetracycline, sulfa, and ampicillin is now common, and treatment should be reserved to those who are ill (39). Antibiotic treatment will shorten the period of fecal excretion of the organism and limit the clinical course of illness. In addition, because colonized persons represent a major reservoir of infection, for public health reasons an argument can be made to treat all persons harboring shigellae in their stool. Treatment of choice where sensitivities are unknown or ampicillin and tetracycline resistance are encountered is trimethoprim-sulfamethoxazole (40,41).

SALMONELLOSIS

Nontyphoidal salmonellosis is among the most common infectious bacterial diseases in the United States. Transmission occurs in human or animal sources, and the disease usually is self-limited. Serologic classification by means of somatic (O) and flagellar (H) antigens has identified more than 1500 serogroups; however, 10 serogroups account for 70% of infection. There are three primary species: *S. typhi, S. choleraesuis,* and *S. enteritidis.*

Epidemiology

The majority of cases of *Salmonella* are acquired from contaminated food or water sources. Rare cases of spread by inadequately sterilized endoscopy instruments have been reported (41,42,43). Salmonellae have been isolated in almost all animal sources, including poultry, fowl, cows, pigs, turtles, snakes, and lizards (44). However, the only known reservoir for *S. typhi* is human beings.

The majority of cases in the United States are sporadic. Once exposed, however, about one-third of family household members will be infected. Similar "outbreaks" can occur in institutional settings, such as acute-care hospitals, nursing homes, and psychiatric hospitals.

Pathogenesis

A large inoculum is required to produce symptomatic infection, often on the order of 10^7 to 10^9 organisms. Small doses may produce asymptomatic carrier states. Most salmonellae are readily killed at gastric pH of 3 or less. Bacteria surviving the acid environment of the stomach are then exposed to the antimicrobial action of short-chain fatty acids produced by normal gut flora. The surviving salmonellae multiply in the small intestines, producing *(a)* an asymptomatic infection with transient excretion of organisms in the stool, *(b)* enterocolitis, *(c)* enteric fever, or *(d)* bacteremia with possible seeding of distant sites. Factors that reduce gastric acidity or alter gut flora enhance the probability of infection. Impaired host defenses such as malnutrition, malignancy, corticosteroids, or immunosuppressive drugs also predispose the patient to infection. Patients with hemolysis, as may occur in sickle cell disease, malaria, and bartonellosis, have increased incidence of *Salmonella* infections.

Salmonella produces diarrhea by mucosal invasion and elaboration of an entertoxin. Once past the mucosa, organisms multiply in the intestinal lymph follicles and progress to invade mesenteric lymph nodes. Bacteremia occurs, with organisms reaching liver, spleen, bone, heart, kidneys, meninges, gallbladder, and bile. The presence of preexisting conditions, such as aneurysms, bone infarcts, and gallstones, predisposes the patient to localized *Salmonella* infections or abscess formation. Gallstones particularly favor chronic biliary infection and a chronic enteric carrier state.

Clinical Manifestations

Salmonella infections result in several clinical syndromes: enterocolitis; enteric fever; bacteremia; chronic carrier states, either urinary or fecal excretors; and localized infections.

Enterocolitis

Acute enterocolitis is the most common form of salmonellosis. Six to 48 hours after ingestion of a contaminated source, the onset of nausea and vomiting, myalgias, headache, and diarrhea occur. Stool may vary from small frequent watery movements to tenesmus and frank dysentery. Abdominal cramps and fever are usually present. Fever usually lasts 2 to 3 days, and diarrhea usually resolves after 5 to 7 days. Colonic involvement is more frequent than suspected (42–45), and sigmoidoscopic examination often shows hyperemia, friability, petechiae, and ulcerations. Biopsy specimens will show inflammation, edema, erosions, and microabscesses.

Thirty to fifty percent of patients will continue to have positive stool cultures 2 or more weeks after clinical symptoms have resolved. Five percent of patients will have positive stool cultures 2 months after onset. Almost all adults' stools will be negative by 6 months. Patients excreting organisms for 1 year or longer are chronic enteric carriers. This is uncommon with nontyphoidal *Salmonella*.

Enteric Fever

S. typhi produces a clinical syndrome of enteric fever manifested by insidious onset of high unremitting fevers, malaise, headache, anorexia, and initial constipation that gives way to profuse watery diarrhea. Cough, myalgias, prostration, chills, and abdominal pains are invariably present. Characteristic rose spots are observed in less than half the cases. Lymphadenopathy, abdominal tenderness, rales, and hepatomegaly are often prominent physical findings (45,46).

Without antibiotic treatment the course of illness is slow, with resolution over 4 to 6 weeks. High fevers, confusion, abdominal pain, and diarrhea are most prominent in the second and third weeks. Treatment will shorten the febrile illness to 3 to 5 days, but response is influenced by the stage of the illness when antibiotics are started (46).

In addition to *S. typhi*, *S. paratyphi A*, *S. schottmülleri*, and *S. hirschfeldii* can produce an enteric fever clinical syndrome. Diagnosis is made by positive blood cultures. Positive stool cultures in the presence of a characteristic clinical course, although of presumptive value, are not diagnostic. Serologic studies are generally not helpful in confirming acute enteric fever. Blood cultures are positive in 80% of untreated patients and may remain so for several weeks if left untreated.

Complications of enteric fever include myocarditis, hemorrhage, abscess, bowel perforation, coagulopathy, meningitis, endocarditis, osteomyelitis, pneumonia, and bone marrow suppression. Relapse occurs in 10% of patients and may be higher in patients treated with antibiotics. One to three percent of patients will become chronic carriers.

Bacteremia

Salmonella can produce a bacteremia in the absence of apparent enterocolitis or enteric fever. This is most characteristic of *S. choleraesuis*, in which there is a 50% incidence of bacteremia that presents clinically as hectic fevers, usually with negative stool cultures.

Chronic Carrier

Excretion of organisms in the stool for greater than 1 year is designated as a chronic carrier state. The incidence in *S. typhi* infection is between 1 and 3% and is rare in nontyphoidal illness. Chronic carriers are asymptomatic. Chronic carriers have a high incidence of biliary tract disease.

Therapy

Patients who are transient intestinal carriers or most patients with acute enterocolitis do not require antibiotics. Patients with prolonged or severe symptoms, bacteremia, or enteric fever require antibiotics. In addition, patients with enterocolitis and concomitant diseases, including lymphoma, sickle cell disease, and immunocompromised hosts, should also receive antibiotics.

Chloramphenicol is still the drug of choice for enteric fever (47). Ampicillin and amoxicillin are alternative therapies in chloramphenicol-resistant infections (48,49,50).

Ampicillin combined with probenecid is the treatment of choice for chronic carriers. A 75% failure rate in patients with gallbladder disease ultimately requires cholecystectomy.

AMEBIASIS

Entamoeba histolytica is acquired by ingestion of food or water contaminated by cysts. Excystation occurs in the small bowel, with trophozoites subsequently infecting the colon. Trophozoites then develop into cysts and are excreted in the stool. When diarrhea occurs trophozoites may also be excreted. There is no intermediate host. *Entamoeba histolytica* must be differentiated from other *Entamoeba* species. *E. histolytica* trophozoites are mobile and ingest red blood cells.

Epidemiology

Modes of transmission commonly involve infected water or vegetable sources. Distribution is worldwide. Venereal transmission is possible and quite common among the homosexual population.

Pathogenesis

Trophozoites invade colonic mucosa with the aid of ameboid motility and production of proteolytic enzymes. Invading amebae cause an inflammatory reaction, resulting in a small mucosal nodule with a microulcer at the center. When cut in cross sections, these form typical flask-shaped necrotic ulcers. Trophozoites spread laterally, undermining the colonic mucosa but generally do not penetrate the muscular layers. Vascular compromise of the mucosa results in 1- to 2-cm ulcerated areas of sloughing mucosa. In severe disease, trophozoites may penetrate through the muscular layers, resulting in perforation.

The most common extraintestinal site of infection is the right lobe of the liver, where trophozoites are delivered via the portal vein. Lung, brain, or skin involvement may occur but less commonly.

Infections are often asymptomatic but when present are a result of tissue invasion by trophozoites. Cramps, fever, and bloody diarrhea may last from days to weeks. Stools are often foul smelling and watery and contain exudate and blood.

Diagnosis

Careful evaluation for amebae should be undertaken in the evaluation of chronic diarrhea. Identification of *E. histolytica* in the stool or in scrapings of rectal ulcers confirms the diagnosis. Use of bismuth, kaolin, barium, or antibiotics may render the feces unsatisfactory for evaluation. Specimens should be obtained prior to the administration of any of these agents. Enema preparations will destroy trophozoites and distort cysts. Adequate specimens may not be obtainable for 10 to 14 days after these substances have been given.

Sigmoidoscopy will show typical 1- to 2-mm well-circumscribed punched-out raised ulcers. Whitish or yellow exudate covers the base of the ulcer. Atypical ulcers with irregular margins occur in 10% of cases. Sigmoidoscopy is invaluable in diagnosis and should be performed without prior preparation to avoid removal of the exudate covering the ulcer base and damage to cysts or trophozoites. Microulcers may be difficult to differentiate from prominent crypts, and small ulcerations may be difficult to see unless surrounded by a rim of inflammation. Sigmoidoscopic appearance may vary from mild diffuse erythema to a picture indistinguishable from ulcerative colitis.

Serologic tests are of limited value in evaluation of diarrheal diseases. These tests are often positive months or years after cure. Serologic tests are valuable, however, in excluding invasive amebiasis.

Prognosis and Treatment

The most serious complication of amebic infection is liver abscess. Colonic strictures, perforation, hemorrhage, and intussusception may also complicate amebiasis. Because immunity does not occur, reinfection is likely. Opinions vary, but probably even asymptomatic amebiasis should be treated.

Metronidazole is the drug of choice in symptomatic intestinal disease. Emetine dihydrochloride alone will not eradicate intestinal infection. Chloroquine phosphate is not effective for intestinal infection and is used only for treatment of liver abscess. After treatment is completed, stools should be examined at monthly intervals for 3 months and repeated again at 6 months to assure treatment success.

CAMPYLOBACTER

Campylobacter is often found as a commensal in the gastrointestinal tracts of both domestic and wild animals. Human infection results from ingestion of infected food sources. Uncooked meats and poultry, unpasteurized milk, surface and municipal water sources, raw shellfish, and contact with infected household pets have all been identified as sources of infection.

Pathogenesis

Campylobacter jejuni multiplies in bile and infects small bowel and colon. Diffuse, bloody, exudative enteritis with biopsies showing an inflammatory infiltrate of neutrophils, mononuclear cells, crypt abscesses, and mucosal ulcerations is characteristic of *Campylobacter* infection. Biopsies are nonspecific and may be indistinguishable from ulcerative colitis or Crohn's colitis (51). The presence of bacteremia in some patients indicates mucosal invasion as one possible mechanism producing diarrhea.

Campylobacter will be present in the stool for 2 to 4 weeks after symptoms resolve. Antibiotic treatment does result in rapid elimination of the organism from the stool. Most cases of bacteremia are caused by *C. fetus* even though *C. jejuni* is a more common pathogen. Most patients infected with *C. jejuni* were previously healthy, whereas infection with *C. fetus* often occurs on the background of impaired immunity, as may occur in alcoholics, diabetics, and patients with malignancies (52).

Acute enteritis lasting from 1 day to 1 to 2 weeks with prodromal symptoms of myalgias, fever, headache, and malaise is common. Diarrhea may be watery or frankly bloody. Abdominal cramps are a prominent manifestation of the illness and are often improved with defecation. Infection is self-limited, and in only 10% of cases do symptoms last longer than one week. Relapse occurs in 5 to 10% of cases (53,54).

Acute colitis is also common and may lead to toxic megacolon (55). Because *Campylobacter* often infects younger patients, symptoms of acute colitis caused by *Campylobacter* may be confused with ulcerative colitis or Crohn's colitis. Acute right lower quadrant pain, in the absence of diarrhea, simulating acute appendicitis as well as mesenteric adenitis and acute ileitis, has been reported (56,57). Bacteremia occurs in less than 1% of *C. jejuni* infections. *C. fetus* infection often produces more pronounced systemic symptoms than infections caused by *C. jejuni.* A variety of local infections, including mycotic aneurysms, endocarditis, septic arthritis, thrombophlebitis, and peritonitis, has been reported as complicating *C. fetus* infections (58–60).

Therapy

Most patients do not require treatment beyond attention to fluid and electrolyte balance. Patients with high fever, bloody diarrhea, or symptoms lasting longer than 1 week may benefit from antibiotic therapy (53,57). Unlike *Salmonella,* antibiotic treatment does not prolong the fecal excretion of the organism and in fact will eliminate fecal carriage within 3 days. Erythromycin is the antibiotic of choice, but tetracycline, clindamyin, chloramphenicol, and aminoglycosides are also effective (61,62). Newer quinolones are also effective and are under investigation as to efficacy and side effects (63,64).

SEXUALLY TRANSMITTED DISEASES

In 1977, Sohn and Robilotti coined the term "gay bowel syndrome" to describe a group of colonic and rectal diseases sharing a common mode of sexual transmission. Although not limited to the homosexual population, male homosexuals appear at greatest risk (65). In addition, to the diseases conventionally considered to be transmitted sexually—syphilis, gonorrhea, lymphogranuloma venereum, and granuloma inguinale—diseases such as amebiasis, shigellosis, condyloma acuminatum, hepatitis, trauma, anal fissures, and abscess also fall under the broad term "gay bowel syndrome." Collectively this term refers to proctologic complications of oral-anal, oral-genital, or proctogenital intercourse and pathologic conditions occurring in high frequency in homosexuals but not exclusive to that group. To this group of diseases, we must now add an entire new spectrum of opportunistic bowel infections affecting a new group of immunocompromised patients—patients with acquired immunodeficiency syndrome (AIDS).

Organisms such as cryptosporidium, isobella, herpes, Histoplasma, Candida, Mycobacterium tuberculosis, atypical myobacterium and cytomegalovirus have a prominent role in producing diarrheal illness in AIDS patients.

Gonorrhea

Gonorrhea is the leading reported venereal disease in the United States (66). Anorectal gonorrhea occurs most commonly in women as a complication of genital infections and in homosexual men. Direct inoculation by rectal intercourse is the most obvious route of infection, but autoinoculation by vaginal secretion may be an alternative mode of transmission in women. Still, 75% of women with anorectal gonorrhea admit to having rectal intercourse (67). In men, anorectal gonorrhea is almost exclusively a result of homosexual or bisexual anal intercourse.

Clinical Manifestations

Stratified squamous epithelium is resistant to invasion by the gonococcus, but columnar or transitional epithelium in the anorectal area is easily penetrated. Two-thirds of anorectal infections are asymptomatic (68).

When symptoms do occur they are nonspecific and more likely related to associated trauma. Rectal itching, burning, tenesmus, and mucoid discharge may occur but in no greater incidence in culture-positive patients than in culture-negative homosexual patients (69). Symptoms more suggestive of gonorrheal infection, such as hematochezia, severe rectal pain, mucopurulent discharge, or ischiorectal abscess, occur in less than 5% of cases. In most cases, symptoms rapidly resolve, and an asymptomatic carrier state results.

Anorectal gonorrhea may simulate a variety of disorders, including ulcer-

ative colitis, Crohn's colitis, radiation proctitis, amebiasis, lymphogranuloma venereum, and syphilis. Only rectal culture is diagnostic. Complications such as fissures, fistulas, strictures, or abscesses are uncommon since the advent of antibiotics. Septicemia and disseminated gonococcemia have been reported after anorectal infection (70).

Diagnosis

Anoscopy is normal in 20% of culture-proven cases. Rectal smears are positive in only 30% of culture-positive cases. Definitive diagnosis is based on culture results. A gram-stained smear is likely to miss 70% of cases, but a positive smear in high-risk patients is an indication for treatment, even in the absence of symptoms.

Cultures can be taken blindly without the use of the sigmoidoscope or anoscope. A cotton swab is placed in the anal canal and rotated side to side. Immediate inoculation will yield the best results. Multiple sites, including urethra, pharynx, and cervix, should also be cultured. False-negative cultures may be as high as 8% in suspicious cases, cultures should be repeated.

Sigmoidoscopic examination shows generalized erythema and friability. Mucopurulent exudate may cover the mucosa, and superficial ulceration limited to the anal canal and rectum may be seen. The distal anal canal is spared because of the stratified squamous epithelium. Patchy erythema, granularity, and pus expressed from the anal crypts and columns of Morgagni may be seen in milder cases, with crypt abscesses seen in more severe infections. The susceptibility of the transitional columnar epithelium in the anal canal area, as well as lack of easy drainage from these blind-end crypts, facilitates infection. Biopsies show neutrophilic, lymphocytic infiltration with vascular engorgement. Patchy disorganization of the surface epithelium and mucosal destruction may occur (71).

Treatment

Penicillin remains the drug of choice. Aqueous procaine penicillin G, 4.8 million units IM, with 1 g of oral probenecid has only a 2% failure rate. Alternative regimens with spectinomycin 2 g IM, ampicillin 3.5 g orally with probenecid, or 4 to 6 g of oral tetracycline or ceftriaxone, cefoxitin, or cefuroxime are equally effective (72, 49).

Careful cultures taken 7 to 14 days after treatment is completed are of utmost importance, as is avoidance of sexual activity until the results of posttreatment cultures are known. Persistent symptoms after culture-proven cure should prompt a search for herpes virus, chlamydiae, enteric pathogens or protozoans.

Syphilis

Patients with both primary and secondary syphilis may have anorectal involvement, with at least 50% of extragenital chancres occurring in homosexual men (73). No single finding is pathognomonic for anorectal syphilis. A primary chancre may be situated at the anal verge or within the anal canal. Chancres rarely occur on the rectal mucosa. Chancres appear at the site of sexual contact within 4 weeks of exposure. In addition to chancres, ulcerations, fissures, polyps, and mucosal friability may occur in anorectal syphilis. The classic indurated painless ulcer seen in primary genital syphilis is less common in anorectal disease. Atypical ulcers may be confused with Crohn's disease, squamous cell cancers of the anus, or adenocarcinomas of the rectum. Inguinal adenopathy is common.

Primary anorectal syphilis may produce mild nonspecific symptoms of itching, soreness, discharge, or painful defecation. Diagnosis is based on serology, anoscopy, and darkfield examination of anal lesions. Serologic tests for syph-

ilis do not become positive for several weeks after the appearance of the primary chancre.

The characteristic anorectal lesion of secondary syphilis is a condyloma latum. Condylomata are multiple oval flat hypertrophic grayish papules frequently associated with a maculopapular rash on the trunk, extremities, palms, and soles; lymphadenopathy; and pharyngeal and palatal ulcers. Nonspecific perianal itching or discomfort may be present but condylomata lata are usually asymptomatic. Anorectal ulcers, especially when associated with inguinal adenopathy, should suggest a diagnosis of syphilis. Serologic tests for syphilis are positive in all cases of secondary syphilis and when the anorectal lesions are teeming with treponemas on darkfield examination. Tertiary syphilis involvement of the anorectal area with gummas is rare.

Diagnosis
The diagnosis of anorectal syphilis is supported by positive serology, demonstration of *Treponema pallidum* by darkfield examination, and occurrence of a Jarisch-Herxheimer reaction after initiation of antibiotics. Silver stain examination of rectal biopsies may demonstrate spirochetes, but the use of immunofluorescent stains increases the sensitivity.

Treatment
Penicillin is the antibiotic of choice, but tetracycline or erythromycin may be substituted in penicillin-allergic patients. Patients must avoid sexual activity until posttreatment follow-up examination confirms noninfectivity. Sexual contacts for the prior 3 months in cases of primary syphilis and 1 year in secondary syphilis must be contacted and tested serologically.

Herpes
Second only to gonorrheal proctitis, herpes proctitis is a leading cause of anorectal disease and is the responsible agent in 30% of male homosexuals with proctitis. Most cases of anorectal herpes are due to anal coitus spreading herpes simplex virus type II. Cases of proctitis caused by herpes simplex virus type I have also been reported and may be spread by oral-anal contact.

The incubation period for herpes proctitis varies from 4 to 20 days. An asymptomatic carrier state known to occur in genital herpes has not been shown for anorectal herpes.

Itching, soreness, and rectal pain are characteristic. Pain may be so severe as to radiate into the buttocks and thighs and may increase with ambulation. Constipation, tenesmus, mucoid rectal discharge, and systemic symptoms of malaise, fever, and chills are frequent. Severe constipation and acute urinary retention may be due to pain-induced reflex spasm of anal and bladder sphincters or as a result of a viral radiculopathy.

Examination of the anal area reveals clusters of vesicles or ulcerations. In one-third of cases only the perianal skin will be involved; in another one-third of cases only the anal canal will be involved; and in the remaining one-third of cases both areas will be affected. Vesicles will rupture after a few days, exposing superficial ulceration that may coalesce to form large irregular ulcers. Sigmoidoscopic evaluation will show friability of the distal 10 cm of the rectum. Tender bilateral inguinal adenopathy is frequent (74). The infection is usually self-limited, resolving in 2 to 3 weeks. Recurrence is the rule, with over 60% experiencing a recurrence within a year.

Diagnosis can be confirmed by observing a characteristic cytopathic effect on appropriately inoculated tissue culture. Scrapings from the base of ulcerated lesions can be observed for the presence of Cowdry type A intranuclear inclusion bodies within multinucleated giant cells. Unless the patient has been previously exposed, serologic tests during acute infection will be negative. Antibodies will appear 2 to 4 weeks after infection.

Treatment

Treatment is predominately supportive with sitz baths, analgesics, and suppositories. Steroid-containing creams are best avoided. Use of acyclovir, which has been beneficial in genital herpes virus infections, has been disappointing in anorectal disease (75,76). Exposed lesions can be treated with photoinactivation. Recurrent attacks are common, and the patient should be advised about the high likelihood of recurrence. All patients with herpetic proctitis should also be tested for syphilis, as there is a high rate of coinfection (77).

Lymphogranuloma Venereum

Lymphogranuloma venereum (LGV) is a rare disorder caused by *Chlamydia trachomatis,* also known to cause trachoma, psittacosis, inclusion conjunctivitis, and genital and perianal infections. Although known since 1932, anogenital LGV is still rarely diagnosed (78).

Small painless vesicular lesions appear at the inoculation site after a 5- to 28-day incubation period. These often remain unnoticed and resolve quickly. Three to 6 weeks after the initial lesion appears, tender fluctuant adenopathy with overlying superficial cellulitis develops. These tender "buboes" are associated with fever, malaise, anorexia, arthralgias, and cephalgia. The organisms spread by way of pelvic lymphatics, resulting in chronic inflammation, pelvic pain, edema, fistulas, and rectal strictures. Rectal discharge, abscess, cryptitis, and hematochezia are frequent (74).

Diagnosis

Physical examination will reveal tender inguinal adenopathy, abdominal and pelvic tenderness, perianal granulomas, fistulas, rhagades, or dependent edema due to lymphatic blockage. Digital rectal examination may be normal in early stages of infection. Strictures develop in later stages of infection and are usually well within reach of the examining finger. Proctoscopic examination shows acute proctitis marked by friability; ulcerations; and characteristic macular, papular, and vesicular lesions occurring together. Frei's test will become positive 7 to 40 days after the onset of adenitis and will remain so for life. Its usefulness in diagnosing acute proctitis caused by LGV is limited by its cross-reactivity to other non-LGV chlamydial strains. A complement fixation test titer is greater than 1:32 in 80% of cases with acute proctitis. A four-fold rise in serum titers is considered evidence of recent infection. Radiation proctitis, ulcerative proctitis, and amebic and tuberculous rectal infections can be differentiated from LGV proctitis by clinical, serologic, sigmoidoscopic, and histologic means. Difficulty may arise in differentiating LGV proctitis and Crohn's proctitis with isolated rectal involvement. Both may histologically reveal granulomata, crypt abscesses, and giant cells. Response to antibiotics may help establish a diagnosis of LGV over Crohn's proctitis.

Treatment

Supportive measures include bowel rest, analgesics, and low-residue diet. Fluctuant buboes should be aspirated, not incised. Tetracycline, erythromycin, and chloramphenicol may help control symptoms. Surgical intervention is reserved for strictures not responsive to dilatation, rectal abscesses, fistulas, or complicating carcinomas.

AIDS AND THE GI TRACT

The virus that causes AIDS, the human immunodeficiency virus (HIV), is a ribonucleic acid (RNA) virus with specific receptors for T-4 lymphocytes. The virus may invade macrophages as well as colonic epithelium. Once inside the T-4 lymphocyte, the virus produces reverse transcriptase, which allows a

deoxyribonucleic acid (DNA) copy of the virus's RNA genome to be produced. Once established, this DNA is incorporated into the native DNA of the lymphocyte and remains there for the life of the lymphocyte. Once infected, the virus will activate, producing daughter copies of its RNA genome, which bud away from the T-4 lymphocyte and infect other cells. As they rupture out of the T-4 lymphocyte, these lymphocytes are destroyed, resulting in an eventual depletion of T-4 lymphocytes. This plays a critical role in producing a defect in cell-mediated immunity. The result is a host with increased susceptibility to cellular rather than humorally mediated infections.

Once exposed to the virus, individuals will develop an acute mononucleosis-like illness, accompanied by diarrhea in 50% of the patients. Symptoms will last about 3 weeks and resolve spontaneously. Seroconversion will occur during this period. Individuals then become asymptomatic, with a latent incubation period often lasting from 2 to 5 years. Patients are infectious during this time.

By 1990, it is estimated that in the United States alone over 240,000 AIDS cases will be diagnosed. The high-risk groups include homosexual or bisexual men, intravenous drug users, and transfusion recipients. About 1% of cases occur in heterosexuals who are not recognized to be in a high-risk group. Today it is estimated that about 200,000 heterosexual contacts have been exposed to the HIV virus. This virus, however, is not very infectious outside of sexual exposure or exposure to blood or blood products. The risk to family members, health care personnel, or casual contacts is very low (79,80,81).

In homosexual men, the most common gastrointestinal infections include rectal gonorrhea, *Chlamydia*, syphilis, *Campylobacter, Shigella* and *Salmonella*. Anorectal herpes, cytomegalic virus, papilloma virus (anal warts), giardiasis, and amebiasis commonly occur in homosexual men (82–87).

Gastrointestinal infections in the immunosuppressed population include these common agents as well as gastrointestinal candidiasis, histoplasmosis, herpes simplex, mycobacteria (including both *Mycobacterium tuberculosis* and *Mycobacterium intracellulare*), cryptosporidiosis, and *Isospora* (88–92).

In AIDS patients presenting with diarrhea, careful investigation and cultures will reveal a causative agent in about half of the cases. In a large group, however, no identifiable pathogen can be determined. Signs and symptoms in AIDS patients are often nondiagnostic and rarely suggest a specific cause. Multiorganism infections are the rule rather than the exception. Difficulty may be encountered in distinguishing true infections from colonization. Cultures and serology often are positive in AIDS patients and do not accurately reflect actual tissue invasion. Symptoms most commonly include diarrhea, dysphagia, weight loss, abdominal pain, jaundice, hepatomegaly, and bleeding (93).

Diarrhea is the most common complaint, occurring in 50 to 90% of patients. Diarrhea usually is watery and secretory, often associated with steatorrhea and hypokalemia. D-xylose tests often are positive, implying mucosal malabsorption. Typically *M. avium-intracellulare* can produce a malabsorption picture similar to Whipple's disease and is the most common cause of malabsorption in AIDS patients. In at least half of the cases of diarrhea, an etiologic agent cannot be identified. These idiopathic cases have coined the term "AIDS enteropathy" (94,95). In patients with true colitis and bloody diarrhea, sigmoidoscopy should be performed, including cultures and biopsies that seek mucosal invasion by cytomegalic virus or herpes virus. Cryptosporidia, *Isospora,* and protozoan infections also may cause an enteritis or a colitis that may be diagnosed by culture and biopsy.

Thrush should always be looked for in cases of chronic diarrhea. Thrush

may be the primary indicator leading the physician to suspect an immuno-deficiency problem. It may be treated with oral Ketoconazole 200 mg twice daily until symptoms resolve or with oral Nystatin. Resistant cases may require treatment with Amphotericin (96). Unfortunately, no effective treatment exists for cryptosporidiae. Support with intravenous fluids and attention to acid-base and electrolyte balance is all that is available at this time (97).

Anal herpes can be treated with intravenous Acyclovir 5 mg per kilogram every 8 hours for 7 to 10 days, then oral Acyclovir one tablet five times daily. Once controlled, recurrences can be suppressed by Acyclovir twice daily.

Microbacterium intracellulare also is very difficult to treat, and a proven effective regimen does not exist. However, care must be taken to differentiate this organism from *Mycobacterium tuberculosis,* which is treatable using a two- or three-drug regimen. Cytomegalic virus is ubiquitous in the immuno-suppressed AIDS population, and no effective treatment exists. Experimental drugs, such as D.H.P.G., are being tested (98).

Microsporidia requires electron microscopy for accurate diagnosis. As yet, no effective treatment exists. Presentation is similar to *Isospora* and crypto-sporidiae with a fulminant diarrheal illness.

Gastrointestinal malignancies also occur in AIDS patients. Kaposi's sarcoma occurs most commonly, but non-Hodgkin's lymphoma, Burkitt's lymphoma, carcinoma of the rectum, and hairy leukoplakia also occur. Kaposi's sarcoma usually is dermatologic, but about 60% of patients with cutaneous Kaposi's also will have gastrointestinal involvement. Endoscopic biopsies of gastrointestinal Kaposi's often are nondiagnostic because of the submucosal location of these lesions. Clinical sequelae from enteric Kaposi's are uncommon, but the prognosis is worse in AIDS patients with gastrointestinal involvement (99).

Risks to health care personnel are small, yet some precautions should be observed. There are no reported cases of antibody conversion after mucosal splashes or any other exposures except for needle-puncture parenteral-type injury. Needles should not be recapped and kept; they should be disposed of in a puncture-proof container. Despite the low risk associated with mucosal exposure, gloves, goggles, masks, and protective gowns are still recommended for physicians and nurses during endoscopic procedures. Double bagging of disposable waste also is recommended. Use of disposable materials, where possible, is advisable. Lens instruments, such as endoscopes or sigmoido-scopes, should be washed with a glutaraldehyde solution and immersed for at least 30 minutes. Gas sterilization is not necessary (100).

References

1. Ammon HV, Soergel KH. Diarrhea. In: Berk JE, ed. Bockus Gastroenterology. Philadelphia: WB Saunders, 1985:125–141.
2. Lifshitz F, Coello-Ramirez R, Gutierrez-Topete G, Cornado-Cornet MC. Carbohydrate intolerance in infants with diarrhea. J Pediatr 1971;79:760–767.
3. Kim K, DuPont HL, Pickering LK. Outbreaks of diarrhea associated with Clostridium difficile and its toxin in day care centers: Evidence of person-to-person spread. J Pediatr 1983;102:376–382.
4. Pickering KL, Evans DG, DuPont HL, Vollet JJ, Evans DJ. Diarrhea caused by Shigella, rotovirus, and Giardia in day care centers. J Pediatr 1981;99:51–56.
5. Harris JC, DuPont HL, Hornick RB. Fecal leukocytes in diarrheal illness. Ann Intern Med 1972;76:697–703.

6. Anand BS, Malhotra V, Bhattacharya SK, Datta P, Datta D, Sen D, Mukherjee PP. Rectal histology in acute bacillary dysentery. Gastroenterology 1986;90:654–660.
7. Sack RB, Cassels J, Mitra R, Merritt C, Butler T, Thomas J, Jacobs B, Chaudhur A, Mondal A. The use of oral replacement solutions in the treatment of cholera and other severe diarrheal disorders. Bull WHO 1970;43:351–360.
8. DuPont HL, Sullivan P, Pickering LK, Haynes G, Ackerman PB. Symptomatic treatment of diarrhea with bismuth subsalicylate among students attending a Mexican university. Gastroenterology 1977;73:715–718.
9. Schiller LR, Davis GR, Santa Ana CA, Morawski SG, Fordtran JS. Studies of the mechanism of the antidiarrheal effect of codeine. J Clin Invest 1982;70:999–1008.
10. DuPont HL, Hornick RB. Adverse effect of lomotil therapy in shigellosis. JAMA 1973;226:1525–1528.
11. Pickering KL, Feldman S, Ericksson CD, Cleary TG. Absorption of salicylate and bismuth from bismuth subsalicylate containing compound. J Pediatr 1981;99:654–656.
12. Lowenstein MS, Balows A, Gangarosa EJ. Turista at an international congress in Mexico. Lancet 1973;1:529.
13. Traveler's diarrhea: National Institutes of Health Concensus Development Report. Rev Infect Dis 1986;8:S109–S227.
14. Kean BH. Travelers' diarrhea: An overview. Rev Infect Dis 1986;8:S111–116.
15. Steffer R. Epidemiologic studies of traveler's diarrhea, severe gastrointestinal infections, and cholera. Rev Infect Dis 1986;8:122–130.
16. Merson MH, Morris GK, Sack DA, Wells JG, Feeley JC. Travelers' diarrhea in Mexico. NEJM 1976;294:1299–1305.
17. Kean BH. Diarrhea of travelers to Mexico. Summary of five year study. Ann Intern Med 1963;59:605–614.
18. Rowe B, Taylor J, Bettelheim KA. An investigation of travelers' diarrhea. Lancet 1970;1:1.
19. Gorbach SL, Kean BH, Evans DG. Travelers' diarrhea and toxigenic E. coli. NEJM 1975;292:933–936.
20. Sack DA, Kaminsky DC, Sack RB, et al. Enterotoxigenic E. coli diarrhea of travelers. A prospective study of American Peace Corps volunteers. Johns Hopkins Med J 1977;141:63–70.
21. Bolivar R, Conklin RH, Vollet JJ. Rotavirus in traveler's diarrhea; Study of adult student population in Mexico. J Int Dis 1978;137:324.
22. Report of Communicable Disease Surveillance Centre and Communicable Disease Unit. Campylobacter infections in Britain. Brit Med J 1978;1:1357.
23. International Conference on the Diarrhea of Travelers. J Int Dis 1978;137:355–369.
24. Kean BH, Schaffner W, Brennan RW. The diarrhea of travelers. Prophylaxis with phthalylsulfathiazole and neomycin sulfate. JAMA 1962;180:367–371.
25. Turner AC Travelers' diarrhea. A survey of symptoms, occurrence, and possible prophylaxis. Brit Med J 1967;4:653.
26. Sack DA, Kaminsky DC, Sack RB. Prophylactic doxycycline for traveler's diarrhea, result of a prospective double-blind study of Peace Corps volunteers in Kenya. NEJM 1978;298:758–763.
27. DuPont HL, Reves RR, Galindo E. Treatment of travelers' diarrhea with trimethoprim sulfamethoxazole and trimethoprim alone. NEJM 1982;307:841–44.
28. Johnson PC, Ericsson CD, DuPont HL, et al. Comparison of loperamide with bismuth subsalicylate for the treatment of acute traveler's diarrhea. JAMA 1986;255:757–760.
29. Reves RR, Johnson PC, Ericsson CD, DuPont HL. A cost-effectiveness comparison of the use of antimicrobial agents of treatment of prophylaxis of travelers' diarrhea. Arch Intern Med 1988; 148:2421–2427.
30. Ericsson CD, DuPont HL, Sullivan P, et al. Bicozamycin, a poorly absorbable antibiotic, effectively treats travellers' diarrhea. Ann Intern Med 1983;98:20–25.
31. Sack RB, Enterohemorrhagic Escherichia coli. Editorial. NEJM 1987;317:1535–1537.
32. Carter AD, Borczyk AA, Carlson JAK, et al. Severe outbreak of Escherichia coli 0157:H7—associated hemorrhagic colitis in a nursing home. N Engl J Med 1987;317:1496–1500.
33. O'Brien AD, Holmes RK. Shiga and shiga-like toxins. Microbiol Rev 1987;51:206–220.
34. Mandell W, Neu HC. Shigella bacteremia in adults. JAMA 1986;255:3116–3117.
35. DuPont HL, Hornick RB, Snyder MJ, et al. Protection induced by oral live vaccine or primary infection. J Infect Dis 1972;125:12–16.
36. Keusch GT. Shigellosis in bacterial infections of humans: Epidemiology and control. Evans AS, Feldman H, eds. New York: Plenum, 1982:487.

37. Sprinz H. Pathogenesis of intestinal infections. Arch Path 1969;87:556–562.

38. DuPont H, Hornick R. Adverse effects of Lomotil therapy in shigellosis. JAMA 1973;226:1525–1526.

39. Weissman J, Gangarosa E, Dupont H. Changing needs in the antimicrobial therapy of shigella. J Infect Dis 1973; 127:611–613.

40. Nelson JD, Kusmiesz H, Jackson LH. Trimethoprim-sulfamethoxazole therapy of shigellosis. JAMA 1976;235:1239–1243.

41. Chmel H, Armstrong D. Salmonella oslo: A focal outbreak in a hospital. Am J Med 1976;60:203–208.

42. Dean AG. Transmission of S. typhi by fiberoptic endoscopy. Lancet 1977;2:134.

43. Dwyer DM, Klein EG, Istre GR, et al. Salmonella newport infections transmitted by fiberoptic colonoscopy. Gastrointest Endosc 1987;33:84–87.

44. Bennett IL Jr, Hook EW. Infectious diseases. Ann Rev Med 1959;10:1.

45. Mandal BK, Mani V. Colonic involvement of salmonellosis. Lancet 1976;1:887–890.

46. Aserkoff B, Bennett JV. Effect of antibiotic therapy in acute salmonellosis on fecal excretion of salmonellae. NEJM 1969;281:636–640.

47. Chin T. Therapy of salmonellosis. Ration Drug Ther 1976;10:1–5.

48. Pillay N, Adams EB, Coombs DN. Comparative trial of amoxycillin and chloramphenicol in treatment of typhoid fever in adults. Lancet 1975;2:333.

49. Goldberg DM. Update on antibiotics I: The cephalosporins. Med Clin North Am 1987;71:(6):1113–1133.

50. Parry MF. Update on antibiotics: The penicillins. Med Clin North Am 1987;71:1093–1112.

51. Lambert ME, Schofield PF, Ironside AG. Campylobacter colitis. Brit Med J 1979;1:857–858.

52. Wright EP, Seager J. Convulsions associated with Campylobacter enteritis. Brit Med J 1980;281:454.

53. Blaser MJ, Berkowitz ID, Laforce FM, et al. Campylobacter enteritis: Clinical and epidemiologic features. Ann Intern Med 1979; 91:179–183.

54. Blaser MJ, Reller B. Campylobacter enteritis. N Engl J Med 1981;305:1444–1452.

55. McKinley MJ, Taylor M, Sangree MH. Toxic megacolon with Campylobacter colitis. Conn Med 1980;44:496–497.

56. Skirrow MB. Campylobacter enteritis. A "new" disease. Brit Med J 1977;2:9–11.

57. Blaser MJ, Reller CB, Luechtefeldmu NW, et al. Campylobacter enteritis in Denver. West J Med 1982;136:287.

58. Franklin B, Ulmer DD. Human infections with Vibrio fetus. West J Med 1974;120:200.

59. Kilo C, Hagemann PO. Septic arthritis and bacteremia due to Vibrio fetus. Am J Med 1965;38:962–971.

60. Lawrence R, Nibbe AF. Lung abscess secondary to Vibrio fetus, malabsorption syndrome and acquired agammaglobulinemia. Chest 1971;60:191–194.

61. Vanhoof R, Vanderlinden MP, et al. Susceptibility of Campylobacter fetus subsp. jejuni to twenty-nine antimicrobial agents. Antimicrob Agents Chemother 1978;14:553–556.

62. Walder M. Susceptibility of Campylobacter fetus to twenty antimicrobial agents. Antimicrob Agents Chemother 1979;16:37–39.

63. Gorbarh SL, ed. Infectious diarrheas. Boston: Blackwell Scientific, 1986.

64. Levine MM. Antimicrobial therapy for infectious diarrhea. Rev Infect Dis 1986;8:S207–S216.

65. Sohn N, Robilotti JG Jr. The gay bowel syndrome. Am J Gastroenterol 1977;67:478–484.

66. Progress toward achieving the national 1990 objectives for sexually transmitted diseases. MMWR 1987;36:2141–2143.

67. Pariser H, Marino AF. Gonorrhea—frequently unrecognized reservoirs. South Med J 1970;63:198–201.

68. Owen RL, Hill JL. Rectal and pharyngeal gonorrhea in homosexual men. JAMA, 1972; 220(10):1315–1318

69. Lebedeff DA, Hochman EB. Rectal gonorrhea in men: Diagnosis and treatment. Ann Intern Med 1980;92:463–466.

70. Holmes KK, Counts GW, Beaty HN. Disseminated gonococcal infection. Ann Intern Med 1971;74:979–993.

71. William DC, Shookhoff HB, Feldman YM, et al. The utility of anoscopy in the rapid diagnosis of symptomtic anorectal gonorrhea in men. Sex Transm Dis 1981 Jan–Mar; 8(1):16–7.

72. Schroeter AL, Reynolds G. The rectal culture as a test of cure of gonorrhea in females. J Infect Dis 1972;125:499–503.

73. Quinn T. AIDS and other medical problems in the male homosexual: Clinical approach to intestinal infection in the homosexual male. Med Clin North Am 1986;70:611–634.

74. Rein MF. AIDS and other medical problems in the male homosexual: Clinical approach to urethritis, mucocutaneous lesions, and inguinal adenopathy in homosexual men. Med Clin North Am 1986;70:587–609.

75. Nahmias AJ, Roizman B. Infections with herpes simplex viruses 1 and 2. N Engl J Med 1973;289:667–673.

76. Rompalo AM, Mertz GJ, Mkrtichian EE. Oral acyclovir vs placebo for treatment of herpes simplex virus proctitis in homosexual men. Clin Res 1985;33:58A.

77. Catteral RD. Sexually transmitted diseases of the anus and rectum. Clin Gastroenterol 1975;4:659–669.

78. Bensaude R, Lambling A. Discussion on the etiology and treatment of fibrous strictures of the rectum. Proc R Soc Med 1935;29:1441–1446.

79. Human immunodeficiency virus infections in the United States: A review of current knowledge. MMWR 1987 (Suppl 5–6):9–12.

80. Selwyn P. AIDS: What is now known. Hosp Pract 1986;21:67–82.

81. Cates W. Epidemiology and control of sexually transmitted diseases: Strategic evolution. Infect Dis Clin North Am 1987;1:1–23.

82. Wexner SD, Smith WB, Milson JW, et al. The surgical management of anorectal diseases in AIDS and pre-AIDS patients. Dis Colon Rect 1986;29:719–723.

83. Quinn TC, Goodell SE, Mkrtchian E, et al. Chlamydia trachomatis proctitis. N Engl J Med 1981;305:195–200.

84. Allason-Jones E, Mindel A, Sargeaunt D, et al. Entamoeba histolytica as a commensal intestinal parasite in homosexual men. N Engl J Med 1986;315:353–356.

85. Goldmeter D, Sargeaunt PG, Price AB, et al. Is Entamoeba histolytica in homosexual men a pathogen? Lancet 1986;1:641–644.

86. Jacobs JL, Gold JWM, Murry HW, et al. Salmonella infections in patients with the acquired immunodeficiency syndrome. Ann Intern Med 1985;102:186–188.

87. Jacobson MA, Mills J. Serious cytomegalovirus disease in acquired immunodeficiency syndrome. Ann Intern Med 1988;108:585–594.

88. Evans P, Goldstein MJ, Sherlock P. Candida infections of the gastrointestinal tract. Medicine 1972;51:367–378.

89. Gillin JS, Urmacher C, West R, et al. Disseminated Mycobacterium avium-intracellulare infection in acquired immunodeficiency syndrome. Lancet 1983;1:956–958.

90. DeHovitz JA, Pape JW, Boncy M, et al. Clinical manifestations and therapy of Isospora belli infection in the patient with acquired immunodeficiency syndrome. N Engl J Med 1986;315:87–90.

91. Holley HP, Dover C. Cryptosporidium: A common cause of parasitic diarrhea in otherwise healthy individuals. J Infect Dis 1986;153:365–367.

92. Janoff EN. Cryptosporidium infections in the immunocompromised host. Immunocomp Host 1988;5:4.

93. Dworkin B, Wormer GP, Rosenthal WS, et al. Gastrointestinal manifestation of the acquired immunodeficiency syndrome. A review of 22 cases. Am J Gastroenterol 1985;80:774–778.

94. Gillin JS, Shike M, Alcock N, et al. Malabsorption and mucosal abnormalities of the small intestine in the acquired immunodeficiency syndrome. Ann Intern Med 1985;102:619–622.

95. Kotler DP, Gaetz HP, Lange M, et al. Enteropathy associated with the acquired immunodeficiency syndrome. Ann Intern Med 1984;101:421–428.

96. Klein RS, Harris CA, Small CB, et al. Oral candidiasis in the high-risk patients as the initial manifestation of acquired immunodeficiency syndrome. N Engl J Med 1984;311:354–358.

97. Navin TR, Juranet DD. Cryptosporidiosis: Clinical, epidemiologic and parasitologic review. Rev Infect Dis 1984;6:313–327.

98. Masur H, Lane HC, Palestine A, et al. Effect of 9-(1,3-dihydroxy-2-propoxymethyl) guanine on serious cytomegalovirus disease in eight immunosuppressed homosexual men. Ann Intern Med 1986;104:41–44.

99. Friedman SL. Gastrointestinal manifestation of AIDS: Gastrointestinal and hepatobiliary neoplasm in AIDS. Gastro Clin North Am 1988;17:465–486.

100. Raufman JP, Straus EW. Gastrointestinal manifestation of AIDS: Endoscopic procedures in the AIDS patient: Risks, precautions, indications and obligations. Gastro Clin North Am 1988;17:495–506.

14

Recognition of Pathology at Flexible Sigmoidoscopy

Melvin Schapiro, M.D.
Glen A. Lehman, M.D.

The editors gratefully acknowledge the following individuals for their kindness in allowing the use of their endoscopic photographs for reproduction in this atlas section:

Sharad Bellapravalu, MD
Sun City, Arizona

G. Peter Bloom, MD
Hartford, Connecticut

Steven Brozinsky, MD
San Diego, California

Peter Chen, MD
Ravenna, Ohio

Florian M. Cortese, MD
Hyde Park, New York

Barry Eisen, MD
Tulsa, Oklahoma

Michael F. Elmore, MD
Indianapolis, Indiana

John R. Hilsabeck, MD
GI Laboratory, St. Joseph's
Hospital of Orange California

Craig A. Johnson, MD
San Francisco, California

Rajinder Kaushal, MD
Valencia, California

N.V. Khaja, MD
Torrance, California

Errol Korn, MD
Chula Vista, California

Gustavo A. Machicado, MD
Northridge, California

James A. Magary, MD
Glendale, Arizona

Joel F. Panish, MD
Los Angeles, California

P.S. Ramanujam, MD
Sun City, Arizona

C.R. Tillman, MD
Natchez, Mississippi

Michael Shiffman, MD
Sherman Oaks, California

Vicente L. Villa, Jr., MD
Glendale, California

Gerald Winnan, MD
Frederick, Maryland

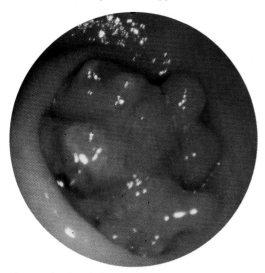

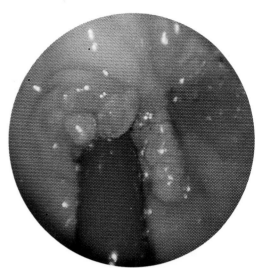

Figure 14.1. Colon cancer. This cancer has an unusual multinodular appearance and occupies the entire lumen. Attachment to the wall cannot be determined by this view.

Figure 14.3. Rectal CA on retroflex rectal view. This invasive colon cancer occupies 50% of the internal anal verge. All anal verge lesions are best viewed by a combination of forward and retroflex viewing. Biopsies are often more successful in the retroflex position.

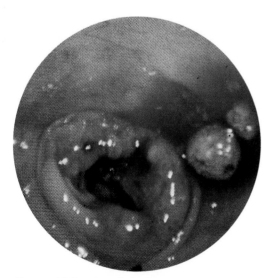

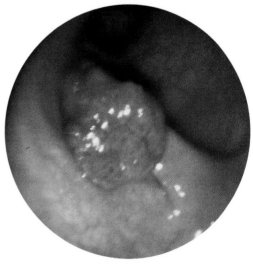

Figure 14.2. Annular adenocarcinoma. This is the most common appearance of carcinoma seen at sigmoidoscopy. The annular lesion has ulceration within the central portions and a typical shoulder, or shelf, at its junction with the normal mucosa.

Figure 14.4. 2-cm pedunculated polyp on a stalk. The lesion had focally invasive carcinoma in the tip of the polyp that did not involve the stalk.

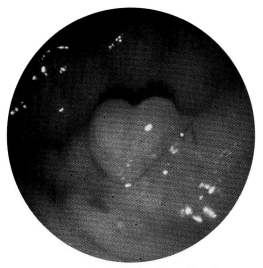

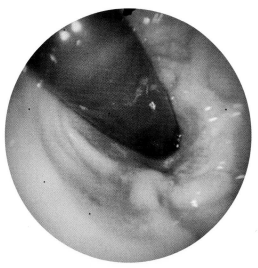

Figure 14.5. Small bilobed sessile adenoma. The pink color suggests an adenoma in contrast to the typical pale color of hyperplastic polyps.

Figure 14.7. Adenocarcinoma on retroflexed rectal view. Such lesions must be differentiated from thrombosed hemorrhoids or other inflammatory lesions.

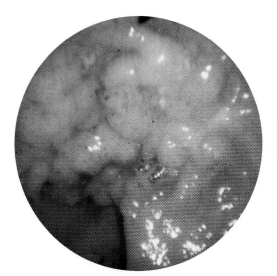

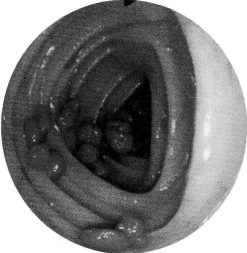

Figure 14.6. Villous adenoma of rectum. This soft pale, multinodular tumor has ill-defined borders that blend with the normal mucosa at the 6 o'clock through 3 o'clock positions.

Figure 14.8. Stool pellets with reddish color simulating polyps. Ingestion of red dye or pigment in foods such as tomatoes, peppers, beets, or red jello may produce such a picture.

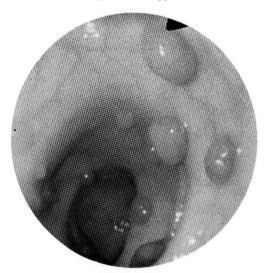

Figure 14.9. Familial polyposis. Numerous adenomatous polyps of varying size are scattered throughout this segment of the colon. Such patients have virtually a 100% chance of developing colon cancer.

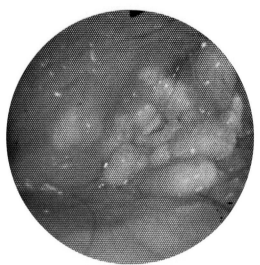

Figure 14.11. Anal canal condyloma accuminata as viewed through the sigmoidoscope. Such venereal warts are generally sexually transmitted and are viral in origin. These are usually restricted to squamous epithelium.

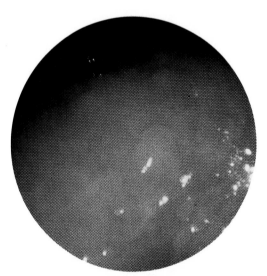

Figure 14.10. Small hyperplastic polyps less than 5 mm in size. These pale mucosal elevations have similar color as the background mucosa. These are more common in the rectum but require biopsy for confirmation of histology. They have no true neoplasm potential.

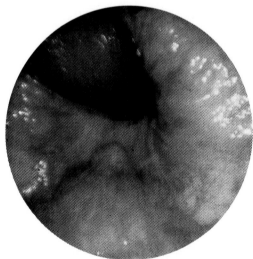

Figure 14.12. Internal hemorrhoids viewed from retroflexed rectal view. The internal sphincter is relaxed to view, and a major portion of the anal canal can be viewed.

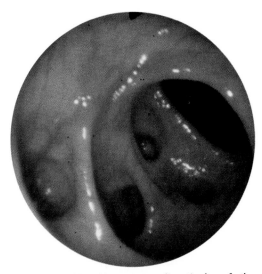

Figure 14.13. Numerous diverticula of the sigmoid colon. There is no evidence of diverticulitis present.

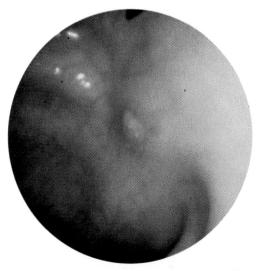

Figure 14.15. Ureterosigmoidostomy orifice. This lesion should not be mistaken for a polyp. Polypectomy, if performed, may result in ureteral obstruction, pyelonephritis, and loss of the kidney. Such patients need to be monitored for development of colon cancer.

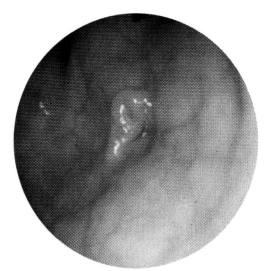

Figure 14.14. Partially inverted diverticulum of sigmoid colon. Diverticula may invert into the lumen and appear as a polypoid lesion. Biopsy or polypectomy may cause perforation. The dimpled tip on the inverted portion is characteristic and a clue to the true nature of the lesion.

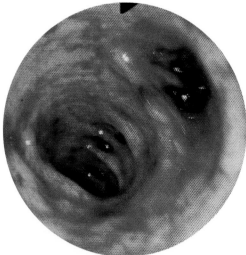

Figure 14.16. Diverticulosis with blood in lumen. Note the scattered blood in the lumen and dark clots within diverticula. Unless active bleeding is observed from a single diverticulum, the examiner is left with only the circumstantial evidence of diverticula and adjacent blood.

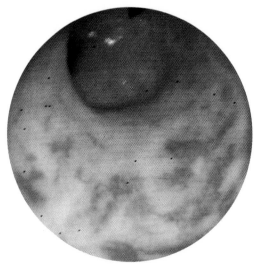

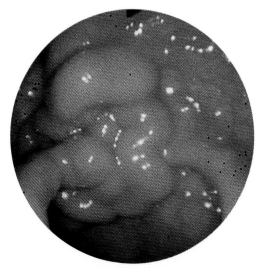

Figure 14.17. Radiation proctitis. The mucosa is somewhat atrophic with retraction of normal rectal valves. Friability is present, and many of the focal red areas are telangectoid vessels.

Figure 14.19. Rectal varices are present in a patient with known portal hypertension and esophageal varices. Such veins may occur with or without liver disease.

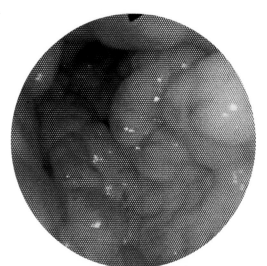

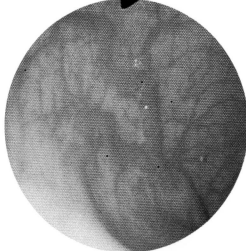

Figure 14.18. Pneumatosis coli. Multiple submucosal nodules are seen, covered by erythematous but otherwise normal mucosa. Biopsy may show gas-filled clefts. Biopsy at rigid sigmoidoscopy may be accompanied by an audible crackle or pop from escaping gas.

Figure 14.20. Prominent, but probably normal, veins in a patient with no history of portal hypertension or vascular disease.

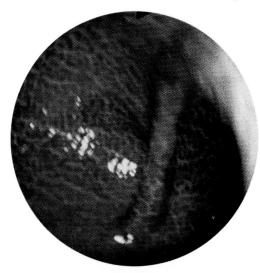

Figure 14.21. Melanosis coli. Note the dark pigment with a pale reticular background. This results from ingestion of anthracene laxatives. There is no pathologic significance.

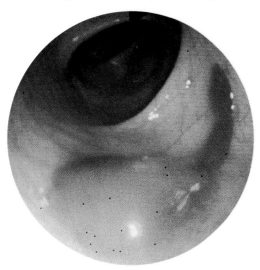

Figure 14.23. Submucosal hemorrhage that has assumed a cystic configuration. The dark color suggests that the hemorrhage is several days old. The endoscopist punctured the overlying mucosa and drained chocolate fluid, confirming the diagnosis.

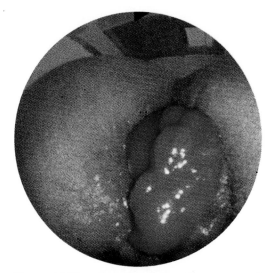

Figure 14.22. Rectal prolapse. The engorged rectal mucosa has prolapsed well beyond the anal canal. Such prolapse should generally be reduced before attempting the sigmoidoscopy.

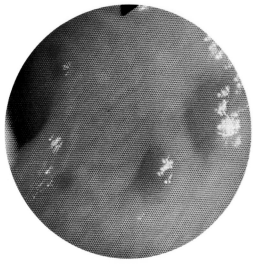

Figure 14.24. Kaposi's sarcoma. Variably sized, red to purple, sessile, plaquelike lesions are seen scattered throughout the visual field in this AIDS patient.

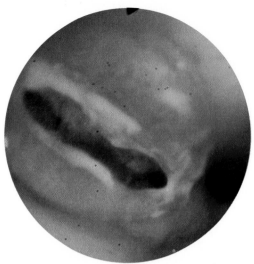

Figure 14.25. Large rectal fistula. The lumen is seen extending to the right, whereas the primary view is into the fistula. Exudate is seen at the fistula rim. The background colonic mucosa is mildly erythematous. Such a lesion would be strongly suggestive of Crohn's disease.

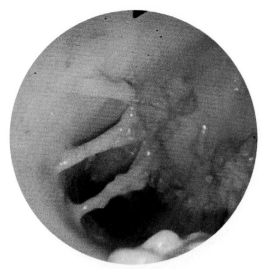

Figure 14.27. Mucosal bridges in a patient with chronic ulcerative colitis. Such bridges result from the healing phase of extensive mucosal ulceration of any etiology. Alternatively, such finger-like projections may be attached at only one end and would then be called filiform pseudopolyps. These have no neoplastic significance.

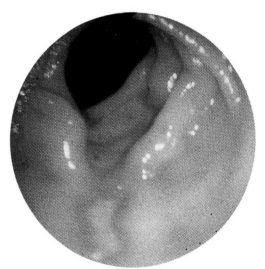

Figure 14.26. Crohn's disease. Linear ulceration with surrounding erythema is seen at the 5 o'clock position. Additional ulceration extends upstream and indents the haustral fold. Background mucosa is nearly normal.

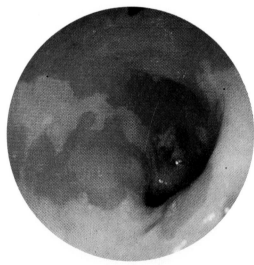

Figure 14.28. Ischemic colitis. Approximately 50% of the luminal view shows erythematous friable mucosa bordering on nearly normal mucosa at the 11 o'clock and 2 o'clock positions. Shallow ulcerations and/or exudate are evident in the 6 o'clock position over the most abnormal mucosa.

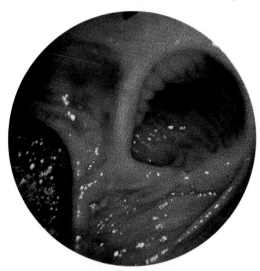

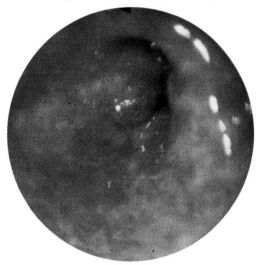

Figure 14.29. Patent ileocolonic anastomosis. The small bowel valvulae are evident as viewed through the anastomosis in the right upper quadrant of the photo.

Figure 14.31. Campylobacter colitis. There is a diffuse inflammatory process with loss of vascular pattern and small amounts of adherent purulent material. Biopsies showed acute inflammation without crypt abscesses or gland architecture distortion.

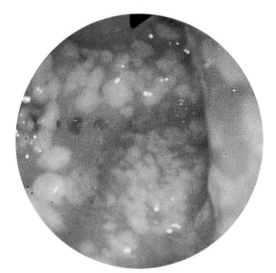

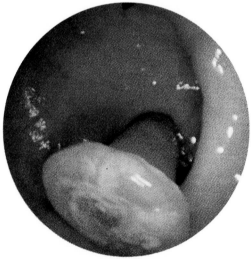

Figure 14.30. Pseudomembranous colitis. There are patchy adherent plaques or islands of exudate. The intervening mucosa may be normal or mildly inflamed. In severe cases the membrane may be confluent.

Figure 14.32. Retained Fleet enema tip. After self-administration of an enema, the enema tip dislodged from the bottle and migrated cephalad into the rectum. Such foreign bodies that are not spontaneously evacuated should be retrieved endoscopically.

15

Screening for Colorectal Cancer and Polyps in Average-Risk Persons

Douglas K. Rex M.D.

INTRODUCTION

The probability of 5-year survival for the patient with colorectal cancer is determined primarily by the extent of tumor invasion of the colon wall at the time of surgical or endoscopic resection. Since Dukes' original description of this critical relationship in 1932 (1), little progress has been made in the treatment of deeply invasive colorectal cancer. Today prevention and early detection are our most promising tools in the battle to improve survival in colorectal cancer.

The ideal preventive approach to cancer is *primary prevention*. This refers to the identification and elimination of environmental carcinogens that lead to the development of cancer. Much work in colorectal cancer has focused on the possible carcinogenic role of dietary fat and on the possible tumor-inhibiting influences of dietary fiber, calcium, vitamins A and C, and selenium (2). Although of great importance, this work has not yet produced an established, validated method of primary prevention of colorectal cancer.

In the past three decades much progress has been made in the *secondary prevention* of colorectal cancer. This approach involves the identification and removal of premalignant lesions (the adenomatous polyps) and of early-staged cancers for which surgical resection is curative. When secondary preventive techniques are applied to detect a disease at an asymptomatic stage the process is called *screening*. In this chapter we will focus on screening for colorectal cancer and colon polyps, with special emphasis on the role of flexible sigmoidoscopy. In the literature on flexible sigmoidoscopy the word "screening" sometimes is used to describe the evaluation of either symptomatic patients or asymptomatic patients who have another positive screening test, usually the fecal occult blood test (FOBT). In these settings the word "screening" is misleading because the yield and cost efficacy of flexible sigmoidoscopy, particularly for cancers, are much different than in asymptomatic patients with unknown or negative FOBT. In our discussion, screening flexible sigmoidoscopy will apply whenever possible to asymptomatic persons not selected for the results of FOBT.

Colorectal cancer is a disease that appears ideally suited to the development of effective screening methods. It is a common disease, with some 145,000 new cases occurring in the United States in 1987 (3), and is uniformly fatal if left untreated. It is a relatively slow-growing cancer, with a long asymptomatic phase. Tumors in asymptomatic persons have less advanced Dukes' stages (Table 15.1), and these persons probably have improved survival (4). However, improved survival because of early detection is not yet proven. Because of factors such as lead time bias (patients with tumors found by screening have longer postdiagnosis survival simply because of earlier discovery) and length bias (screening detects a disproportionate number of slow-growing tumors), only large randomized trials can prove survival benefit from screening (5). Two such trials of FOBT in screening for colorectal cancer are now in

Table 15.1.
Survival Distribution of Dukes' Classes in Symptomatic and Asymptomatic Patients

Dukes' Stage	Extent of Cancer	Symptomatic Patients (%)	Asymptomatic Persons (%)*	5-year Survival (%)
A	Mucosa	10	50	91
B	Bowel wall	30	25	64
C	Lymph nodes	40	20	30
D	Distant metastases	20	5	<5

*From Wihawer et al. Current status of fecal occult blood testing in screening for colorectal cancer. Cancer 1982;32:101–112.

progress in the United States (6,7) (see Chapter 1). Until the results of these trials are available, we will not be certain whether screening affects survival in colorectal cancer.

Of critical importance to the rationale for screening in colorectal cancer is the concept of the adenoma-carcinoma sequence. This concept is based on a series of indirect arguments (8) but is widely accepted by experts (9). According to this theory, greater than 90% of colorectal cancers arise within previously benign adenomatous polyps. Approximately 5% of adenomas will transform into malignancy over a typical interval of 5 to 10 years (10). In a landmark study, Gilbertsen demonstrated that regular proctoscopic removal of all rectal adenomas reduced the incidence of rectal cancer by 85% from expected (11). Gilbertsen's study design has been criticized (12), but the results suggest that identification and removal of colorectal adenomas actually prevents colorectal cancer. Given a choice between cancer prevention and cancer detection, prevention would seem preferable. This is of crucial importance to the role of flexible sigmoidoscopy in colorectal cancer screening, since endoscopic techniques are far superior to other screening methods for the detection of adenomatous polyps.

SCREENING IN THE AVERAGE-RISK PATIENT

About 20% of persons with colorectal cancer have an identifiable disease or inherited disorder associated with increased risk for development of colorectal cancer (see Chapter 1). These conditions can be easily screened for in the physician's office by routine use of a written patient questionnaire. Persons with these conditions require an aggressive screening program, which may begin at an early age and which should be tailored to the specific condition (see Chapter 1). The remaining 80% of persons with colorectal cancer have no identifiable genetic or disease factor that would increase the risk of developing colorectal cancer. Such persons are considered to have been at "average risk." In Western countries the incidence of colorectal cancer in average-risk persons begins to rise at age 40, rises rapidly after age 50, and continues to rise with increasing age until approximately age 85. Thus, virtually everyone in the United States age 40 or over has at least average risk for development of colorectal cancer. To emphasize this point, about 5% of persons in the United States will eventually develop colorectal cancer if current trends continue, and recent studies indicate that as many as 25% of the population over age 50 harbor an adenomatous polyp (13).

In 1980 the American Cancer Society issued guidelines for screening average-risk persons with colorectal cancer (Table 15.2). The most widely accepted and used aspect of these screening guidelines is the FOBT using guaiac impregnated slides. The use of guaiac slide tests has been reviewed in detail

Table 15.2.
American Cancer Society Guidelines for Screening in Average-Risk Persons

Age ≥ 40	Annual fecal occult blood test plus annual digital rectal examination
Age ≥ 50	Above *plus* annual sigmoidoscopy for 2 years and if negative sigmoido-scopy every 3–5 years thereafter

elsewhere (5) and in Chapter 1, and only a few practical points regarding implementation of the FOBT will be summarized here.

Clinicians planning to offer the FOBT to their patients do well to prepare a brief instruction sheet for home use. The sheet should include general information about the signs and symptoms of colorectal cancer, the purpose and limitations of FOBT, instructions for mailing the slide tests after completion, medications to be avoided during testing (iron, vitamin C, and aspirin if possible), and dietary instructions if desired. Companies providing home screening kits may have such instruction sheets available for inclusion with the kits. Our own practice is not to restrict the diet, since there is little evidence that diet restriction influences results as long as the slides are not rehydrated (14). Rehydration improves sensitivity but drops the positive predictive value for neoplasia from 50% to about 20% (5). If rehydration is used, it is important to restrict red meat intake in order to avoid an even lower positive predictive value.

Fecal material for slide testing commonly is obtained by one of two methods; one is by home collection, and the other is by digital rectal examination in the physician's office. In the first case, the screenee is instructed to collect samples from two different portions of stool on 3 consecutive days for a total of six samples. Collection of feces from areas that look obviously bloody is appropriate. Nearly all literature on the FOBT is derived from this type of home screening. One common error we encounter is that when a positive FOBT is obtained, the clinician elects to repeat the FOBT with the plan that if subsequent FOBT are negative the initial positive test may be ignored. In fact, bleeding from cancers usually is associated with only one or two positive samples out of six (15). Thus, a single positive FOBT should signal the need for full colon evaluation in the patient over age 40.

In the absence of an established home colorectal cancer screening program, many FOBT are performed by using feces obtained by the clinician during the digital rectal examination. A positive FOBT during rectal examination has theoretical disadvantages in that trauma might induce bleeding and because diet is less likely to be controlled. This question is of importance in some settings. At the Indiana University Medical Center, for example, a rectal examination is performed routinely on all patients admitted to the medical and surgical services. Thus, patients with a positive FOBT obtained during rectal examination constitute a major fraction of referrals for colonoscopy. During a recent prospective study of 332 patients at our institution, including both asymptomatic and symptomatic subjects with suspected lower gastrointestinal (GI) bleeding, most of whom were found by positive FOBT during rectal examination, 8% of those undergoing colonoscopy had cancer, and 38% had colon polyps (16). Thus, until further data are forthcoming, a positive FOBT obtained at the time of rectal examination should be followed by full colon evaluation.

The guaiac slide test as used for home colorectal cancer screening offers the advantages of simplicity, safety, and good acceptability to screenees and the materials needed to perform the tests are relatively inexpensive. Major problems with the slide tests are their imperfect sensitivity for colorectal cancer (70%), their poor sensitivity for polyps (<25%), and the considerable expense of evaluating the approximately 50% of persons with positive slide tests who have no colorectal neoplasm (polyp or cancer) when colonoscopy is performed (5).

Table 15.3 demonstrates the yield of FOBT and flexible sigmoidoscopy in a hypothetical population of 1000 asymptomatic, average-risk persons. The yields for FOBT are based on an expected positive slide rate of 2 to 4%. The positive predictive value of the slide test is assumed to be 10% for cancer and 35% for polyps (6,7).

The data in Table 15.3 regarding flexible sigmoidoscopy are taken from Table 15.4, which is a summary of the literature on flexible sigmoidoscopy in screening asymptomatic average-risk persons with 60-cm or longer scopes. Yields with 30- or 35-cm scopes would be expected to be only slightly less (17) (see Chapter 5). Note that flexible sigmoidoscopy detects few cancers in the asymptomatic population. In our hypothetical group of 1000 screenees, the actual yield of cancers detected by flexible sigmoidoscopy is similar to that detected using the FOBT. However, each screening modality will detect some cancers that the other technique misses. This is primarily because right-sided colon cancers bleed more than left-sided cancers and are more likely to produce a positive FOBT (32). Thus, the two tests should be considered complimentary in the detection of colorectal cancer. Table 15.3 demonstrates that the power of flexible sigmoidoscopy over occult blood screening lies in the detection of colon polyps. Here flexible sigmoidoscopy far exceeds the sensitivity of the FOBT. Several reports have found the sensitivity of the Hemoccult assay to be in the range of 3 to 19% for polyps (21,33). Thus, the FOBT clearly is not a sensitive technique for the detection of colon polyps. Although not all authors reporting the yield of flexible sigmoidoscopy for polyps (Table 15.4) provided a breakdown of the number of patients with adenomas versus hyperplastic polyps, the great majority of patients with polyps had adenomas in studies providing this data (18,23,26–28,31). Detection of patients with adenomas in the range of flexible sigmoidoscopy and enrollment of these patients into regular screening programs should have a positive effect on colorectal cancer survival, since these patients must constitute a significant fraction of persons destined to develop cancer.

It is interesting to consider the impact of screening with flexible sigmoidoscopy on cancer and polyp detection relative to the era of rigid sigmoidoscopy. In 1966 Moertel summarized a number of reports of rigid sigmoidoscopy (34). In 47,207 asymptomatic patients undergoing routine rigid sigmoidoscopy there were 55 (0.12%) with cancer. In 149,007 (many symptomatic), 7.2% had polyps detected by rigid sigmoidoscopy. This may not be substantially different from the number of polyps in asymptomatic persons, since the yield of polyps

Table 15.3.
Yield of Fecal Occult Blood Testing and Flexible Sigmoidoscopy in a Hypothetical Population of 1000 Asymptomatic Average-Risk Persons

	Persons with Cancers	Persons with Polyps
Occult blood	2–4*	7–14*
Flexible sigmoidoscopy	2†	130†

*Assumes that 2–4% of persons have positive FOBT, and of these 10% have cancer and 35% have adenomas (6,7).
†Taken from Table 15.4.

Table 15.4.
Yield of 60-cm (or longer) Flexible Sigmoidoscopy in Average-Risk Screenees

Reference	No. Patients	No. Patients with Cancers	No. Patients with Polyps	No. Patients with Adenomas
17 Dubow	225	1	27	NS
18 Foley	500	3	180	86
19 Goldsmith	1000	0	53	NS
20 Hoff	324	0	112	NS
21 Lipshutz	200	0	39	NS
22 Marks	203	0	26	NS
23 Meyer	122	1	25	25
24 O'Connor	395	2	73	NS
25 Pearl	370	0	43	NS
26 Smith	211	0	28	28
27 Ujszaszy	3863	11	328	308*
28 Vellacott	13	0	3	3
29 Weiner	457	1	47	"most"
30 Wherry	417	0	52	NS
31 Yarborough	435	1	104	104
Total	8735	20 (0.23%)	1140 (13%)	

*94% of 402 total polyps were adenomas.
NS: Not stated.

in asymptomatic and symptomatic persons is usually comparable (23). Comparable numbers of persons screened by flexible sigmoidoscopy are not yet available (Table 15.4). Several studies have established that when flexible sigmoidoscopy and rigid sigmoidoscopy are compared in the same usually symptomatic patients, flexible sigmoidoscopy detects about three times more cancers and polyps than does rigid sigmoidoscopy (22,35–39). However, the yield of screening flexible sigmoidoscopy today for both cancers and polyps (Table 15.4) is only 1.7 times that noted by Moertel for rigid sigmoidoscopy 20 years ago. This is presumably the result of a rightward or proximal shift in the distribution of colon neoplasms in the past 2 decades (40).

Major problems with flexible sigmoidoscopy as a screening test concern its acceptability to the general population and its cost. Factors influencing acceptability (willingness to undergo screening) and compliance (adherence to instructions regarding screening) are complex (41). Acceptability of colorectal cancer screening usually decreases with increasing age (5). Thus, those most likely to have a positive screening test are the least likely to undergo it. Acceptability and compliance are greatly influenced by who offers the screening test (42). The best results occur when the patient's own physician or nurse practitioner approaches the screenee and the worst when a non-health care worker offers testing. In general, the acceptability of flexible sigmoidoscopy is worse than for FOBT. Poor acceptability of flexible sigmoidoscopy to screenees is related to the cost of the procedure, fear of discomfort and injury, and a still prevalent negative stigma associated with sigmoidoscopy in the general population. Part of this stigma dates to the discomfort associated with rigid sigmoidoscopy and the indignity of the knee-chest position used for that procedure. Physicians offering colorectal cancer screening should be aware of several additional negative attitudes that may underlie failure to participate or comply in colorectal screening programs. These include anxiety regarding or fear of cancer, denial (refusal of the screenee to even consider his or her chance of developing cancer), and fatalism (the belief that screening for cancer or treatment of it cannot alter the outcome) (43). A recent fear we have encountered is that of acquiring AIDS from the procedure. Improvements in acceptability probably will not occur until the public is more knowledgeable about colorectal cancer. To this end the American Cancer Society and the Memorial Sloan Kettering-Strang Clinic group have organized a nationwide campaign to educate the public about colorectal cancer.

An additional factor influencing acceptability is how the patient perceives the doctor's own attitude toward screening. Primary care physicians and even gastrointestinal specialists are often not aware of recent developments in colorectal cancer and its management (44) and may not regularly identify and approach candidates for flexible sigmoidoscopy screening or even believe in its value. In addition, an insufficient number of physicians are currently trained in the performance of flexible sigmoidoscopy. This was a factor in the American Board of Internal Medicine's decision to require training in sigmoidoscopy for certification. For the already practicing physician who wishes to develop independence in the performance of flexible sigmoidoscopy, a significant investment in time and money is required (see Chapters 4 and 17).

Another major concern regarding the widespread implementation of flexible sigmoidoscopy for colorectal cancer screening has been its cost. This issue is addressed in Chapter 16.

EVALUATION OF THE POSITIVE SCREENING TEST

The Positive FOBT

Patients with positive FOBT should undergo imaging of the entire colon. A variety of strategies employing various combinations of rigid proctosigmoidoscopy, flexible sigmoidoscopy, air contrast barium enema (ACBE), and/or colonoscopy have been advocated for this purpose (45). In our opinion, strategies employing rigid sigmoidoscopy and ACBE are not appropriate, since several studies have found that the sensitivity of ACBE for neoplasm detection in the sigmoid is impaired by diverticulosis and overlap of bowel loops (46–48). Thus, ACBE should be accompanied by endoscopic examination of at least the sigmoid colon.

The two most widely used strategies for evaluation of the positive FOBT are total colonoscopy and the combination of flexible sigmoidoscopy plus ACBE, often performed on the same day. Colonoscopy is more sensitive than ACBE for detecting polyps less than 1 cm in size and for detecting inflammation and vascular malformations. Colonoscopy offers the capacity to take biopsies and perform polypectomies at the time of the diagnostic examination. ACBE is more sensitive for detection of diverticulosis and is associated with fewer complications than colonoscopy. Also, the combination of flexible sigmoidoscopy plus ACBE is generally less expensive than colonoscopy. The question of relative cost-efficacy of these strategies is addressed in Chapter 16.

In addition to costs, several other factors affect the choice of colonoscopy versus flexible sigmoidoscopy plus ACBE. One factor is the compliance of the patient population. Noncompliant patients may not return for colonoscopy after polyps are found at flexible sigmoidoscopy or ACBE. In such populations colonoscopy may be the best first test because it affords the chance to perform polypectomy at the same setting.

Another factor that should influence the decision is the use of the single-contrast barium enema. Although the single-contrast study still has specific indications, it has poor sensitivity for detection of polyps and nonobstructing cancer. In hospitals where the single-contrast study is used routinely, patients with positive FOBT should be referred for colonoscopy.

A variable to consider is the skill of local colonoscopists. Success rates for reaching the cecal tip of more than 90% have been reported by centers with great experience. However, success rates of 75% and below are also common (49). A low success rate in reaching the cecum does not favor the use of colonoscopy as the initial test because many patients will need ACBE to complete colon evaluation at considerable expense. All of these factors, in addition to procedural and X-ray charges, influence the choice of diagnostic strategy.

Some alternative strategies for evaluation of the positive FOBT and their relative cost-effectiveness are discussed in Chapter 16.

The Positive Screening Flexible Sigmoidoscopy

There is general agreement that when an adenoma is discovered at flexible sigmoidoscopy the patient should undergo colonoscopy and polypectomy, since about one-third of such patients will have one or more adenomas in the proximal colon. The incidence of proximal adenomas increases with increasing size of the index polyp found at flexible sigmoidoscopy.

One problem for the sigmoidoscopist is to determine which polyps detected at flexible sigmoidoscopy are adenomas rather than nonneoplastic (hyperplastic) polyps. Although a red color to the polyp seen endoscopically favors an adenoma, whereas a pale color makes hyperplastic more likely, accurate differentiation of hyperplastic from adenomatous polyps by visual inspection at the time of flexible sigmoidoscopy is not possible (50). The most useful characteristic in this regard is the size of the polyp. Estimation of polyp size improves with operator experience. Persons with less experience in flexible sigmoidoscopy can improve their estimates of polyp size by comparing the polyp to an object of known size, such as an open biopsy forceps. Polyps ≥ 1 cm in size are nearly all adenomas and carry a significant risk of containing invasive cancer (51). There is little point in taking a biopsy of a polyp ≥ 1 cm at the time of screening flexible sigmoidoscopy. Such a biopsy could miss a focus of cancer and thereby generate a false sense of security. The sigmoidoscopist should note the size and location of polyps ≥ 1 cm, withdraw the sigmoidoscope, and arrange for colonoscopy and polypectomy. The excisional biopsy performed at the time of colonoscopy allows thorough pathologic examination of the polyp. If the polyp was biopsied at the time of screening flexible sigmoidoscopy a useless double pathologic examination (and fee!) was generated for the same polyp.

Similarly, it is unlikely to be cost-effective to take biopsies of polyps 6 to 9 mm in size discovered at screening flexible sigmoidoscopy. About 85% of such polyps are adenomas, and 1% contain invasive carcinoma (52–54). Again, the sigmoidoscopist should, after withdrawal of the instrument, arrange for colonoscopy and polypectomy.

There is some controversy about how to approach the patient with only diminutive polyps (≤ 5 mm in size) detected at flexible sigmoidoscopy. This question is of considerable importance, since this is the most common size range encountered. These polyps have been previously thought to be largely hyperplastic. This misconception was based largely on autopsy studies (55–56). Examination of endoscopically removed diminutive polyps has shown that half or more of these polyps are adenomas (52–54, 57–61). Grandqvist subdivided diminutive polyps by size and found that when a polyp reaches 4 mm in size there is a greater than 50% chance it is adenomatous (62). Diminutive polyps of equal size are more likely to be hyperplastic if found in the rectosigmoid than in the right colon. However, the endoscopist must be aware that the diminutive polyp, even if found in the rectosigmoid, may well be an adenoma.

Cold pinch biopsies of diminutive polyps usually will reflect the entire histology of the polyp accurately, despite the fact that mixed adenomatous-hyperplastic polyps have been reported (59). The important question for the sigmoidoscopist who detects only diminutive polyps at flexible sigmoidoscopy is whether a biopsy of the polyp should be taken to differentiate an adenomatous from a hyperplastic polyp. In other words, what is the significance of finding only hyperplastic polyps at flexible sigmoidoscopy? The finding of carcinoma in a hyperplastic polyp is quite rare. Hyperplastic polyps need not be considered malignant precursors, although they appear to be associated with a somewhat increased risk of colorectal adenomas and cancer. Does a hyperplastic polyp detected at flexible sigmoidoscopy indicate a significantly increased likelihood of finding an adenoma or carcinoma in the more proximal colon? Such a likelihood would imply the need for colonoscopy in screenees with only hyperplastic polyps at flexible sigmoidoscopy. Several recent studies have addressed this issue (Table 15.5). Four reports have shown that the incidence of proximal colon adenomas is substantial in persons with only hyperplastic polyps at flexible sigmoidoscopy and not significantly different from the incidence in persons with adenomas at flexible sigmoidoscopy (63–66). In two of these studies persons with hyperplastic polyps only in the rectosigmoid had a significant incidence of proximal colon cancers (63,65). Proximal colon adenomas in these reports may reflect the background incidence that would be found if colonoscopy were performed on screenees with no polyps at flexible sigmoidoscopy. Winawer, reporting data from the National Polyp Study, noted only a 1.25-fold increased risk of adenomas in the proximal colon in patients with only hyperplastic polyps in the rectosigmoid when compared to persons with no polyps in the rectosigmoid (67). However, the 19% incidence of proximal colon adenomas noted in the National Polyp Study in persons with only hyperplastic polyps detected in the rectosigmoid could be considered clinically important.

Currently, there are two acceptable approaches to the patient with diminutive polyps only at screening flexible sigmoidoscopy. One approach used at some institutions is to perform pinch biopsy of the polyp at the time of flexible sigmoidoscopy. If the polyp is an adenoma, colonoscopy is indicated. One advantage of this initial biopsy is that occasionally the diminutive polyp is

Table 15.5.
Incidence of Proximal Colon Adenomas in Patients with Hyperplastic Only Versus Adenomas in the Rectosigmoid

Reference	Asymptomatic	Procedure Used to Identify RS Polyp	Findings in RS	% of Patients with Proximal Colon Adenomas
63	Yes	35-cm FS	Diminutive AP	27
			Diminutive HP only	22
64	Yes	35-cm FS	AP	33
			HP only	34
65	NS	Colonoscopy		*
66	NS	Proctosigmoidoscopy	AP	66%
			HP only	50%
67	No	Colonoscopy	AP	31
			HP only	19

RS: Rectosigmoid.
FS: Flexible sigmoidoscopy.
NS: Not stated.
AP: Adenomatous polyp.
HP: Hyperplastic polyp.
*Exact number of patients not clear, but the number of synchronous neoplasms was higher in patients with rectosigmoid HP than those with rectosigmoid AP.

difficult to find at subsequent colonoscopy. If the polyp is hyperplastic, colonoscopy would not be performed. At the Indiana University Medical Center we use a different approach that has been advocated by others (63–66). We do not perform pinch biopsies of diminutive polyps detected at screening flexible sigmoidoscopy. Based on the data in Table 15.5, we perform and recommend colonoscopy on persons with polyps at screening flexible sigmoidoscopy regardless of size or histology. The biopsy taken at the time of flexible sigmoidoscopy generates an additional charge for pathologic examination, which at our institution exceeds the charge for flexible sigmoidoscopy. This charge is duplicated when the polyp is completely removed at colonoscopy. Certainly more data will soon be available to clarify this important matter further.

THE FUTURE OF COLORECTAL CANCER SCREENING

The future of colorectal cancer screening depends on many factors. Physicians need to project a positive outlook to the public regarding the progress that has been made in the secondary prevention of colorectal cancer. Public knowledge regarding colorectal cancer and physician awareness and performance of screening techniques must increase. The number of trained sigmoidoscopists and colonoscopists must increase to meet the demand for screening large numbers of persons. Concern about the enormous cost of full implementation of screening must be answered. Immunochemical tests for stool occult blood and stool blood assays such as Hemoquant (68) offer hope for more sensitive and specific screening tests. Colonoscopy of large numbers of asymptomatic average-risk volunteers in a research setting will help determine the background incidence of adenomas in the general population. This information will help tell us whether any of the occult blood tests or flexible sigmoidoscopy are adequate to detect a high percentage of persons with colorectal neoplasms. Meanwhile, advances in our understanding of environmental and genetic factors that lead to development of colonic adenomas and cancers will continue to take place. We have both reason to believe that the goal of eliminating colorectal cancer can be reached and much work to do toward achievement of this goal.

References

1. Dukes, CE. The classification of cancer of the rectum. J Pathol Bacteriol 1932;35:323–332.
2. Ron E, Lubin F. Epidemiology of colorectal cancer and its relevance to screening. In: Rozen P, Winawer SJ, eds. Frontiers gastrointestinal research Vol. 10. Karger, Basel, 1986:1–34.
3. Silverberg E, Lubera J. Cancer statistics 1987. CA 1987;37:2–19.
4. Hertz RL, Deddish MR, Day E. Value of periodic examination in detecting cancer of the rectum and colon. Postgrad Med 1960;27:290–294.
5. Simon JB. Occult blood screening for colorectal carcinoma: A clinical review. Gastroenterology 1985;88:820–837.
6. Winawer SJ, Fleischer M, Baldwin M, Sherlock P. Current status of fecal occult blood testing in screening for colorectal cancer. Cancer 1982;32:101–112.
7. Gilbertsen VA, McHugh RB, Schuman LM. A preliminary report of the results of the occult blood study. Cancer 1980;45:2899–2901.
8. Hill MJ, Morrison BC, Bussey HJR. Aetiology of adenoma-carcinoma sequence in the large bowel. Lancet 1978;1:245–247.
9. Waye JD. Colon polyps: Problems, promises, prospects. Am J Gastroenterol 1986;81:101–103.
10. Shinya H, Wolff WI. Morphology, anatomic distribution and and cancer potential of colonic polyps. Ann Surg 1979;190:679–683.
11. Gilbertsen VA. Proctosigmoidoscopy and polypectomy in reducing the incidence of rectal cancer. Cancer 1974;34:936–939.

12. Chuong JJH. A screening primer: Basic principles, criteria and pitfalls of screening with comments on colorectal carcinoma. J Clin Gastroenterol 1983;5:229–233.
13. Johnson D, Gurney M, Volpe R, et al. A prospective study of the prevalence of colonic neoplasms in asymptomatic patients with an age-related risk. Am J Gastroenterol 1987;82:957 (abstract).
14. Macrae FA, St. John DJB, Caligiere P, Taylor L, Legge J. Optimal dietary conditions for Hemoccult testing. Gastroenterology 1982;82:899–903.
15. Niv Y. Positive hemoccult tests and colonoscopic results. Ann Intern Med 1986;105:470.
16. Rex DK, Weddle RA, Lehman GA, et al. A prospective randomized comparison of cost efficacy for colonoscopy (CS) versus fiberoptic sigmoidoscopy plus air contrast barium enema (F + A) in the management of suspected lower gastrointestinal bleeding (LGIB). Gastrointest Endosc 1987;33:165 (abstract).
17. Dubow RA, Katon RM, Benner KG, VanDijk CM, Koval G, Smith SW. Short (35-cm) versus long (60-cm) flexible sigmoidoscopy: A comparison of findings and tolerance in asymptomatic screening for colorectal neoplasia. Gastrointest Endosc 1985;31:305–308.
18. Foley DP, Dunne P, O'Brien M, et al. Left-sided colonoscopy as screening procedure for colorectal neoplasia in asymptomatic volunteers ≥ 45 yrs. Gut 1987;28:A1367 (abstract).
19. Goldsmith O, Frankel H, Gerety D. Fiberoptic sigmoidoscopy in an asymptomatic population. Gastrointest Endosc 19778;23:228 (abstract).
20. Hoff G, Vath M, Gjone E, Larsen S, Savar J. Epidemiology of polyps in the rectum and sigmoid colon. Design of a population screening study. Scan J Gastroenterol 1985;20:351–355.
21. Lipshutz GR, Kata RM, McCool MF, et al. Flexible sigmoidoscopy as a screening procedure for neoplasia of the colon. Surg Gynecol Obstet 1979;148:19–22.
22. Marks G, Boggs HW, Castro AF, Gathright JB, Ray JE, Salvati E. Sigmoidoscopic examinations with rigid and flexible fiberoptic sigmoidoscope in the surgeon's office: A comparative prospective study of effectiveness in 1,012 cases. Dis Colon Rect 1979;22:162–168.
23. Meyer CT, McBride W, Goldblatt RS, et al. Clinical experience with flexible sigmoidoscopy in asymptomatic and symptomatic patients. J Biol Med 1980;53:345–352.
24. O'Connor K, Flynn J, Rex D, Hawes R, Crabb D, Lehman G. Fiberoptic sigmoidoscopy—Is longer better? Gastroenterology 1988;94:A328 (abstract).
25. Pearl RK, Nelson RL, Abcarian H, Nyhus LM. Establishing a flexible sigmoidoscopy/colonoscopy program for surgical residents. Amer Surg 1986;52:577–580.
26. Smith LE. Flexible fiberoptic sigmoidoscopy: An office procedure. Can J Surg 1985;28:233–236.
27. Ujszaszy L, Pronay G, Nagy GY, Kovice J, Libor S, Minik K. Screening for colorectal cancer in an Hungarian county. Endoscopy 1985;17:109–112.
28. Vellacott KD, Hardcastle JD. An evaluation of flexible fiberoptic sigmoidoscopy. Br Med J 1981;283:1583–1586.
29. Weiner RS. Free flexible sigmoidoscopy on Kauai. Hawaii Med J 1986;45:131.
30. Wherry DC. Screening for colorectal neoplasia in asymptomatic patients using flexible fiberoptic sigmoidoscopy. Dis Colon Rec 1981;24:521–522.
31. Yarborough GW, Waisbren BA. The benefits of systematic fiberoptic flexible sigmoidoscopy. Arch Intern Med 1985;145:95–96.
32. Macrae FA, St. John DJB. Relationship between patterns of bleeding and Hemoccult sensitivity in patients with colorectal cancers or adenomas. Gastroenterology 1982;82:891–898.
33. Demers RY, Stawick LE, Demers P. Relative sensitivity of the fecal occult blood test and flexible sigmoidoscopy in detecting polyps. Prev Med 1985;14:55–62.
34. Moertel CG, Hill JR, Dockerty MB. The routine proctoscopic examination: A second look. Mayo Clin Proc 1966;41:368–374.
35. Bohlman TW, Katon RM, Lipshutz JGR, McCool MF, Smith FW, Melnyk CS. Fiberoptic pansigmoidoscopy: An evaluation and comparison with rigid sigmoidoscopy. Gastroenterology 1977;72:644–649.
36. Leicester RJ, Pollet WG, Hawley PR. Flexible fiberoptic sigmoidoscopy as an outpatient procedure. Lancet 1982;1:34–35.
37. McCallum R, Covingten S, Berci G. Flexible fiberoptic proctosigmoidoscopy vs. rigid proctosigmoidoscopy as a routine diagnostic procedure. Gastrointest Endosc 1977;23:235 (abstract).
38. Winawer SJ, Leidnen SD, Boyle C, Kurtz RC. Comparison of flexible sigmoidoscopy with other diagnostic techniques in the diagnosis of rectocolon neoplasia. Dig Dis Sci 1979;24:277–281.

39. Winnan G, Berci G, Panish J, Talbot TM, Overholt B, McCallum RW. Superiority of the flexible to the rigid sigmoidoscope in routine proctosigmoidoscopy. N Engl J Med 1980;302:1011–1012.

40. Greene FL. Distribution of colorectal neoplasms: left to right shift of polyps and cancer. Amer Surg 1983;49:62–65.

41. Goulston KJ, Dent O, St. John DJB. Physician awareness and patient compliance for colon tumor screening. In: Rosen P, Winawer SJ. Secondary prevention of colon cancer. Vol. 10, Frontiers Gastrointestinal Research. Karger, Basel, 1986:46–54.

42. Sontag SJ, Durczak C, Aranha GV, Chejfec G, Frederick W, Greenlee HB. Fecal occult blood screening for colorectal cancer in a veterans administration hospital. Am J Surg 1983;145:89–94.

43. Dent O, Goulston K. A short scale of cancer knowledge and some sociodemographic correlates. Soc Sci Med 1983;16:235–240.

44. Dent O, Bassett M, Goulston KJ. Knowledge and attitudes of gastroenterologists in colorectal cancer. Aust N Z J Surg 1978;48:331–336.

45. Brandeau M, Eddy D. The workup of the asymptomatic patient with positive fecal occult blood tests. Med Dec Making 1987;7:32–46.

46. Baker SR, Alterman DD. False-negative barium enema in patients with sigmoid cancer and coexistent diverticula. Gastrointest Radiol 1985;10:171–173.

47. Williams CB, Macrae FA, Bartram CI. A prospective study of diagnostic methods in adenoma follow-up. Endoscopy 1982;14:74–75.

48. Vellacott KD, Amar SS, Hardcastle JD. Comparison of rigid and flexible fiberoptic sigmoidoscopy with double contrast barium enemas. Br J Surg 1982;69:399–400.

49. Gilbert DA, Shaneyfelt SL, Silverstein FE, Mahler AK, Hallstrom AP, and 674 Members of the ASGE. The National ASGE Colonoscopic Survey—analysis of colonoscopic practices and yields. Gastrointest Endosc 1984;30:143 (abstract).

50. Norfleet RG, Ryan ME, Wyman JB. Adenomatous and hyperplastic polyps cannot be reliably distinguished by their appearance through the fiberoptic sigmoidoscope. Dig Dis Sci 1988;33:1175–1177.

51. Muto T, Bussey HJR, Morson BC. The evolution of cancer of the colon and rectum. Cancer 1975;36:2251–2270.

52. Feczko PJ, Bernstein MA, Halpert RD, Ackerman LV. Small colonic polyps: a reappraisal of their significance. Radiology 1984;152:301–303.

53. Tedesco FJ, Hendrix JL, Pichams CA, Brady PG, Mills LR. Diminutive polyps: Histopathology spatial distribution and clinical significance. Gastrointest Endosc 1982;28:1–5.

54. Waye JD, Frankel A, Braunfeld SF. The histopathology of small colon polyps. Gastrointest Endosc 1980;26:80.

55. Lane N, Kaplan H, Pascal RR. Minute adenomatous and hyperplastic polyps of the colon: divergent patterns of epithelial growth with specific associated mesenchymal changes. Gastroenterology 1971;60:537–551.

56. Arthur JF. Structure and significance of metaplastic nodules in the rectal mucoas. J Clin Pathol 1968;21:735–743.

57. Grimmel RS, Lane N. Benign and malignant adenomatous polyps and papillary adenomas of the colon and rectum: An analysis of 1,856 tumors in 1,335 patients. Int Abstr Surg 1958;106:519–538.

58. Pagtalunan RJG, Dockerty MB, Jackman RJ. The histopathology of diminutive polyps of the large intestine. Surg Gynecol Obstet 1965;120:1259–1265.

59. Estrada RG, Spjut HJ. Hyperplastic polyps of the large bowel. Am J Surg Pathol 1980;4:127–133.

60. Fork FT, Lindstrom C, Ekelund GR. Reliability of routine double-contrast examination of the large bowel in polyp detection: A prospective clinical study. Gastrointest Radiol 1983;8:163–172.

61. Gottlieb LS, Winawer SJ, Sternberg S, et al. National polyp study (NPS): The diminutive colon polyp. Gastrointest Endosc 1984;30:143.

62. Grandqvist S, Gabrielson N, Sundelin B. Diminutive colonic polyps: Clinical significance and management. Endoscopy 1979;11:36–42.

63. Stoltenberg PH, Kirtley DW, Culp KS, LeSage GD, White JG. Are diminutive colorectal polyps (DCP) clinically significant? Gastrointest Endosc 1988;34:172 (abstract).

64. Blue M, Sivak MV, Achkar E, Matzen R, Stahl R. Colonoscopy as treatment of all polyps found at screening flexible proctosigmoidoscopy. Gastrointest Endosc 1988;34:193 (abstract).

65. Rauf A, Levendoglu H. Significance of diminutive colonic polyps with reference to hyperplastic rectosigmoid polyps. Am J Gastro 1988;83:1057.

66. Meziere T, Kastens D, Guild R, Welsh J. Colonoscopy in patients with polyp(s) on proctosigmoidoscopy. Am J Gastro 1988;83:1054 (abstract).

67. Zauber A, Winawer SJ, Diaz B, et al. The National Polyp Study (NPS): The association of colonic hyperplastic polyps and adenomas. Am J Gastro 1988;83:1060 (abstract). Data used includes data presented orally at the American College of Gastroenterology annual meeting in New York, October, 1988.

68. Ahlquist DA, McGill DB, Schwartz S, Taylor F, Ellefson M, Owen RA. Hemoquant, a new quantitative assay for fecal hemoglobin. Ann Intern Med 1984;101:297–302.

Cost Considerations in the Use of Flexible Sigmoidoscopy

Thomas L. Gross M.D.
Douglas K. Rex M.D.

INTRODUCTION

Decades of increasing expectations of health care, in conjunction with technologic advances that have provided an array of expensive tools at the physician's disposal, have resulted in U.S. health care costs consistently rising more rapidly than the economy as a whole. In response to rising health care costs, cost-containment strategies such as the Health Maintenance Organization and Diagnostic Related Groups have appeared. Despite the unknown effect these and other cost-containment strategies will have on the quality of health care, there is every reason to expect that the pressure to "contain" medical costs will continue to increase.

Therefore, it is important to know what costs are incurred through the use of flexible sigmoidoscopy and what benefits are realized from the expenditure. In the case of flexible sigmoidoscopy, the potential benefits may vary, depending on the indication for which it is being used. In this chapter we will discuss the costs and benefits of flexible sigmoidoscopy in two settings: *(a)* screening asymptomatic individuals and *(b)* evaluation of an individual with a positive fecal occult blood test.

SIGMOIDOSCOPY COSTS

To discuss sigmoidoscopy costs, a distinction must first be made between costs and charges. Costs are the actual expenses incurred in performing a procedure, whereas charges are what is billed for that procedure. Charges for endoscopic procedures are highly variable. For example, charges for upper endoscopy have been reported to vary up to six-fold within the same region of the United States (1). Determining the actual cost of an endoscopic procedure to everyone's satisfaction is difficult. Most facets of cost accounting are open to debate, i.e., depreciation rates for equipment, number of personnel required for office operation, cost of physician labor, and so on. In Table 16.1 we present a cost analysis of flexible sigmoidoscopy as performed by a primary care physician using an approach similar to that used by Overholt for upper endoscopy (1). The derived cost for flexible sigmoidoscopy is less important than the algorithm from which it was derived, which allows the reader to formulate his or her own opinion regarding sigmoidoscopy costs. In regard to the formula in Table 16.1, assumed costs could be changed in a manner to alter the derived sigmoidoscopy cost at least two-fold in either direction.

As one would expect, the largest component of sigmoidoscopy cost is physician labor. In our estimate, physician labor comprised almost 36% of total costs. Clearly, if sigmoidoscopy costs are to be minimized, containing physician labor costs is the most obvious target. One possibility would be to use technician or nursing labor for physician labor. This could be approached in several ways, including having the nurse initially advance the instrument and the physician either withdraw or observe as the nurse withdraws; having

Table 16.1.
Estimation of Sigmoidoscopy Costs in a Primary Care Physician's Office

Assumptions
  1/20 of income generated from sigmoidoscopy
  1/20 of nursing/secretary time devoted to endoscopic procedures
  Sigmoidoscope lifespan: 2000 procedures
  130 sigmoidoscopies performed per year

	Costs	(% of Total Costs)
Fixed Costs		
Labor		
MD ($120,000) × .05 sigmoidoscopy	$6000.00	(35.9%)
RN ($30,000) × .05 sigmoidoscopy	$1500.00	(9.0%)
LPN ($20,000) × .05 sigmoidoscopy	$1000.00	(6.0%)
Sec.($15,000) × .05 sigmoidoscopy	$700.00	(4.2%)
Space 585 sq ft at $2.00/sq ft/mo × .05		
sigmoidoscopy	$702.00	(4.2%)
Equipment (all devoted full time to		
sigmoidoscopy)		
1 light source	$3000.00	(17.9%)
1 patient cart	$800.00	(4.8%)
1 endoscopic cart	$300.00	(1.8%)
1 suction machine	$300.00	(1.8%)
[Items depreciated at 10% per yr over 10 yr +		
10%/yr interest expense]	$4600.00	(27.5%)
Overhead $25,000 × .05 sigmoidoscopy	$1250.00	(7.4%)
Total fixed costs ($15,752)/130 sigmoidoscopies/yr	$121.17	
Variable costs		
Supplies	$5.00	(3.9%)
Sigmoidoscopy depreciation ($5000 sigmoido-		
scope cost)/(2000 procedures per scope)	$2.50	(1.9%)
Total variable costs	$7.50	
Total costs	$128.67	

the nurse perform the entire procedure, only calling in the physician if abnormalities are detected; or having the nurse perform the entire procedure on videotape for later inspection by the physician.

COST EFFECTIVENESS OF SCREENING FLEXIBLE SIGMOIDOSCOPY IN AN ASYMPTOMATIC POPULATION

A large number of strategies employing various combinations of occult blood testing, rigid or flexible sigmoidoscopy, and air contrast barium enema or colonoscopy are available for colorectal cancer screening. There are few data available on the cost-effectiveness of these strategies for colorectal cancer screening. Ideally, data on cost-effectiveness of screening would come from randomized controlled trials comparing various screening strategies. The enormous size and cost of such trials, however, prohibit the comparison of any significant fraction of the available strategies by such trials. Some guidelines regarding cost-effectiveness of various strategies can be gleaned from studies using mathematical models and computer assistance, such as that performed by Eddy et al. (2). As pointed out by Eddy et al., these models require a wide range of assumptions regarding the natural history of colorectal adenomas and cancers, the effectiveness and complication rates of screening procedures, and the effectiveness of therapy. Some of these assumptions are well established and based on firm data available in the literature, whereas others can only be subjectively estimated. Therefore, the results of these studies can only be considered to serve as guidelines regarding cost-effectiveness.

Eddy et al.'s study was directed to asymptomatic high-risk subjects with

Table 16.2.
**Effect of Screening Strategies on an Asymptomatic
High-Risk Man. Increase in Life Expectancy and Net
Financial Cost**

Strategy	Days of Life Expectancy Increase	Cost
FB/3	39	$ 79
FB/2	51	125
FB/1	69	286
FS/5	60	461
FS/3	71	774
FS/1	98	2426
FB/1, FS/5	116	754
FB/1, FS/3	123	1072
FB/1, FS/1	140	2749
FB/1, FS/5, AC/5	205	1470
FB/1, AC/5	184	819
FB/1, CS/5	184	2100

The digits following each abbreviation signify the frequency (years between examinations).
FB = fecal occult blood test
FS = 60-cm flexible sigmoidoscopy
AC = air-contrast barium enema
CS = colonoscopy
Data from Eddy DM, Nugent FW, Eddy JF, et al. Screening for colorectal cancer in a high-risk population. Gastroenterology 1987; 92:682–692.

an 11% chance of developing colorectal cancer and a 5.5% chance of dying of the disease. It was estimated that if this risk could be completely eliminated, each such screenee on average would have an increased life expectancy of approximately 0.67 years, whereas the individual destined to colorectal cancer would live an additional 6 to 7 years. Table 16.2 displays selected data from Eddy et al.'s study that are of relevance to the individual performing colorectal cancer screening using flexible sigmoidoscopy.

Current recommendations for screening high-risk persons do not include strategies such as 1 to 9 in Table 16.2, since they do not examine the full colon and are thus considered insufficiently sensitive for detection of colorectal neoplasms in such persons. In fact, Eddy et al. favored strategies 11 or 12 as cost-effective strategies for use in high-risk persons. However, for average-risk persons (who constitute 80% of the population) there is no general consensus among experts that full colon screening is cost-effective. Thus, strategies 1 to 9 are particularly relevant to average-risk persons. "High-risk" persons in Eddy et al.'s study were assumed to have twice the average risk. Thus, we may extrapolate that screening average-risk persons would produce one-half the increase in life expectancy shown for each strategy in Table 16.2.

In regard to the data of Eddy et al.'s study, several points emerge that are relevant to the cost-effective use of flexible sigmoidoscopy for screening average-risk persons. These are consistent with information available from the literature and with the experience of many gastroenterologists and surgeons.

1. Screening with flexible sigmoidoscopy at regular intervals may reduce colorectal cancer mortality by 30 to 40%. To understand this we need only recall that although flexible sigmoidoscopy detects 55 to 60% of colon cancers, about one-half of persons detected at an asymptomatic stage would have been cured by treatment when they presented at a symptomatic stage.
2. The recommended interval between endoscopic screening is tending to increase. Annual screening in average-risk and most high-risk persons (ex-

cluding conditions such as long-standing ulcerative colitis) is unnecessary and excessively expensive. For average-risk persons, performing flexible sigmoidoscopy every 5 years as opposed to every 3 years results in an approximately 14% decrease in life expectancy (an average of 5 days per screenee) and a 40% decrease in cost.

3. Addition of an annual fecal occult blood test to flexible sigmoidoscopy performed every 3 years or every 5 years increases effectiveness substantially at a relatively small increase in cost.

Based on this information, our own suggestion is that a cost-effective approach to screening asymptomatic persons with two- to three-fold increased risk is annual occult blood testing at age 30 to 35 and colonoscopy every 5 years to begin at age 40. Obviously earlier or more intensive screening may be indicated by certain hereditary cancer or polyposis syndromes or by ulcerative colitis. For persons at average risk, annual occult blood testing at age 40 (as recommended by the American Cancer Society) and flexible sigmoidoscopy every 5 years beginning at age 50 appears to be a cost-effective approach.

How does the cost of using flexible sigmoidoscopy to screen for colorectal cancer in asymptomatic persons compare with other accepted medical practices? For our own calculation of the costs incurred in using flexible sigmoidoscopy for a screening program, we assume that regular screening by flexible sigmoidoscopy would begin at age 50 and continue every 5 years until age 75. Thus, at most, six examinations would be performed per screenee. Our calculation does not take into account that many screenees would need fewer examinations because of death from other causes or the finding of polyps or cancer, which would result in further screening by colonoscopy. We assume a charge for flexible sigmoidoscopy of $130, that the practice would result in a 30% improvement in colorectal cancer survival, and that each individual benefiting would live an additional 6 years. Using these assumptions the cost of flexible sigmoidoscopy per additional year of life expectancy is $15,758. This cost is greater than the cost extrapolated from Eddy et al.'s study, which also considered the cost *savings* of terminal cancer care avoided. Our calculated cost also compares favorably with costs of other accepted medical practices listed in Table 16.3, suggesting that screening flexible sigmoidoscopy may be a cost-effective concept.

We suspect that the trend toward more extensive endoscopic screening of high-risk and average-risk persons will continue. In a recent editorial (9), serious consideration was given to screening the entire population by colonoscopy every 7 years, beginning at age 40. Although this approach was not recommended, an argument was given for its cost-effectiveness, and a suggestion was made to initiate randomized controlled trials. Until more data is

Table 16.3.
Estimates of Costs of Currently Accepted Medical Practices*

Treatment	Cost/Year of Increased Life Expectancy	Ref
Coronary artery bypass grafting	$10,000	4
Screening and treatment of mild hypertension	30,000	5
Hemodialysis for end-stage renal disease	32,000	6
Heart transplantation	23,000	7
Heart transplantation	33,700	8

*Derived from Casscells, W. Heart transplantation. Recent policy developments. N Engl J Med 1986; 315:1365–1368.

forthcoming regarding the role of colonoscopy in screening average-risk persons, screening flexible sigmoidoscopy, which has half the efficacy but at about one-fifth the cost, will continue to seem like a good buy.

THE EVALUATION OF THE INDIVIDUAL WITH A POSITIVE FECAL OCCULT BLOOD TEST

There is a general consensus that the patient with symptoms of colorectal cancer and the individual with a positive fecal occult blood test must undergo complete colon visualization. Experts are divided between those who advocate sigmoidoscopy and barium enema (10–13) and those who favor colonoscopy (14–16) as the initial workup.

Advocates of double-contrast barium enema cite the relative ease with which the colon can be examined, the generally good sensitivity for lesions greater than 1 cm in size, the lower cost, and the minimal risk of procedure-related complications. Those favoring colonoscopy emphasize its greater sensitivity, particularly for lesions less than 1 cm in size, and the opportunity it provides to combine diagnosis and therapy into a single session, avoiding additional bowel preps and therapeutic delays. Because neither technique is clearly superior with regard to all characteristics, i.e., safety, sensitivity, and cost, a case can be made for either technique, depending on which aspects one chooses to emphasize.

In addition to fundamental differences between endoscopy and barium enema, other issues exist to confuse the decision on an optimal strategy for evaluating the colon. First, colonoscopy and barium enema are interdependent in that each technique will prompt the subsequent use of the other in a certain fraction of patients. Individuals in whom cancers or polyps are detected on barium enema will then require follow-up colonoscopy for biopsy or removal of the lesions. Likewise, a fraction of individuals undergoing colonoscopy as the initial diagnostic procedure will require follow-up barium enema to examine the proximal colon because the endoscopist is unable to reach the cecum.

Second, several options are available for performing sigmoidoscopy and barium enema. Sigmoidoscopy can be performed with either a rigid or a flexible instrument. When flexible sigmoidoscopy is done, options include using either a 60-cm or a 35-cm sigmoidoscope. Individuals undergoing barium enema can be studied by either single- or double-contrast techniques.

Also, there are factors that vary locally that must be considered. Both barium studies and endoscopy are dependent on operator skill for the ultimate sensitivity of the procedure. Availability of individual procedures in terms of how quickly they can be scheduled or how far the patient must travel to have it performed can become important considerations. Finally, the local charges for the individual procedures can vary widely.

Clinical Trials

The many issues involved in choosing a strategy for colon evaluation, as described above, make clinical trials difficult, time consuming, labor intensive, and expensive to perform. The number of different procedures available and the various sequences in which they might be performed result in a large number of potential strategies that might be evaluated. At the Indiana University Medical Center, we recently conducted a prospective randomized comparison of the cost-effectiveness of two of the most widely used initial strategies for the evaluation of patients with suspected lower GI bleeding: *(a)* diagnostic colonoscopy and *(b)* flexible sigmoidoscopy plus air-contrast barium enema. Three hundred thirty-two patients age $\geq$ 40 were randomized and completed their diagnostic studies (see ref. 17, manuscript in preparation). Colonoscopy detected significantly more patients with polyps <9 mm and more patients with arteriovenous malformations, whereas flexible sigmoidoscopy plus barium enema detected significantly more patients with diverticulosis. There were no statistically significant differences between strategies in detection of cancers or of polyps ≥9 mm in size. Patients undergoing initial colonoscopy were referred for ACBE if the colonoscopy was incomplete. Likewise patients with polyps discovered at initial flexible sigmoidoscopy or ACBE were referred for colonoscopy and polypectomy. The charges for these follow-up procedures were added to the charges for the initial procedures to determine total costs for the two strategies. If all patients with polyps detected at flexible sigmoidoscopy and/or barium enema are referred for colonoscopy and polypectomy, then the charge ratio of diagnostic colonoscopy to flexible sigmoidoscopy plus ACBE leading to equal total costs for the two strategies was 1.86. Thus, if the charge for diagnostic colonoscopy is less than 1.86 times the sum of the charges for flexible sigmoidoscopy and air-contrast barium enema, then this study suggested that total costs would be lower if diagnostic colonoscopy was the initial diagnostic strategy for patients with suspected lower GI bleeding. The similar charge ratio (diagnostic colonoscopy to flexible sigmoidoscopy plus ACBE) leading to equal costs per patient determined to have either a colorectal cancer of a polyp ≥5 mm was 2.61. However, the study indicated that different initial strategies may be preferable from a cost-effective standpoint, depending on the patient's age. Thus, initial colonoscopy appeared to be particularly cost-effective for patients age ≥55 in whom the incidence of polyps and cancers was substantially higher than in younger patients. Because of the lower incidence of polyps in younger patients (and thus the decreased need for follow-up colonoscopy and polypectomy), flexible sigmoidoscopy plus ACBE appeared more cost-effective for patients <55 years.

Evaluation of Strategies by Decision Science

The techniques of decision science, i.e., decision analysis and computer simulation, allow comparison of multiple strategies in a relatively effortless fashion in comparison to clinical trials. Strategy variables such as procedure sensitivities, morbidities, and costs are not only explicitly stated but can be systematically varied. This allows identification of those parameters that significantly affect results and thus require closer scrutiny. The process also identifies variables whose values may be controversial, e.g., procedure sensitivity, but that may not dramatically affect results when varied over a wide range. Also, the ability to vary system parameters such as costs allows a generalization of results to the many different cost relationships present throughout the country. Small differences in parameter values and large numbers of potential strategies are not limiting features for either decision analysis or computer simulation.

Overview of Recent Analytical Models

The applicability of decision science for comparing strategies for evaluation of individuals with positive fecal occult blood tests is attested to by the appearance of three different studies on the subject in 1987. Two of these studies—Barry et al. (18) and Brandeau and Eddy (19)—used decision analysis, whereas the third, Gross et al. (20), employed computer simulation. Although the studies varied somewhat in their approach, i.e., in strategies analyzed and measurements of strategy effectiveness, the underlying assumptions regarding procedure sensitivities, cost, and morbidity were relatively similar.

A common finding was that any strategy in which patients received a minimum of either sigmoidoscopy and barium enema or colonoscopy yielded at least an 89% cancer detection rate and most frequently a 90 to 95% cancer detection rate. Because each study found little difference in complication rates between strategies, the tradeoff was sensitivity for cost, with additional sensitivity generally requiring additional expenditures. Given this almost universal tradeoff, no optimal strategy was identified. A summary of the findings of these three studies is presented below.

Strategy Sensitivity.   Procedure sensitivities used in the three models are shown in Table 16.4. Sensitivities in Barry's model are presented as the fraction of all lesions in the colon that are detected by a procedure. In the other two models, sensitivity is defined as the fraction of lesions within the anatomic range of the examination that are detected. Direct comparison of model sensitivities is further complicated by the subdivision of polyp sensitivities by Gross and the use of low, medium, and high sensitivities for sigmoidoscopy by Brandeau.

Although a positive fecal occult blood test warrants complete colon examination, it is controversial whether barium enema alone is sufficient. An appreciation for the additional sensitivity gained by combining barium enema and sigmoidoscopy can be found in the model results.

All three studies evaluated strategies in which no further workup was performed if barium enema was negative (Table 16.5). The fraction of cancers detected (disregarding disseminated cancer in Barry's's study) ranged from 80 to 96.7% among the studies. The addition of rigid or flexible sigmoidoscopy

Table 16.4.
Procedure Sensitivities

	Sensitivity*		
	Localized Cancer	Disseminated Cancer	Polyps >5 mm
Barry et al.			
Procedure			
Rigid sigmoidoscopy	0.20	0.20	0.10
Flexible sigmoidoscopy (60 cm)	0.50	0.50	0.50
Air-contrast barium enema	0.80	1.00	0.60
Colonoscopy	0.95	1.00	0.90

	Sensitivity†	
	Cancer	Polyps
Brandeau & Eddy		
Procedure		
Rigid sigmoidoscopy	0.40/0.51/0.58‡	0.36/0.44/0.51
Flexible sigmoidoscopy (60 cm)	0.62/0.77/0.89	0.62/0.77/0.89
Air-contrast barium enema	0.95	0.92
Colonoscopy w/o barium enema	0.90	0.90
Colonoscopy after barium enema	0.95	0.95

	Sensitivity†			
		Polyps		
	Cancer	>10 mm	6–10 mm	<5 mm
Gross et al.				
Procedure				
Flexible sigmoidoscopy (60)	0.95	0.95	0.90	0.90
Air-contrast barium enema	0.90	0.90	0.80	0.45
Colonoscopy	0.95	0.95	0.90	0.90

*Fraction of lesions present in the colon detected by a procedure.
†Fraction of lesions within range detected by a procedure.
‡Low, medium, and high estimates.

Table 16.5.
Sensitivity of Barium Enema vs Barium Enema and Sigmoidoscopy

	BE	BE + RSig	BE + FSig	Additional Ca Yield Due to Sigmoidoscopy
Cancer sensitivity				
Barry et al. (local ca)	0.80	0.84		0.04
Barry et al (local ca)	0.80		0.90	0.10
Gross et al.	0.895		0.935	0.04
Brandeau & Eddy	0.967			
	BE	BE + RSig	BE + FSig	Additional Polyp Yield Due to Sigmoidoscopy
Polyp sensitivity*				
Barry et al.	0.60	0.64		0.04
Barry et al.	0.60		0.80	0.20
Gross et al.	0.911		0.887	0.024
Brandeau & Eddy	0.910			

*Polyps >5 mm in Barry's and Gross's studies. Size unspecified in Brandeau's study.

Strategy details

Barry et al.

BE

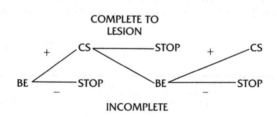

BE + Rigid/Flex Sig

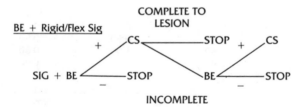

Gross et al.

BE

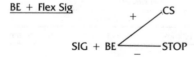

BE + Flex Sig

SIG + BE

Brandeau & Eddy

BE

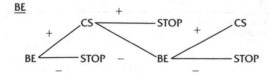

increased cancer yield from 80 to 84% and 90% respectively in Barry's study. In Gross's study, the addition of flexible sigmoidoscopy increased cancer yield from 89.5 to 93.5%. (Comparable strategies were not present in Brandeau's analysis.) The sensitivities of these strategies for polyps over 5 mm are also listed. Thus, these studies would suggest an additional 4% yield of cancers with the addition of rigid sigmoidoscopy to barium enema and between 4 and 10% additional cancers detected when flexible sigmoidoscopy is added to barium enema. The incremental increase in polyps greater than 5 mm detected with the addition of sigmoidoscopy was 4% for rigid sigmoidoscopy and 1.9 to 20% for flexible sigmoidoscopy.

Those that advocate colonoscopy as the initial workup for a positive fecal occult blood test emphasize the increased sensitivity of colonoscopy over barium enema. Again, it is possible from model results to get an appreciation for the additional sensitivity gained by starting with colonoscopy as opposed to sigmoidoscopy and barium enema (Table 16.6). Two of the studies examined strategies in which colonoscopy was the initial test performed, and no further evaluation was performed if colonoscopy was negative. In both strategies, barium enema was performed whenever initial colonoscopy was incomplete. Initial colonoscopy resulted in a 95% sensitivity for localized cancer in Barry's study and 94.8% or cancers in Gross's study. Similarly, the respective sensitivities of initial colonoscopy for polyps greater than 5 mm were 90 to 91.1%. The incremental increases in sensitivities for colon detection using initial colonoscopy were 11% (versus rigid sigmoidoscopy plus barium enema) and 5% (versus flexible sigmoidoscopy plus barium enema) in Barry's study and 1.3% over flexible sigmoidoscopy plus barium enema in Gross's study. Initial colonoscopy increased the yield for polyps over 5 mm by 26% (versus rigid sigmoidoscopy plus barium enema) and 10% (versus flexible sigmoidoscopy plus barium enema) in Barry's study and by 2.4% over flexible sigmoidoscopy plus barium enema in Gross's study.

Strategy Costs. Procedure costs are shown in Table 16.7. The most obvious difference in costs was that in Gross's model the combined costs of sigmoidoscopy and barium enema were approximately $100 greater than in the other two studies, and the average cost of colonoscopy was roughly $60 less than in the other two studies.

Comparing the resultant strategy costs is somewhat difficult because different models used different cost measurements. In Barry's study, strategy costs were measured in terms of costs required to screen 10,000 65-year-olds with occult blood testing, assuming all those with positive test were evaluated with a given strategy. In Brandeau's and Gross's models, strategy costs were measured in terms of average cost for each individual with a positive fecal occult blood test evaluated by a strategy.

In all three studies, initial evaluation with barium enema was the least expensive of the strategies in which all individuals had the entire colon examined, using the authors' best estimates of procedure costs (Table 16.8). In terms of costs to screen 10,000 65-year-olds for occult fecal bleeding, evaluating all those with positive tests with a minimum of barium enema cost $211,040 in Barry's model. Evaluating all patients with positive fecal occult blood tests with barium enema cost an average of $734 in Gross's's study and $687 in Brandeau's study.

As would be expected, the addition of sigmoidoscopy to barium enema increased costs. In Barry's model, the addition of rigid sigmoidoscopy increased screening costs from $211,040 to $237,177, and the addition of flexible sigmoidoscopy to barium enema increased screening costs to $287,580. In terms of average cost per patient, adding flexible sigmoidoscopy to barium enema increased the cost from $734 to $900 in Gross's model.

Table 16.6.
Sensitivity of Colonoscopy vs Sigmoidoscopy and Barium Enema

	BE + RSig	BE + FSig	CS	Additional Ca Yield Due to Colonoscopy
Cancer sensitivity				
Barry et al. (local ca)	0.84		0.95	0.11
Barry et al. (local ca)		0.90	0.95	0.05
Gross et al.		0.935	0.948	0.013
	BE + RSig	BE + FSig	CS	Additional Polyp Yield Due to Colonoscopy
Polyp sensitivity*				
Barry et al.	0.64		0.90	0.26
Barry et al.		0.80	0.90	0.10
Gross et al.		0.887	0.91	0.023

*Polyps >5 mm

Strategy details

Barry et al.

 BE + Rigid/Flex Sig

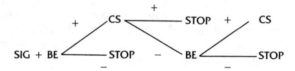

 CS

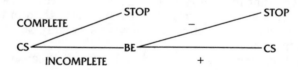

Gross et al.

 BE + Flex Sig

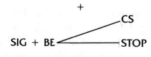

 CS

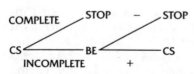

Table 16.7.
Procedure Costs ($)

Procedure	Barry	Brandeau	Gross
Rigid sigmoidoscopy	50.00	49.00	
Flexible sigmoidoscopy	114.00	105.00	154.00
ACBE	199.00	175.00	250.00
Colonoscopy	524.00	680.00	508.00
Colonoscopy w/biopsy	756.00		
Colonoscopy w/polypectomy	860.00		730.00

Maybe less intuitive, both Barry and Gross found that starting with colonoscopy was less expensive than performing flexible sigmoidoscopy and barium enema in all patients with positive fecal occult blood tests. In Barry's study, evaluating all patients with positive fecal occult blood tests with colonoscopy resulted in costs of $281,697 per 10,000 screened, compared to $287,580 for flexible sigmoidoscopy and barium enema. By comparison, rigid sigmoidoscopy was still clearly less expensive at $237,177. In Gross's study, starting with colonoscopy resulted in an average cost per patient of $758, which was $142 less per patient than starting with flexible sigmoidoscopy and barium enema ($900) and only $24 more per patient than evaluating with barium enema alone ($734).

Unfortunately, all of these cost calculations are highly dependent on the relative costs of the individual procedures. Because procedure costs can vary widely, even between different institutions in the same city, conclusions drawn from a cost analysis derived from a single set of procedure costs often has little applicability to a significant number of practitioners. In Barry's study, it was pointed out that reducing the cost of diagnostic colonoscopy by 15% from $524 to $445 would reduce the cost of initial evaluation with colonoscopy to that of initial evaluation with rigid sigmoidoscopy and barium enema.

In an effort to allow the reader to evaluate the cost of different strategies in his or her community, Gross et al. examined strategy costs at different ratios of colonoscopy cost and combined flexible sigmoidoscopy and barium enema costs (Fig. 16.1). Excluding barium enema alone because of its decreased sensitivity, starting with colonoscopy remained the least expensive workup until average colonoscopy cost rose to approximately twice the combined costs of flexible sigmoidoscopy and barium enema.

When average colonoscopy cost rose above twice the combined costs of sigmoidoscopy and barium enema, it was less expensive to use a strategy in which all patients underwent either sigmoidoscopy or barium enema with the intention that the other would be performed if the initial test was normal but that the patient would avoid the second test and go directly to colonoscopy if a cancer or polyp was seen on the first test. Although the sequence of barium

Table 16.8.
Strategy Costs ($)

	BE	RSIG + BE	FSIG + BE	CS
Barry et al.*	211,040	237,177	287,580	281,697
Gross et al.†	734		900	758
Brandeau & Eddy†	687			

*Costs required to screen 10,000 65-year-olds with fecal occult blood testing if all positive tests are evaluated with a certain strategy.
†Cost per individual with a positive fecal occult blood test evaluated with a certain strategy.
See Tables 16.5 and 16.6 for details of strategies.

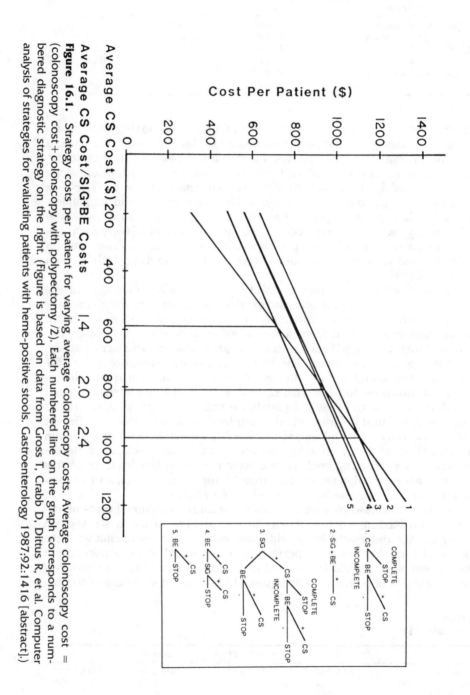

Figure 16.1. Strategy costs per patient for varying average colonoscopy costs. Average colonoscopy cost = (colonoscopy cost + colonscopy with polypectomy /2). Each numbered line on the graph corresponds to a numbered diagnostic strategy on the right. (Figure is based on data from Gross T, Crabb D, Dittus R, et al. Computer analysis of strategies for evaluating patients with heme-positive stools. Gastroenterology 1987;92:1416 [abstract].)

enema followed by either colonoscopy or sigmoidoscopy appeared slightly less expensive than sigmoidoscopy followed by either colonoscopy or barium enema, in reality the opposite is likely to be true. Starting with barium enema required a second bowel cleansing prep for all patients. When the indirect costs associated with bowel cleansing preps are included, i.e., transportation costs and additional time off work, starting with sigmoidoscopy followed by either colonoscopy or barium enema was the least expensive of the two strategies.

Strategy Morbidity.   Procedure-related morbidity rates used in the three studies are shown in Table 16.9. Advocates of barium enema cite its lower risk of morbidity in comparison to colonoscopy. However, the differences in strategy morbidity rates are much less than that of the individual procedures because of the frequent use of multiple procedures in the same patient. Most important, individuals with neoplasms detected on sigmoidoscopy or barium enema require subsequent colonoscopy for biopsy or removal of these lesions. Also, a fraction of individuals without colon lesions will undergo follow-up colonoscopy because of false-positive barium enema.

Although these interactions do not completely mitigate the increased risk of colonoscopy, the absolute difference in morbidities between strategies that start with colonoscopy and those that start with barium enema is much less than the morbidity rates for the individual procedures would suggest (Table 16.10). The largest difference in complication rates was found with Barry's model, in which there was a 1.87-fold increase in complication rates when starting with colonoscopy instead of barium enema. In Gross's study, starting with barium enema resulted in a 1.06% complication rate versus 1.33% for initial colonoscopy, for a difference in overall complication rate of 0.27%. An even smaller difference in complication rates is suggested by Brandeau's results. Although no strategy was evaluated in which no further workup was performed if initial colonoscopy was negative, a strategy of follow-up barium enema if initial colonoscopy was negative was evaluated and found to have a morbidity rate of 0.3%, which was only 0.07% higher than initial barium enema.

None of the decision analyses discussed here evaluated a potentially im-

Table 16.9.
Procedure Morbidity Rates

Procedure	Barry*	Brandeau†	Gross†
Rigid sigmoidoscopy	0.0001	0.0001	
Flexible sigmoidoscopy	0.0010	0.0001	0.00034
Air contrast barium enema	0.0000	0.0002	0.00017
Colonoscopy	0.0035	0.0028	0.00278
Colonoscopy w/biopsy	0.0230		
Colonoscopy w/polypectomy			0.02220

*Cardiovascular event, perforation, or bleeding.
†Bleeding or perforation.

Table 16.10.
Strategy Morbidity Rates

	BE	RSIG + BE	FSIG + BE	CS
Barry et al.*	2.51	2.72	3.70	4.69
Gross et al.†	0.0106		0.0108	0.0133
Brandeau & Eddy†	0.0023			

*Number of cardiovascular events, perforations, and bleeding for every 10,000 65-year-olds screened with fecal occult bleeding test, when positive tests are evaluated with a given strategy.
†Likelihood of bleeding or perforation occurring when evaluated with a given strategy.
See Tables 16.5 and 16.6 for details of strategies.

portant variable addressed by the clinical study (17) discussed earlier, i.e., the influence of the patient's age on which strategy is most cost-effective. Considering the decision analysis alone, our opinion is that the use of barium enema alone, although it is the least expensive strategy in certain cases, is not acceptable because of its decreased sensitivity. Initial colonoscopy is very sensitive and less expensive than flexible sigmoidoscopy plus barium enema whenever the charge for colonoscopy is less than about twice the combined charges of flexible sigmoidoscopy and barium enema. When colonoscopy charges are higher, starting with flexible sigmoidoscopy is the least expensive strategy. Flexible sigmoidoscopy serves a triage function, and patients with lesions seen on sigmoidoscopy then go on to colonoscopy. Those with normal sigmoidoscopies go on to barium enema.

References

1. Overholt BF. Gastrointestinal endoscopy in the 1980s: Cost, challenge, and change. Gastrointest Endosc 1984;30:325–328.
2. Eddy DM, Nugent FW, Eddy JF, et al. Screening for colorectal cancer in a high-risk population. Gastroenterology 1987;92:682–692.
3. Cassells W. Heart transplantation. Recent policy developments. N Engl J Med 1986;315:1365–1368.
4. Weinstein MC, Stason WB. Cost-effectiveness of coronary artery bypass surgery. Circulation 1982;66(Suppl 3):III-56-III-66.
5. Stason WB, Weinstein MC. Allocation of resources to manage hypertension. N Engl J Med 1977;296:732–739.
6. Roberts SD, Maxwell DR, Gross TL. Cost-effective care of end-stage renal disease: a billion dollar question. Ann Intern Med 1980;92:243–248.
7. Evans RQ, Manniken DL, Overcast TD, et al. The National Heart Transplantation Study: Final report. Seattle: Battelle Human Affairs Research Centers, 1984.
8. Cassells W. Estimated costs of heart transplantation. Clin Res 1985;33:245A (abstract).
9. Neugut AI, Forde KA. Screening colonoscopy: Has the time come? Am J Gastro 1988;83:295–297.
10. Tedesco F, Waye J, Raskin J, Morris S, Greenwald R. Colonoscopy evaluation of rectal bleeding . Ann Int Med 1978;89:907–909.
11. Miller R. Barium enema versus colonoscopy (editorial). Gastrointest Endosc 1982;28:40–41.
12. Abrams J. A second look at colonoscopy. Arch Surg 1982;117:913–917.
13. Ott D, Gelfand D, Chen Y, Munitz H. Colonoscopy and the barium enema: A radiologic viewpoint. South Med J 1985;78:1033–1035.
14. Spiegel M, Johannes R, Hendrix T. Clinical decision analysis approach to patients with a positive fecal occult blood test. Gastrointest Endosc 1984;30:145–146.
15. Stroehlein J, Goulston K, Hunt R. Diagnostic approach to evaluating the cause of a positive fecal occult blood test. CA 1984;34:148–157.
16. Gilbertsen V. Colon cancer screening. The Minnesota experience. Gastrointest Endosc 1980;26(Supp.):31S–32S.
17. Rex DK, Weddle, R, Lehman G, et al. A prospective randomized comparison of cost efficacy for colonoscopy (CS) versus fiberoptic sigmoidoscopy plus air contrast barium enema (F + A) in the management of suspected lower gastrointestinal bleeding (LGIB). Gastro Endosc 1987;33:165 (abstract).
18. Barry MJ, Mulley AG, Richter JM. Effect of workup strategy on the cost-effectiveness of fecal occult blood screening for colorectal cancer. Gastroenterology 1987;93:301–310.
19. Brandeau ML, Eddy DM. The workup of the asymptomatic patient with a positive fecal occult blood test. Med Decis Mak 1987;7:32–46.
20. Gross T, Crabb D, Dittus R, et al. Computer analysis of strategies for evaluating patients with heme-positive stools. Gastroenterology 1987;92:1416 (abstract).

Training in Flexible Sigmoidoscopy and Quality Assurance

Robert H. Hawes, M.D.

Flexible sigmoidoscopy has been used on a regular basis only since the early 1980s, and as a result, most primary care physicians did not receive training in this technique during internship or residency periods. Primary care physicians must assume a major role in colon cancer screening, which includes flexible sigmoidoscopy. One of the greatest challenges regarding colon cancer screening involves the development of training of primary care physicians in the cognitive and technical skills needed to perform independent flexible sigmoidoscopy. In this regard, this chapter will address five issues:

1. Development of a thorough standardized training technique;
2. The number of supervised examinations required to assure competency;
3. Establishment of programs within residency training institutions that will assure that all trainees who anticipate entering a primary care practice are trained in flexible sigmoidoscopy;
4. Development of postgraduate programs to provide flexible sigmoidoscopy training to all primary care physicians already in practice;
5. Accreditation and quality assurance programs for physicians performing flexible sigmoidoscopy.

TRAINING TECHNIQUES

Many institutions and organizations have established training programs for flexible sigmoidoscopy. Although different approaches to training fiberoptic sigmoidoscopy exist, the complete training program usually includes the following:

1. Written materials (syllabi, reprints, books) (Table 17.1);
2. Slide materials (normal and abnormal anatomy, lesion recognition);
3. Instructional lectures;
4. Instrument orientation;
5. Practice on a rubber colon model;
6. Observation of examinations;
7. Supervised examinations.

Once preliminary training has been completed (steps 1 through 6), hands-on training may begin with a variety of techniques:

- Trainee manipulates the directional controls and instructor controls instrument shaft for insertion and withdrawal.
- Trainee controls shaft insertion and instructor controls directional dials.
- Instructor inserts instrument and trainee withdraws manipulating directional controls with instructor controlling the insertion shaft.
- Trainee allowed 5 to 10 minutes for attempts at independent insertion. Instructor observes for safety and initially gives verbal instruction only. Instructor then assists as needed to complete examination.

Table 17.1.
Published Training Materials for Flexible Sigmoidoscopy

A. Complete books
  1. Schapiro M, Lehman GA, eds. Flexible sigmoidoscopy: Utilization and techniques (this text).
  2. Katon RM, Keeffe EB, Melnyk CS. Flexible sigmoidoscopy. Orlando, Florida: Grune & Stratton, 1985.
  3. Dutta SK, Kowalewski EJ. Flexible sigmoidoscopy for primary care physicians. New York: Alan R. Liss, 1987.
  4. W MacMillian Rodney, ed. Flexible sigmoidoscopy for the family physician. Copyright 1985 by the American Academy of Family Physicians and the American Society for Gastrointestinal Endoscopy.
B. Texts with chapters on flexible sigmoidoscopy
  1. Cotton PB, Williams CB. Practical gastrointestinal endoscopy. 2nd ed. London: Blackwell Scientific Publication, 1982.
  2. Sivak MV. Gastroenterologic endoscopy. Philadelphia: W.B. Saunders, 1987.
  3. Winawer SJ, Shotlenfeld D, Sherlock PL, eds. Colorectal cancer: Prevention epidemiology and screening. New York: Raven Press, 1980.
C. Atlases with colorectal sections
  1. Blackstone MO. Endoscopic interpretation. New York: Raven Press, 1984.
  2. Silverstein F, Tytgat GNJ. Atlas of gastrointestinal endoscopy. Philadelphia: W.B. Saunders, 1987.
D. Video
  1. Routine anorectal and sigmoidoscopic examination with differential diagnosis. Malcolm R. Hill, M.D. Audio-Video Digest Foundation. Glendale, CA 91206.
  2. Flexible sigmoidoscopy—Why, when and how? Part I and Part II. John P. Christie, M.D. Audio-Video Digest Foundation. Glendale, CA 91206.
  3. An introduction to flexible sigmoidoscopy. Dennis R. Sinar, M.D. Pentax Precision Instrument Corporation. Orangeburg, NY 10962.
  4. A teaching tape on sigmoidoscopy. Fujinon, Inc. Wayne, NJ 07470.
  5. Fiberoptic sigmoidoscopy. John F. Morressey, M.D. Olympus Corporation, Lake Success, NY. Available through local Olympus representative.
  6. Flexible sigmoidoscopy—The vital difference. Jeffrey Shaps, M.D. Olympus Corporation, Lake Success, NY. Available through local Olympus Corporation of America representative.

We prefer the third alternative. Once proficiency at directional control is established, the trainee is allowed to attempt insertion independently, with the instructor assisting to complete insertion and observing on withdrawal to assure that good visualization is obtained and lesions are recognized. The final step is to allow the trainee to do the examinations entirely independently with a trained endoscopist merely observing. The trainee is certified for independent examinations when competence is established with regard to safe insertion and the ability to visualize the lumen and recognize lesions.

COMPETENCY

Variability exists in published reports regarding the number of supervised examinations necessary for an individual to become competent in flexible sigmoidoscopy. McCray (1) found that it took an average of 50 examinations for four out of five trainees to become competent in the performance of independent flexible sigmoidoscopy with 60-cm instruments. Johnson (2) reported on their experience in training family practice residents and concluded that with close supervision, most residents are competent after performing 20 examinations. Baskin (3) states that a minimum of 25 one-on-one supervised cases is necessary to achieve basic competence. Our own data (4) reveal that when trainees are entered into a program as outlined in the previous section, 80% of trainees will be competent to perform independent flexible sigmoidoscopy with 60-cm instruments after 26 to 30 supervised examinations (Table 17.2). We found that previous experience with rigid sigmoidoscopy was beneficial when learning the technique of flexible sigmoidoscopy and that those with

Table 17.2.
Percentage of Trainees Achieving Overall Competence Versus Total Number of Examinations Performed during a 1- or 2-Month Training Period

	Total Number of Examinations Performed by Each Trainee				
	15	16–20	21–25	26–30	>30
Number of trainees competent	0	0	5	4	8
Number of trainees not competent	2	2	2	1	1
Percent competent	0	0	71	80	89

this experience performed 85% cf their examinations in a competent manner after 21 to 24 examinations (Figs 17.1 and 17.2). In the training program established jointly by the American Academy of Family Physicians (AAFP) and American Society for Gastrointestinal Endoscopy (ASGE), trainees are expected to do at least 15 supervised examinations before independent examinations are begun. Because individuals learn at different rates, the number of supervised procedures necessary may vary. An additional point that

FIGURE II

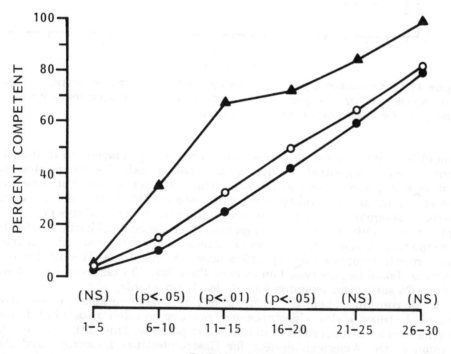

Figure 17.1. Percent of competent examinations versus examination number for trainees with (triangles) and without (solid circles) prior rigid sigmoidoscopy experience. Open circles represent all trainees combined. For each group of five examinations, the symbol represents the percent of examinations grade 4 (competent) or above. The p values reflect the differences in percent competent scores between groups with and without prior rigid sigmoidoscopy experience.

ALL TRAINEES COMBINED

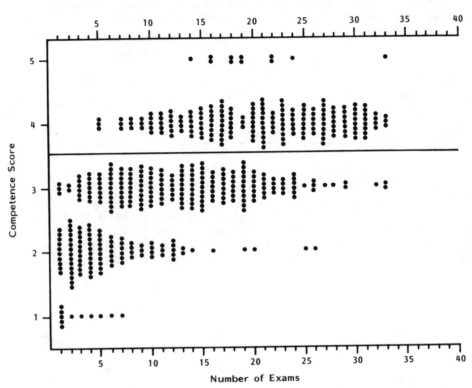

Figure 17.2. Cumulative experience of 495 graded flexible sigmoidoscopic examinations as performed by 25 resident trainees. Each solid circle represents the competence score given the trainee for that individual examination.

should be emphasized is that most papers regarding competence in flexible sigmoidoscopy concentrate on determining how quickly one can master the skill of safe insertion and withdrawal. This, however, is only one aspect of the examination. The ability to recognize abnormalities and identify them correctly is equally important. In determining the number of supervised examinations required to become competent, it should be a sufficient number to give the trainee adequate exposure to various colonic disorders such that they are correctly recognized during independent examinations. Toward this end trainees should be supervised on at least their first 15 examinations, and we believe 25 supervised examinations is clearly preferable.

Debate continues about the adequacy of 1- or 2-day "weekend courses" that provide lectures, slides, videotapes, and practice on colon models but do not provide hands-on supervised examinations of patients. This author shares the opinion of the American Society for Gastrointestinal Endoscopy and the American College of Physicians (5,6,7) that such programs are inadequate to assure competency in flexible sigmoidoscopy. Although the cognitive skills may be taught effectively in these short courses, the technical skills cannot. In our own program, the trainees' initial instruction (steps 1 through 5) is not dissimilar to that presented at weekend courses. In our study, we looked carefully at the development of cognitive and technical skills by trainees early in the fiberoptic sigmoidoscopy training. We designed a competency scoring system ranging from totally unskilled and possibly dangerous (Score = 1) to skills sufficient to perform independent flexible sigmoidoscopy (Score = 4). Each examination performed by the trainees was proctored, evaluated, and then scored by an experienced endoscopist. As Figure 17.2 reveals, nearly all of the first 15 examinations performed by the trainees were scored as incompetent (Score ≤ 3), with several examinations considered totally unskilled and potentially dangerous. We feel this data provides strong evidence that the initial 15 examinations performed by any trainee should be closely supervised by an experienced endoscopist. Therefore, short courses that do not assure proctoring for actual patient examinations should not be considered adequate to grant hospital privileges for performance of independent flexible sigmoidoscopy.

RESIDENT TRAINING PROGRAMS

If the medical community is to follow the American Cancer Society's recommendations (8) in screening for colorectal cancer, it will be necessary for primary care physicians, including family practitioners, general internists and general surgeons, to be trained adequately to perform independent flexible sigmoidoscopy. Toward this end, it will be necessary for resident training programs to incorporate preparation for and supervised performance of flexible sigmoidoscopy. In The American Board of Internal Medicine booklet on Essentials of Accredited Residencies in the section titled "Special Requirements For Residency Training in Internal Medicine" under Procedures and Technical Skills it states that "the training program must provide opportunities for the trainees to learn the indications, contraindications, complications and limitations of flexible sigmoidoscopy and the technical skills necessary to perform it." This policy seems appropriate because if graduating residents expect to gain hospital privileges to perform flexible sigmoidoscopy, they will likely need to show proof of their competence. The Health and Public Policy Committee of the American College of Physicians has been specific in their recommendations for level of training in flexible sigmoidoscopy stating that "a minimum number of 15 supervised examinations be done to gain hospital privileges (5). This committee goes on to state that all flexible sigmoidoscopy training should include:

1. Adequate preexamination instructional material and availability of colon models;
2. Close supervision of all examinations by trained endoscopists;
3. Mandatory minimal requirements of 15 flexible sigmoidoscopy examinations per trainee prior to graduation;
4. Documentation of the trainee's experience for each performance to include date, patient, identification number, patient age, indications, findings, complications, duration of the procedure, therapeutic plans based on results, and signature of the supervisor;
5. A letter from the head of the training program indicating that the trainee is competent to perform independent flexible sigmoidoscopy.

Training programs must be designed to ensure that participating physicians will obtain supervision for their initial examinations. Unless adequate postcourse supervision is attained, hospital privileges should not be granted based on short-course experience alone.

We instituted such a residency training program at Indiana University Medical Center in 1985. We require all internal medicine trainees who anticipate a career in general internal medicine to perform at least 25 flexible sigmoidoscopies under supervision during their 3 years of internal medicine training.

Although we advocate making flexible sigmoidoscopy training compulsory in primary care residency programs, this does not guarantee that resident physicians will actually use the procedure once they leave the training program. We polled our primary care trainees from 1984 to the present (9). We were able to reach 107/131 former residents (82%). Of these, 55 entered primary care, and 52 entered subspecialties. Of the 55 physicians in primary care, 42 had hands-on training in flexible sigmoidoscopy during their residencies. Of these, 27 (64%) were currently using flexible sigmoidoscopy. We found, however, that only 25 of these physicians were in a traditional private practice, 8 entered hospital maintenance organizations or multispecialty clinics, and 9 entered academic general medicine. In the latter two circumstances, subspecialty expertise in flexible sigmoidoscopy is readily available, therefore, the need for primary care physicians to perform the procedure is not as great. Of the 25 physicians in traditional private practice, 24 were performing flexible sigmoidoscopy (96%).

Of the 52 physicians entering subspecialties, 28 were trained in flexible sigmoidoscopy, but only 1 (4%) was using the technique. These data indicate that training in flexible sigmoidoscopy is used most frequently by primary care physicians entering traditional private practices; those who enter subspecialties rarely use it. Because hands-on training in this technique is labor intensive and can be limited by the number of patients available for trainees, we believe compulsory cognitive and technical competence in flexible sigmoidoscopy should be reserved for those anticipating a career in primary care, whereas learning the cognitive aspects will suffice for those entering subspecialties. This position appears consistent with policy set forth by the American Board of Internal Medicine.

TRAINING OF PRIMARY CARE PHYSICIANS CURRENTLY IN PRACTICE

The majority of primary care physicians now in practice are not trained in flexible sigmoidoscopy. The training of this group poses more difficult problems, including:

1. Education of primary care physicians regarding the importance of screening for colorectal cancer and the role of flexible sigmoidoscopy in this endeavor;
2. Demonstration to primary care physicians that flexible sigmoidoscopy can be a cost-effective use of their time even if the cost of flexible sigmoidoscopy is kept in the range of twice that of rigid sigmoidoscopy;
3. Provision of training programs that include readily available instructional material and the opportunity to practice on a rubber colon model;
4. Provision of a proctoring system so that physicians can be supervised during their training examinations;
5. Recruitment of patients on which to perform the initial supervised examinations (10).

In response to this need, a joint program was developed in 1985 by the American Society for Gastrointestinal Endoscopy (ASGE) and the American Academy of Family Physicians (AAFP) to provide such a system for practicing family practitioners. An initial $200 fee to offset costs for instructional materials and to provide incentive for physicians to complete the program is assessed each physician who signs up for the program. Each participant is sent a set of instructional materials that includes a multiauthored syllabus

Table 17.3.
Cognitive and Technical Skills to be Evaluated during Flexible Sigmoidoscopy Examinations

Informed consent
Instrument check out
Digital rectal
Patient positioning
Physician to patient communication during examination
Instrument insertion technique
Insertion beyond anus
Air insufflation
Suctioning
Torquing
Attention to patient discomfort
Rectal retroflection
Diagnostic accuracy
Patient plan and management

Table 17.1) and is required to take a written examination to assure that the material was reviewed. Approximately 1000 volunteer preceptors were recruited from the ASGE membership and AAFP training programs. All primary care physicians (both AAFP members and non-members) have been invited to enroll. As of 1989, 395 family practice physicians from across the country have registered for the course, and 255 have completed the program. It is the responsibility of the primary care physicians to contact potential preceptors in their vicinity to work out arrangements for supervision of training examinations. The primary care physician then performs at least 15 examinations under the supervision of an experienced endoscopist, who evaluates the cognitive and technical skills of each examination based on a number of observations (Table 17.3). The proctor is asked to evaluate the competency of each examination and then determine when the trainee is competent to do independent flexible sigmoidoscopy. In each category the examination was rated as a) very limited, b) fair but not in full control, or c) good-appropriate for performing independent examinations. The preceptor then assigns an overall competency rating for the examination. Review of the data submitted on the first 110 trainees indicates that greater than 90% of the trainees were rated as competent on their 15th examination. Torquing and retroflection in the rectum are the most difficult tasks to master. The Postgraduate Courses Subcommittee of The American College of Physicians is planning the development of a hands-on tutorial for practitioners for learning flexible sigmoidoscopy as well.

Although participation in these programs organized on a national level is encouraged and early results are promising, an alternative approach is to organize similar programs on a local level. A community gastroenterologist or surgeon skilled in endoscopy can organize a 1- to 2-day course in conjunction with a local endoscope manufacturer's representative, who provides sigmoidoscopes and rubber colon models for practice. A seminar may be presented in the local hospital that includes instructional material, slide pathology presentations, video tapes, and practice on rubber colon models. The primary care physicians are then encouraged to begin performing examinations under the proctorship of the skilled endoscopist, who has agreed to certify them when examinations are consistently done in a competent manner. Such a relationship mutually benefits both parties. The primary care physician obtains the necessary skills in an important aspect of his or her primary care duties, and in return the cooperating endoscopist is most likely asked to perform colonoscopy and polypectomy in patients with polyps.

To date, such programs have occurred in eight communities in Indiana. Over 200 primary care physicians have completed the 1-day course. Sixty-three percent of physicians answering a mailed questionnaire indicated that they had followed through the recommendations to obtain supervision for their initial examinations. Twenty-four percent bought sigmoidoscopes for office use or applied for hospital privileges without further training. The remainder had not yet initiated further training or examinations.

CREDENTIALING AND QUALITY ASSURANCE

Gaining hospital privileges in flexible sigmoidoscopy is often simply a matter of completing required hospital forms for the person who has received appropriate training. Persons leaving training programs should carry a letter of qualification from their training director. Persons completing training under the private supervision of a skilled gastroenterologist or other endoscopist should obtain letters of certification from that instructor. Certificates of completion of short courses should be presented but should not serve as adequate documentation for privileging. Persons with past experience in flexible sigmoidoscopy who believe they qualify for hospital privileges or physicians who are relocating and wanting to transfer privileges from one hospital to another should be willing to perform examinations under the direct observation of the skilled endoscopist to determine levels of skill before they are granted privileges. Physicians are encouraged to maintain the same standard of medical care for their office setting as is required for hospital privileges. Because of the difference in expertise required to do colonoscopy and polypectomy, flexible sigmoidoscopy credentialing should be clearly separated from colonoscopy credentialing.

The Joint Commission on Accreditation of Health Care Organizations (JCAHO) requires hospitals to develop and implement quality assurance programs. The programs are designed to "objectively and systematically monitor and evaluate the quality and appropriateness of patient care, pursue opportunities to improve patient care and resolve identified problems" and must include "a written plan that describes the program's objectives, organization, scope and mechanisms for overseeing the effectiveness of monitoring, evaluation and problem-solving activities." (11).

The development of a Quality Assurance Program for Sigmoidoscopy involves the establishment of parameters of the examinations. Parameters might include indications for the procedure, complications associated with the procedure and management plan after the procedure. (6). Standards of thresholds should be established as acceptable levels for the parameters. Those cases that exceed an acceptable level should be reviewed and discussed.

The tallying of the data can be performed on a daily basis and evaluated and reported on a monthly or quarterly basis. The major elements of data collection include procedure reports, an endoscopic unit record and procedure review that logs the number of procedures performed during the period and the volume of complications. A second section can consist of a case review in which specific cases are discussed and evaluated, such as complications. The final section includes conclusions, recommendations, anticipated changes, and methods to implement changes. A problem or area of concern should continue to be monitored and documented until an improvement or resolution has been found. The year-end report summarizes the quarterly reports and makes program changes for the upcoming year. Such a quality assurance program should be initiated in the office setting, as well as the hospital.

As in any technical procedure, continued competence requires regular performance. Occasional use may lead to missed diagnoses and higher complication rates. The American College of Physicians Committee on Clinical Privileges states that physicians need to perform at least 15 examinations per year with 60-cm instruments to maintain competence in flexible sigmoidoscopy (5). As a part of quality assurance programs, the Health and Public Policy Committee for the American College of Physicians recommends random sampling of flexible sigmoidoscopies done by physicians requesting continued privileges to confirm the appropriateness of indications and management plans and to make sure complication rates are acceptable (5). It must be emphasized that these measures should not be viewed as punitive; rather they assure that patients receive the highest quality of medical care possible within acceptable safety limits.

CONCLUSION

The need for quality training of flexible sigmoidoscopy is clear. Components of a quality training program have been outlined. Although the number of examinations required to become competent in flexible sigmoidoscopy is not fully defined, approximately 25 supervised examinations are recommended for most trainees. Short courses on sigmoidoscopy give familiarity but not competence in this area. Quality assurance programs should help establish and maintain quality work in the area of fiberoptic sigmoidoscopy.

Bibliography

1. McCray RS. A fiberoptic sigmoidoscopy training program for cancer screening physicians [Abstract]. Gastrointest Endoscopy 1981;27:137.
2. Johnson RA, Quan M, Rodney W. Flexible sigmoidoscopy in primary care: The procedure and its potential. Post Graduate Medicine 1982;72:151–156.
3. Baskin WN, Greenlaw RL, Fraker JT, Vidican DE, Lewan RB. Flexible sigmoidoscopy training for primary care physicians. Gastrointest Endoscopy 1984;30(2):141.
4. Hawes RH, Lehman GA, Hast J, O'Connor KW, Crabb DW, Lui A, Christiansen PA. Training resident physicians in fiberoptic sigmodoscopy: How many supervised examinations are required to achieve competence? Amer J Med 1986;80:465–470.
5. Health and Public Policy Committee, American College of Physicians. Clinical competence in the use of flexible sigmoidoscopy for screening purposes. Ann Int Med 1987;107:589–591.
6. Appropriate use of gastrointestinal endoscopy. A Consensus Statement from the American Society for Gastrointest Endoscopy. Manchester, MA, June 1986.
7. American Society for Gastrointestinal Endoscopy. Statement on role of short courses in endoscopic training: The standards of training and practice committee. Manchester, MA: American Society for Gastrointest Endoscopy, 1983.
8. American Cancer Society. Cancer of the colon and rectum. CA 1980;30:208–215.
9. Pound D. Do internal medicine (IM) and family practice (FP) physicians trained in sigmoidoscopy during residency use that skill in practice? [Abstract] Gastrointest Endoscopy 1988;34(2):198–199.
10. Schapiro M, Auslander MO, Getzug SJ, Klasky I. Flexible fiberoptic sigmoidoscopy training of non-endoscopic physicians in the community hospital [Abstract]. Gastrointest Endoscopy 1983;29:186.
11. Accreditation Manual for Hospitals. JCAHO, 1989. Quality Assurance Section p 219.

Index

Page numbers in italics denote *figures*; those followed by "t" denote tables.